M
Ab viations
pocket

E /F

G

H

I/J

K/L

M/N

O/P

Q/R

S

T

U/V

W/X

Y/Z

Symbols

Index

Börm
Bruckmeier
Publishing

Author: Adrian Padurean, M.D., padurean@media4u.com
Cover Illustration: Franka Krueger, Jaqueline Kuehne-Hellmessen
Publisher: Börm Bruckmeier Publishing LLC, www.media4u.com

68 17th Street, Hermosa Beach, CA 90254
www.media4u.com
Second Edition

Printed in China
ISBN 1-59103-221-0

Preface to the Second Edition

Our medical literature suffers from the terrible disease called TLA. You don't know what TLA is? It is the Three-Letter Abbreviation syndrome! I have been affected by it ever since I started reading medical texts. The continuity of the reading and the logic of the sentence were disturbingly interrupted by an overuse of abbreviations and acronyms.

The idea of itemizing all of the abbreviations I found within a certain article or book seemed to be the only practical solution to boil down the load of the unknowns I came across while preparing my medical exams. But the list never stopped growing! I made my list available on the web in the hope it might help others. Thus, I added even more items at the suggestion of some of the curious visitors of my site.

Medical Abbreviations pocket is divided into two sections for your convenience. The first part lists the abbreviations and acronyms alphabetically, while the second one is an index of the expanded terms for reverse searching. The PDA version is even easier to use.

Medical Abbreviations pocket is also available on the web at **www.media4u.com.** From here you can download the entire database to your Palm Pilot or Pocket PC as well.

Although this pocket dictionary is not a comprehensive source of medical abbreviations in use today, I do hope it will give you all the basics that you need to navigate through the ocean of medical terminology.

Adrian Padurean, M.D.
padurean@media4u.com

September 2005

PDA and free Website Version:
www.media4u.com

Additional titles in this series:
Anatomy pocket
Canadian Drug pocket 2006-2007
Differential Diagnosis pocket
Drug pocket 2006
Drug Therapy pocket 2006-2007
Drug pocket plus 2006-2007
ECG pocket
EMS pocket
Homeopathy pocket
Medical Classifications
Medical Spanish pocket
Medical Spanish Dictionary pocket
Medical Spanish pocket plus
Normal Values pocket
Respiratory pocket

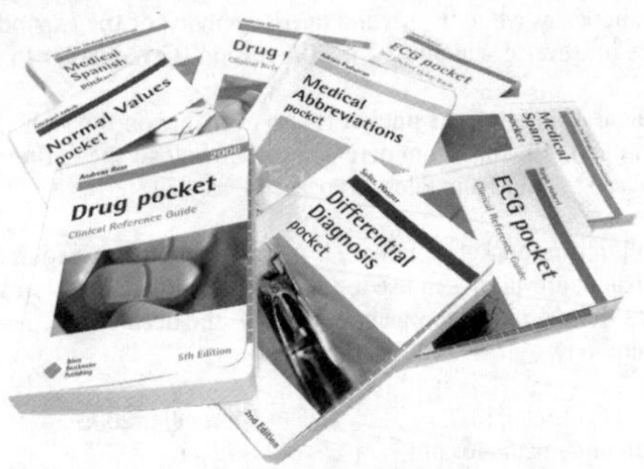

Börm Bruckmeier Publishing LLC on the Internet:
www.media4u.com

A

a artery
autopsy
before

A adenine
alanine
anemia
arteria
arteriole
asymptomatic
no symptoms

A1 aortic first sound

A2 aortic second sound

aa arteries
of each (Greek: Ana)
equal part of each

A–a gradient alveolar to arterial gradient

AA affected area
African-American
Alcoholics Anonymous
arachidonic acid
reactive (secondary) amyloidosis

AAA abdominal aortic aneurysm
adenine-adenine-adenine codon for lysine
diagnostic arthroscopy, operative arthroscopy, and possible operative arthrotomy

AAAASF American Association for Accreditation of Ambulatory Surgery Facilities

AAAP activity of antiactivator in plasma

AABB American Association of Blood Banks

AAC adenine-adenine-cytosine codon for asparagine

AACPDM American Academy for Cerebral Palsy and Developmental Medicine (also: AAOS Specialty Societies)

AACR American Association for Cancer Research

Aad aminoadipic acid

AADC amino acid decarboxylase

AAE American Association of Endodontists

AAETS American Academy of Experts in Traumatic Stress

AAF 2-acetylaminofluorene
anterior auditory field
astrocytoma with atypical/anaplastic foci

AAF/OL anaplastic astrocytomas/oligodendrogliomas

AAFP American Academy of Family Physicians

AAG adenine-adenine-guanine codon for lysine

AAHKS American Association of Hip and Knee Surgeons (also: AAOS Specialty Societies)

AAHS American Association for Hand Surgery (also: AAOS Related Organizations)

AAI fixed-rate atrial single-chamber systems

AAIR age-adjusted incidence rate, single chamber rate responsive atrial pacing

AAL acute lymphoblastic leukemia
anterior axillary line

AAMC Association of American Medical Colleges

AAMI Association for the Advancement of Medical Instrumentation

AAMT American Association for Medical Transcriptionists

AAN American Academy of Neurology

AANA Arthroscopy Association of North America (also: AAOS Related Organizations)

AANOS The American Academy of Neurological and Orthopaedic Surgeons
AANS American Association of Neurological Surgeons
A-a O2 alveolo-arterial oxygen tension
AAo ascending aorta
AAO American Academy of Ophthalmology
AAOC antacid of choice
AAofA Ambulance Association of America
AAOFAS American Association of Orthopaedic Foot and Ankle Surgeons
AAOHN American Association of Occupational Health Nurses
AAOM American Academy of Oral Medicine
AAOO American Academy of Ophthalmology and Otolaryngology
AAOP American Academy of Oral Pathology
American Academy of Orthotists and Prosthetists
AAOPP American Association of Osteopathic Postgraduate Physicians
AAOS American Academy of Orthopaedic Surgery
AAOT Asociacion Argentina de Ortopedia y Traumatologia (Argentinian Orthopaedic Association)
AAOx3 awake, alert and oriented x 3 (to person, place and time)
AAP air at atmospheric pressure
American Academy of Pediatrics
American Academy of Pedodontics
American Academy of Periodontology
American Academy of Psychoanalysis

AAP (cont.) American Academy of Psychotherapists
American Association of Pathologists
aminoantipyrine
Association for the Advancement of Psychoanalysis
Association of Academic Physiatrists
Association of American Physicians
AAPA American Academy of Physician Assistants
American Association of Pathologist Assistants
AAPB American Association of Pathologists and Bacteriologists
AAPC antibiotic-associated pseudomembranous colitis
AAPCC adjusted annual per capita cost
adjusted average per capita cost
American Association of Poison Control Centers
AaPco2 alveolo-arterial carbon dioxide tension difference
(A-a)Pc02 alveolo-arterial carbon dioxide tension difference
AAPF anti-arteriosclerosis polysaccharide factor
AAPH 2,2'-azobis-(amidinopropane) dihydrochloride
AAPHD American Association of Public Health Dentists
AAPHP American Association of Public Health Physicians
AAPL American Academy of Psychiatry and the Law
AAPM American Association of Physicists in Medicine
AAPMC antibiotic-associated pseudo-membranous colitis
AAPMR American Academy of Physical Medicine and Rehabilitation

AAPM+R American Academy of Physical Medicine and Rehabilitation
AaPO2 alveolo-arterial oxygen tension difference
(A-a) PO2 alveolo-arterial oxygen tension difference
AAPOS American Association for Pediatric Ophthalmology and Strabismus
AAPP American Academy on Physician and Patient
AAPPO American Association of Preferred Provider Organizations
AAPS American Association of Plastic Surgeons
Arizona Articulation Proficiency Scale
Association of American Physicians and Surgeons
AAPSM American Academy of Podiatric Sports Medicine
aar against all risks
AAR active avoidance reaction
acute articular rheumatism
antigen-antiglobulin reaction
AARC American Association for Respiratory Care
AARDA American Autoimmune Related Diseases Association
AARE automobile accident, rear end
AAROM active assertive range of motion
active assisted range of motion
AARP American Association of Retired Persons
AAS Aarskog-Scott (syndrome)
acid aspiration syndrome
acute abdominal series
alcoholic abstinence syndrome
American Academy of Sanitarians
American Analgesia Society
aneurysm of atrial septum
anthrax anti serum
aortic arch syndrome

AAS (cont.) atomic absorption spectrophotometry
AASD American Academy of Stress Disorders
aa seq amino acid sequence
AASH adrenal androgen stimulating hormone
American Association for the Study of Headache
AASK African American Study of Kidney Diseases and Hypertension Pilot Study
AASP acute atrophic spinal paralysis
American Association of Senior Physicians
ascending aorta synchronized pulsation
AASS American Association for Social Security
AAST American Association for the Surgery of Trauma
a1AT alpha-1-antitrypsin
AAT Aachen Aphasia Test
academic aptitude test
alanine aminotransferase
alkylating agent therapy
alpha-1-antitrypsin
atrial triggered (pacemaker)
auditory apperception test
automatic atrial tachycardia
American Association for Thoracic Surgery
AAU acute anterior uveitis
adenine-adenine-uracil codon for asparagine
AAV adeno-associated virus
AAVMC Association of American Veterinary Medical Colleges
AAVP American Association of Veterinary Parasitologists
AAVPT American Academy of Veterinary Pharmacology and Therapeutics

AAW anterior aortic wall
AAWD American Association of Women Dentists
AAWM American Academy of Wound Management
ab abortion
antibody
aB azure B
Ab abortion
antibiotic
antibody
AB abortion
abdominal
abnormal
Ace bandage
active bilaterally
aid to the blind
alcian blue
alertness behavior
antibiotic
antibody
antigen binding
apex beat
asbestos body
asthmatic bronchitis
axiobuccal
Bachelor of Arts *(Lat: Artium Baccalaureus)*
blood group AB
3AB 3-aminobenzamide
A/B acid-base ratio
A+B apnea and bradycardia
A>B air greater than bone (conduction)
ABA abscisic acid
allergic bronchopulmonary aspergillosis
American Board of Anesthesiologists
antibacterial activity
arrest before arrival
Arthroscopie Belge - Belgian Arthroscopy Association
ABAT American Board of Applied Toxicology
Abb abbreviations
ABB Albright-Butler-Bloomberg syndrome
American Board of Bioanalysis
Asea Brown Boveri
ABBQ Acquired Immunodeficiency Syndrome Beliefs and Behavior Questionnaire
abbr abbreviated
abbreviation
ABc autoantibodies to collagen
ABC absolute basophil count
absolute bone conduction
acalculous biliary colic
acid balance control
aconite-belladonna-chloroform
advanced breast cancer
airway, breathing, circulation
alternative birth center
alum, blood and charcoal (purification and deodorizing method)
alum, blood and clay (sludge deodorizing method)
American Blood Commission
aneurysmal bone cyst
antigen-binding capacity
apnea, bradycardia, cyanosis
aspiration biopsy cytology
aspiration needle biopsy
assessment of basic competency
atomic, biological and chemical (warfare)
avidin-biotin complex
axiobuccocervical
A+BC air and bone conduction
ABCC Atomic Bomb Casualty Commission
ABCD airway, breathing, circulation, differential diagnosis (or

defibrillate) in cardiopulmonary resuscitation

ABCD (cont.) asymmetry, borders irregular, color variegated, diameter > 6 mm (assessment of melanoma)

ABCDE airway, breathing, circulation, disability, exposure/environmental control - trauma protocol
botulism toxin pentavalent

ABCDEFGH air ways, bones, cardiac shadow, diaphragm, effusions, fields (pulmonary), gastric, hardware (chest X-ray reading mnemonic)

ABCDES abnormal alignment, bones-periarticular osteoporosis, cartilage joint space loss, deformities, marginal erosions, soft tissue swelling (x-ray features in rheumatoid arthritis)
adjust medication, bacterial prophylaxis, cervical spine disease, deep vein thrombosis prophylaxis, evaluate extent and activity of disease, stress-dose steroid coverage

Abd (abdere) abdomen
abdominal
abduction

abd, ABD abdomen, abdominal

ABE acetone-butanol-ethanol
acid-base equilibrium
activity before exercise
actual base excess
acute bacterial endocarditis
acute bacterial exacerbations of chronic bronchitis
Adult Basic Education Programs
American Board of Endodontics
aminobenzoate
anode-break excitation
antisheep beta-endorphin
atypical bronchial epithelium

ABE (cont.) autoantibodies to elastin
average bioequivalence
Averrhoa bilimbi
estradiol bound to albumin
trivalent botulinic antitoxin

ABE-1 a strain of the psychophilic marine bacterium Vibrio ABE-1

ABE-I anion-binding exosite I

ABE-II anion-binding exosite II

Abeta beta-amyloid (component of Alzheimer's disease plaques)

ABF alpha-L-arabinofuranosidases

ABG arterial blood gases
autogenous bone graft

ABI ankle to brachial index

ABJS Association of Bone and Joint Surgeons (AAOS Specialty Societies)

ABMA anti-basement membrane antibody disease (Goodpasture's syndrome)

ABMS American Board of Medical Specialties

ABMT autologous bone marrow transplant

abn abnormal
abnormality of a chromosome (e.g.abn 12p)

Abn abnormal(ity)

AbN ablation nephropathy
antibody nitrogen
antibody to the N terminus (of a protein or peptide)

ABN abducens nucleus
abnormal
active bulimia nervosa (BN)
acute bacterial nephritis
acute brachial neuritis
acute brachial neuropathy
alkali-treated bound niacin
anterior BNST lesions (BNST, bed nucleus of the stria terminalis)

ABN (cont.) arched-back nursing (about laboratory rats)
artificial background noise
aseptic (avascular) bone/bone marrow necrosis
Association of British Neurologists
endo-1,5-alpha-L-arabinase
The Brazilian Academy of Neurology

Abn-cbd abnormal cannabidiol

ABO blood grouping system

ABOS American Board of Orthopaedic Surgery

ABP American Board of Pathology
American Board of Pediatrics
androgen binding protein
arterial blood pressure

ABPA allergic bronchopulmonary aspergillosis

ABPB abductor pollicis brevis (also APB)

ABPL abductor pollicis longus (also APL)

ABR auditory brainstem response audiometry

abs absent

ABS American Back Society
arterial blood pressure

AbT applied biotechnology

ABT autologous blood transfusion

ABTA American Brain Tumor Association

ABVD adriamycin, bleomycin, vinblastine, and dacarbazine (regimen used to treat Hodgkin's disease)

ABW actual body weight

Abx antibiotics

ac, a.c. ante cenam, before meal/s

Ac acute

AC abdominal circumference
acromioclavicular joint
adrenal cortex
air conduction
alternating current
anterior chamber

ACA adenine-cytosine-adenine codon for threonine
American Chiropractic Association
Amputee Coalition of America (also: AAOS Related Organizations)

AcAAP N-acetylaminoantipyrine

acc accident

ACC adenine-cytosine-cytosine codon for serine
adenine-cytosine-cytosine codon for threonine
American College of Cardiology
anodal closure contraction

ACCME Accreditation Council for Continuing Medical Education

accom. accommodation

Accom accommodation

ACCP American College Of Chest Physicians

ACCx anterior cingulate cortex

ACD absorbent cover dressing
acid-citrate-dextrose
allergic contact dermatitis
anemia of chronic disease
anterior cervical discectomy
asymmetrical cortical degeneration syndromes
Available Chemical Directory

ACDF adult children from dysfunctional family
anterior cervical discectomy and fusion

ACDM Association for Clinical Data Management

ACE angiotensin converting enzyme

ACEI, ACE-I angiotensin-converting enzyme inhibitors

ACF anterior cervical fusion

ACFAS American College of Foot and Ankle Surgeons

ACG adenine-cytosine-guanine codon for threonine
angiocardiography
ACh acetylcholine
AChR acetylcholine receptor
ACI acute coronary insufficiency
acid phos. acid phosphate
ACILS American Center for International Labor Solidarity
ACIP Advisory Committee on Immunization Practices
ACJ acromioclavicular joint (also AC joint)
ACJT acromioclavicular joint
ACl aspiryl chloride
ACL Achievement Check List
acromegaloid features, cutis verticis gyrata, corneal leukoma (syndrome)
anterior clavicular line
anterior cruciate ligament
anticardiolipin (antibody)
ACLA American Clinical Laboratory Association
ACLC Assessment of Children's Language Comprehension
ACLD Association for Children with Learning Disabilities
ACLF adult congregate living facility
ACLI American Council on Life Insurance
aCLL atypical chronic lymphocytic leukemia
ACLM American College of Legal Medicine
ACLPS Academy of Clinical Laboratory Physicians and Scientists
ACLR anterior capsulolabral reconstruction
ACLS advanced cardiac life support
AcLV avian acute leukemia virus
ACM acetaminophen
acute cerebrospinal meningitis

ACM (cont.) Adriamycin, cyclophosphamide, methotrexate
albumin-calcium-magnesium
alveolar capillary membrane
anticardiac myosin
Arnold-Chiari malformation
ACMA American Occupational Medical Association
ACMC Association of Canadian Medical Colleges
ACMD associate chief medical director
ACME Advisory Council on Medical Education
Automated Classification of Medical Entities
ACMF arachnoid cyst of the middle fossa
ACMI American College of Medical Informatics
ACML atypical chronic myeloid leukemia
ACMP alveolar-capillary membrane permeability
ACMR Advisory Committee on Medical Research
ACMS American Chinese Medical Society
ACMSF Advisory Committee on the Microbiological Safety of Food (UK)
ACMT artificial circus movement tachycardia
ACMV assist-controlled mechanical ventilation
ACN acute conditioned neurosis ventilation
Ambulatory Care Network ventilation
American College of Neuropsychiatrists ventilation
American College of Nutrition
ACNM American College of Nuclear Medicine Nutrition
American College of Nurse-Midwives

A

ACNP acute care nurse practitioner Midwives
American College of Nuclear Physicians

ACO acute coronary occlusion
alert, cooperative, oriented
anodal closure odor

ACoA anterior communicating artery

ACOA adult children of alcoholics

ACOAs collegiate adult children of alcoholics

ACOEM American College of Occupational and Environmental Medicine

ACOEP American College of Osteopathic Emergency Physicians

ACOG American College of Obstetricians and Gynecologists

ACOHA American College of Osteopathic Hospital Administrators

ACO-HNS American Council of Otolaryngology-Head and Neck Surgery

ACOI American College of Osteopathic Internists

· **ACOM** American College of Occupational Medicine
anterior communicating (artery)

AComA anterior communicating artery

ACOMS American College of Oral and Maxillofacial Surgeons

ACOOG American College of Osteopathic Obstetricians and Gynecologists

ACOP American College of Osteopathic Pediatricians
approved code of practice

ACORDE A Consortium on Restorative Dentistry Education

ACOS American College of Osteopathic Surgeons
associate chief of staff

ACOS/AC associate chief of staff for ambulatory care

Acous acoustics
acoustic

AcP acid phosphatase

ACP accessory conduction pathway
acid phosphatase
acyl carrier protein
American College of Pathologists
American College of Pharmacists
American College of Physicians
American College of Prosthodontists
American College of Psychiatrists

ACPA American Cleft Palate Association

ACPC aminocyclopentane carboxylic (acid)

ACPE American College of Physician Executives

AC-PH ac phos acid phosphatase

ACPM American College of Preventive Medicine

ACPOC Association of Children's Prosthetic-Orthotic Clinics (AAOS Specialty Societies)

ACPP adrenocortical polypeptide
prostate-specific acid phosphatase

ACPS acrocephalopolysyndactyly

Acr acrylic

ACR abnormally contracting region
absolute catabolic rate
acriflavine
adenomatosis of colon and rectum
adjusted community rate
ambulance call report
American College of Radiology
American College of Rheumatology
anticonstipation regimen
axillary count rate

ACRF ambulatory care research facility

ACRI Africa Crisis Response Initiative

ACRM American Congress on Rehabilitation Medicine

ACRPI Association of Clinical Research for the Pharmaceutical Industry
ACS acrocallosal syndrome
acrocephalosyndactyly
acute chest syndrome
acute confusional state
acute coronary syndrome
Alcon Closure System
American Cancer Society
American Chemical Society
American College of Surgeons
anodal closure sound
antireticular cytotoxic serum
aperture current setting
Association of Clinical Scientists
acute cervical strain
acute cervical sprain
ACSA adenylate cyclase-stimulating activity
ACSE association control service element
ACSF artificial cerebrospinal fluid
AC/SIUG ambulatory care special-interest user group
ACSM American College of Sports Medicine
ACSP adenylate cyclase-stimulating protein
Australian College of Sports Physicians
ACSV aortocoronary saphenous vein
ACSVBG aortocoronary saphenous vein bypass graft
act actinomycin
activity
active
AcT acceleration time
ACT achievement through counseling and treatment
actin
actinomycin
activated clotting time
active motion
ACT (cont.) advanced coronary treatment
anterocolic transposition
antichymotrypsin
anticoagulant therapy
anxiety control training
asthma care training
atropine coma therapy
ACTA American Cardiology Technologists Association
automatic computerized transverse axial (scanning)
Act-C actinomycin C
Act-D actinomycin D
ACTe anodal closure tetanus
ACTG AIDS Clinical Trial Group
ACTH adrenocorticotropic hormone
ACTH-LI adrenocorticotropin-like immunoreactivity
ACTHR adrenocorticotropic hormone receptor
ACTS acute cervical trauma syndrome
ACTZ acetazolamide
ACU adenine-cytosine-uracil codon for threonine
ambulatory (acute) care unit
ACVB aortocoronary venous bypass
ACVD acute cardiovascular disease
arteriosclerotic cardiovascular disease
AD Action for Democracy
admission and discharge
admitting diagnosis
adult disease
alternating days
Alzheimer's disease
atopic dermatitis
auris dextra (right ear)
ADA American Dental Association
American Diabetes Association
anterior descending artery
ADADS Alcohol and Drug Abuse Data System

A

ADAS-Cog	Alzheimer's Disease Assessment Scale-Cognitive Subscale
ADASP	Association of Directors of Anatomic and Surgical Pathology
ADC	AIDS dementia complex
ADCC	antibody-dependent cell-mediated cytotoxicity
ADD	addiction
	adduct
	adduction
	attention deficit disorder
	average daily dose
ADEA	Association for the Development of Education in Africa
ADEM	acute disseminated encephalomyelitis
	acute disseminated encephalopathy
adeno-Ca	adenocarcinoma
ADF	acid detergent fiber
	actin depolymerizing factor
ADG	average daily gain
ADH	antidiuretic hormone
	atypical ductal hyperplasia
	vasopressin
ADHD	attention deficit hyperactivity disorder
ADI	acceptable daily intake
ADJ	adjacent
	adjoining
	adjunct
	adjust
	adjuvant chemotherapy
ADL	activities of daily living
ad lib	at liberty
	as desired
adm, adm.	admission
ADM	admission
	adult onset diabetes mellitus
ADP	abductor pollicis
	adenosine diphosphate
	Agricultural Development Program
ADR	adverse drug reaction
Adria	Adriamycin (trade name for doxorubicin)
ADS	anterior dynamized system
ADT	admission-discharge-transfer
	automated defibrillator technician
ADV	advised
	arterial deep venous
	Aujeszky's Disease Virus
AE	above the elbow
	active and equal
	adverse effect
	adverse event
AEA	above elbow amputation
	Asociación Española de Artroscopia (Spanish Arthroscopy Association - only Spanish)
	auricular electroacupuncture
AEB	as evidenced by
AEC	5-amino 9 ethyl carbazol
AED	automated external defibrillator
AEEC	attaching and effacing Escherichia coli
AEH	atypical endometrial hyperplasia
AEI	acetyleethyleneimine
AER	auditory evoked response
	average evoked response
AERC	African Economic Research Consortium
AET	2-aminoethylisothiouronium bromide hydrobromide
AF	acid-fast
	adult female
	amniotic fluid
	aortic flow
	atrial fibrillation
	atrial flutter
AFB	acid fast bacilli
AFB1	aflatoxin B1
AFB2a	aflatoxin B2a
AFC	amniotic fluid cortisol

AFDC Aid to Families with Dependent Children
aFGF acidic fibroblast growth factor
AFI amniotic fluid index
Afib, A-fib atrial fibrillation
AFIP Armed Forces Institute of Pathology
AFL aflatoxicol
artificial limb
atrial flutter
AFLP acute fatty liver of pregnancy
AFM atomic force microscope
AFLM1 aflatoxicol M1
AFNOR French Standardization Institute
AFO ankle-foot orthoses
AFP acute flaccid paralysis
alpha-fetoprotein (expressed by germ cell tumors and other cancers)
AFSI Africa Food Security Initiative
AFTR atrophy, fasciculation, tremor, rigidity
AFX atypical fibroxanthoma
AG anion gap
antigen
A/G albumin/globulin ratio
aga agropinic acid
AGA adenine-guanine-adenine codon for arginine
appropriate-for-gestational age
AGCT adult granulosa cell tumor
AGF angle of greatest flexion
AGG adenine-guanine-guanine codon for arginine
aggravation
AGI Academy for Guided Imagery
AGL acute granulocytic leukemia
AGN acute glomerulonephritis
a-GPA alpha-D-glucose pentaacetate
AGTT abnormal glucose tolerance test
AGU adenine-guanine-uracil codon for serine
AGUS atypical glands of unknown significance
AH abdominal hysterectom
accidental hypothermia
acute hepatitis
arterial hypertension
AHA American Heart Association
American Hospital Association
AHB alpha-hydroxybutyric acid
AHC academic health care
academic health center
acute hemorrhagic conjunctivitis
acute hemorrhagic cystitis
amygdalohippocampal complexes
antihemophilic factor C
AHCA Agency for Health Care Administration
American Health Care Association
AHCD acquired hepatocellular degeneration
AHCPR Agency for Health Care Policy and Research
AHCy adenosyl homocysteine
AHD acquired hepatocerebral degeneration
acute heart disease
antihyaluronidase
antihypertensive drug
arterio-hepatic dysplasia
atherosclerotic heart disease
autoimmune hemolytic disease
AHDMS automated hospital data management system
AHDP azacycloheptane diphosphonate
AHDS Allan-Herndon-Dudley syndrome
AHE acute hazardous events (database)
acute hemorrhagic encephalomyelitis
AHEA area health education activity
AHEC area health education center
AHES artificial heart energy system
acute heart failure

AHES (cont.) American Health Foundation
American Hepatic Foundation
American Hospital Formulary
antihemophilic factor
Argentinian hemorrhagic fever
Associated Health Foundation

AHFS American Hospital Formulary Service

AHG aggregated human globulin
antihemophilic globulin factor
antihemophilic globulin
antihuman globulin

AHGG aggregated human gammaglobulin
antihuman gammaglobulin

AHGS acute herpetic gingival stomatitis

AHH alpha-hydrazine analog of histidine
anosmia and hypogonadotropic hypogonadism (syndrome)
arylhydrocarbon hydroxylase
Association for Holistic Health

AHI active hostility index
Animal Health Institute
apnea-plus-hypopnea index

AHIMA American Health Information Management Association

AHIP assisted health insurance plan

AHIS automated hospital information system

AHJ artificial hip joint

AHL acquired hypertrichosis lanuginosa
acute hemorrhagic leukoencephalitis
apparent half-life

AHLE acute hemorrhagic leukoencephalitis

AHLG antihuman lymphocyte globulin

AHLS antihuman lymphocyte serum

AHM Allied health manpower
ambulatory Holter monitor

AHMA American Holistic Medicine Association
antiheart muscle autoantibody

AHMC Association of Hospital Management Committees

AHN Army Head Nurse
assistant head nurse

AHNMD associated clonal hematopoietic non-mast cell lineage disorder

AHO Albright hereditary osteodystrophy

AHP accountable health plan or partnership
acute hemorrhagic pancreatitis
after hyperpolarization
air at high pressure
analytic hierarchy process
approved health plan
Assistant House Physician

AHPA American Health Planning Association

AHPO anterior hypothalamic preoptic (area)

AHR antihyaluronidase reaction
Association for Health Records
atrial heart rate

AHRA American Hospital Radiology Administration

AHRF acute hypoxemic respiratory failure
American Hearing Research Foundation

AHRQ Agency for Healthcare Research and Quality

AHS Academy of Health Sciences
African horse sickness
alveolar hypoventilation syndrome
American Hearing Society
American Hospital Society
area health service
assistant house surgeon

AHSA American Health Security Act

AHSDF area health service development fund

AHSG alpha-2HS-glycoprotein

AHSN Assembly of Hospital Schools of Nursing

A

AHSP	AIDS Health Services Program (of the Robert Wood Johnson Foundation)
AHSR	Association for Health Services Research
AHT	aggregation half time
	antihyaluronidase titer
	arterial hypertension
	augmented histamine test
	autogenous hamster tumor
AHTG	antihuman thymocyte globulin
AHTP	antihuman thymocyte plasma
AHTS	antihuman thymus serum
AHU	acute hemolytic uremic (syndrome)
AHU	arginine, hypoxanthine, uracil
AHuG	aggregated human IgG
AHV	avian herpes virus
a.k.	above knee
al	active ingredient
AI	accidental injury
	accidentally incurred
	adiposity index
	aggregation index
	allergy and immunology
	amylogenesis imperfecta
	anaphylatoxin inactivator
	angiogenesis inhibitor
	angiotensin I
	anxiety index
	aortic incompetence
	aortic insufficiency
	apical impulse
	articulation index
	artificial insemination
	artificial intelligence
	atherogenic index
	atrial insufficience
	autoimmune
	autoimmunity
	axio-incisal
	first meiotic anaphase
A+I	allergy and immunology
AIA	allylisopropylacetamide
	amylase inhibitor activity
	anti-immunoglobulin antibody
	anti-insulin antibody
	aspirin-induced asthma
	automated image analysis
AIB	airflow-induced bronchospasm
	aminoisobutyrate
	avian infectious bronchitis
AIBA	aminoisobutyric acid
AIBS	American Institute of Biological Sciences
AIC	Akaike's information criterion (a goodness-of-fit measure)
	aminoimidazole carboxamide
	Association des Infirmières Canadiennes
A-IC	average integrated concentration
AICA	anterior inferior cerebellar artery
	anterior inferior communicating artery
AI-CAH	autoimmune-type chronic active hepatitis
AICAR	aminoimidazole carboxamide ribonucleotide
AICD	automatic implantable cardioverter defibrillator
AICE	angiotensin I converting enzyme
AICF	autoimmune complement fixation
AI/COAG	artificial intelligence hemostasis consultant system
AID	acquired immunodeficiency disease
	acute infectious disease
	acute ionization detector
	Agency for International Development
	argon ionization detector
	artificial insemination by donor
	autoimmune deficiency
	autoimmune disease
	automatic implantable defibrillator
	average interocular difference

A

AIDP acute inflammatory demyelinating polyradiculoneuropathy
AIDS acquired immunodeficiency syndrome
AIDSDRUGS clinical trials of acquired immunodeficiency drugs
AIDS-KS acquired immune deficiency syndrome with Kaposi's sarcoma
AIDSLINE on-line information on acquired immunodeficiency syndrome
AIDS-OI acquired immune deficiency syndrome with opportunistic infection
AIDSTRIALS clinical trials of acquired immunodeficiency syndrome drugs
AIIS anterior inferior iliac spine
AIL angioimmunoblastic lymphadenopathy
AIMBE American Institute for Medical and Biological Engineering
AIN anterior interosseous nerve
Aind indicative dosage
AIOD Association Internationale pour l'Ostéosynthèse Dynamique
AIOM Italian Association for Medical Oncology
AION anterior ischemic optic neuropathy
AIOSM American Institute of Orthopaedic and Sports Medicine
AIP acute interstitial pneumonia (Hamman-Rich disease)
AIRO Associazione Italiana di Radioterapia Oncologica
AIS adenocarcinoma in situ
adolescent idiopathic scoliosis
AIT acute intensive treatment
AJ ankle jerk
AJAO American Juvenile Arthritis Organization
AJCC American Joint Committee on Cancer
AJKS American Journal of Knee Surgery
AJNR American Journal of Neuroradiology
AJO American Journal of Orthopaedics
AK above knee
above the knee (amputation)
aka alcoholic ketoacidosis, also known as
AKA above knee amputation
also known as
AKS American Knee Society
Al porous alumni
AL idiopathic (primary) amyloidosis
left ear
Ala alanine
ALAT alanine aminotransferase / alanine transaminase
alb. albumin
ALB albendazole
alc. alcohol
ALC alternative level of care
anaplastic large cell
approximate lethal concentration
ALD alcoholic liver disease
ALIP atypical localization of immature precursors
ALK anaplastic lymphoma kinase
automated lamellar keratoplasty
alk phos alkaline phosphatase
Alk Phos alkaline phosphatase
ALL allergy
acute lymphoblastic leukemia
acute lymphocytic leukemia
AlloSCT allogeneic stem-cell transplantation
ALMI anterior lateral myocardial infarction
Aloc allyloxycarbonyl
ALOC altered level of consciousness
amphetamine-induced locomotion
ALP alkaline phosphatase
alpha-MPT alpha-methyl-p-tyrosine

alpha 2,6-ST alpha 2,6 sialyltransferase
alpha-T7 transgenic line of mice
ALRI antero-lateral rotatory instability
ALS advanced life support
amyotrophic lateral sclerosis
anterolateral sclerosis
acute lumbar strain
Alt aluminum tartrate
ALT alanine aminotransferase (formerly SGPT)
alternate
altitude
argon laser trabeculoplasty
autolymphocyte therapy
avian laryngotracheitis
ALTB acute laryngotracheobronchitis
ALTE acute life-threatening event
ALTEE acetyl-L-tyrosine ethyl ester
alt hor alternate hours
every other hour
ALTS acute lumbar trauma syndrome
ALVF acute left ventricular failure
am morning
AM adult male
aerospace medicine
alveolar macrophages
anteromedial
before noon
AMA against medical advice
American Medical Association
antimitochondrial Ab
AMAN acute motor axonal neuropathy
amb ambulate, ambulation
amb. ambulating, ambulatory
AMB ambulate
ambulatory
AMG acceleromyography
alpha-2-macroglobulin
AMI acute myocardial infarction
AMIA American Medical Informatics Association
AML acute myeloblastic leukemia
AML (cont.) acute myelogenous leukemia
AMM agnogenic myeloid metaplasia
AMM+M agnogenic myeloid metaplasia with myelofibrosis
amnio amniocentesis
amp ampere
ampoule
amp. amputation, ampoule
AMP amphetamine
amputation
AMPLE allergies, medication, previous illnesses, last meal, events preceding incident
AMS American Medical Systems Inc Amsterdam
aseptic meningitis syndrome
AMSAN acute motor sensory axonal neuropathy
AMSSM American Medical Society for Sports Medicine
amt amount
AMV alfalfa mosaic virus
anterior medullary velum
apical membrane vesicles (about lung)
AMV-RT avian myeloblastosis virus reverse transcriptase
AMY2 alpha-amylase 2
ANA anesthesia
antinuclear antibody (test; see also FANA)
ANAL analgesic
ANC absolute neutrophil count
ANCA antineutrophil cytoplasmic antibodies
AND algoneurodystrophy
anterior nasal discharge
ANED alive no evidence of disease
anes., ANES anesthesia
ANG angle
ANHE acute necrotizing hemorrhagic encephalopathy

ANI	acute nerve irritation
ANLL	acute non-lymphocytic leukemia
ann. fib.	annulus fibrosis
ANO	amiodarone neuropathy of the optic nerve
ANOVA	analysis of variance
ANP	atrial natriuretic peptide
ANPs	advanced nurse practitioners
ANRF	Arthritis National Research Foundation
ANRI	acute nerve root irritation
ANS	autonomic nervous system
AN69-S	Biospal
ANSI	American National Standards Institute
ant, ANT	anterior
ante	before
anti-OJ	anti-isoleucyl-tRNA synthetase
ANUG	acute necrotizing ulcerative gingivitis
ANV	anticipatory nausea and vomiting symptoms
ANX	anxiety
Anxty	anxiety
A+O	alert and oriented
AO	angle of aorta Arbeitsgemeinschaft fuer Osteosynthesefragen inbred strains of rats [AO(RT1u/AgB2)]
A/O	alert and orientated
AOA	American Orthopaedic Association (also: AAOS Related Organizations) American Osteopathic Association Asian Orthopaedic Association Australian Orthopaedic Association
AOAC	Association of Official Analytical Chemist
AO ASIF	AO (Arbeitsgemeinschaft fuer Osteosynthesefragen) Association of the Study of Internal Fixation
AOB	Abteilung für Orthopädische Biomechanik (Orthopaedic Biomechanics Division) alcohol on breath
AOD	arteriosclerotic occlusive disease
AODA	alcohol and other drugs of abuse
AODM	adult onset diabetes mellitus
AOFAS	American Orthopaedic Foot and Ankle Society (also: AAOS Related Organizations)
AOI	AO (Arbeitsgemeinschaft fuer Osteosynthesefragen) International
AOLF	Association des Orthopédistes de Langue Française
AOM	acute otitis media
AOPA	American Orthotic and Prosthetic Association
AOQ	l'Association d'Orthopédie du Québec
AORFA	American Orthopaedic Rugby Football Association
AORN	Association of Perioperative Registered Nurses
AOS	Academic Orthopaedic Society (also: AAOS Specialty Societies) Alaska Orthopaedic Society Arizona Orthopaedic Societ
AOSSM	American Orthopaedic Society for Sports Medicine (Journal) (also: AAOS Related Organizations)
AOx4	alert and oriented in 4 questions asked in evaluation of metal status
A-P	anteroposterior
ap	attachment point before dinner
Ap, AP	abdominal - perineal acute phase aminopurine angina pectoris ante partum (before delivery)

Ap, AP(cont.) antipyrine
apex
assessment and plans
access permit
accessory pathway
accounts payable
acid phosphatase
acinar parenchyma
action potential
active pepsin
acute pancreatitis
acute pneumonia
acute proliferative
adenomatous polyposis
adolescent psychiatry
aerosol pentamidine
after parturition
alkaline phosphatase
alum precipitated
aminopeptidase
amyloid p-component
angina pectoris
anterior pituitary
anteroposterior (view in X-rays)
antidromic potential
antral peristalsis
aortic pressure
aortopulmonary
apical pulse
apothecary
appendectomy
appendicitis
appendix
apurinic acid
area postrema
arithmetic progression
arterial pressure
artificial pneumothorax
aspiration pneumonia
association period
atherosclerotic plaque
atrial pacing

Ap, AP (cont.) atrioventricular pathway
Australian pharmacist
axiopulpal
before delivery *(Lat: ante partum)*

AP resection abdominal perineal resection of the rectum

A+P anterior and posterior
auscultation and palpation
auscultation and percussion

APA Abrus precatorius agglutinin
American Paralysis Association
American Psychiatric Association

APAAP alkaline phosphatase anti-alkaline phosphatase

APACHE acral pseudolymphomatous angiokeratoma of childhood

APAP acetaminophen (paracetamol)

APB abductor pollicis brevis (also ABPB)
atrial premature beat

APC activated protein C
adenomatous polyposis coli (gene on 5q21)
allophycocyanin
Ambulatory Patient Classification
anterior polar cataract
antero-posterior compression
antigen presenting cells
Argon Plasma Coagulation
aspirin, phenacetin, caffeine
atrial premature contraction

APCI atmosphere pressure chemical ionization

APD acquired perforating dermatosis
acute peritoneal dialysis
animal-based low-protein diet
antero-posterior diameter
anti-cholinergic antiparkinsonian drugs
automated peritoneal dialysis
pamidronate (a drug widely used for the treatment of hypercalcemia of malignancy)

APF assigned protection factor
APGAR American Pediatric Gross Assessment Record
aph aphasia
APH anterior pituitary hormone
aphasia
APHIS USDA's Animal and Plant Health Inspection Service
API Association for Pathology Informatics
APKD autosomal (dominant adult) polycystic kidney disease
APKD1 gene on chromosome 16 affected in 90% of cases of autosomal dominant polycystic kidney disease
APKD2 gene on chromosome 4 affected in 10% of cases of autosomal dominant polycystic kidney disease
APL abductor pollicis longus (also ABPL)
AP + L anteroposterior and lateral
APLAR Asian Pacific League of Association for Rheumatology
APLS advanced pediatric life support
APMA American Podiatric Medical Association
ApMV apple mosaic virus
APP Alzheimer amyloid precursor protein
appears
appendix
appointment
approximate
ApPC anthrylvinyl-labeled phosphatidylcholine
APPc cytoplasmic tail of the amyloid precursor protein
APPC aorto-pericardial pouch conduit
apalcillin
apoptotic cells
APPC (cont.) knee arthroplasty with polyethylene patellar components
p-aminophenylphosphorylcholine
APTA American Physical Therapy Association
APTT automated partial thromboplastin time
APUD amine precursor uptake and decarboxylation
APVOD arteriosclerotic peripheral vascular occlusive disease
APX ascorbate peroxidase
AQ water
aq, aq. water
AQL acceptance quality level
AR active resistance
admitting room
apical rate
artificial respiration
assessment report
assisted respiration
at risk
ARA-C cytarabine
ARC AIDS related complex
American red cross
ARD acute respiratory disease
atheroembolic renal disease
ARDS acute/adult respiratory distress syndrome
adult respiratory distress syndrome
ARE active-resistance exercise
ARF acute renal failure
acute respiratory failure
acute rheumatic fever
Arg arginine
ARI anxiety reaction, intense
ARIC atherosclerosis risk in communities
ARM allergy relief medicine
anxiety reaction, mild
arteriovenous malformation
ARNP advanced registered nurse practitioner

AROM active range of motion
artificial rupture of membranes

ARP absolute refractory period
American Registry of Pathology

ARRT American Registry of Radiologic Technologists

art arterial

ART absolute retention time (chromatography)
Achilles' tendon reflex test
artery
articulation
artificial

ARTH arthritic

ARVD arrythmogenic right ventricular dysplasia

AS alpha-synuclein
anal sphincter
aortic stenosis
arteriosclerosis
auris sinistra (left ear)
ankylosing spondylitis

ASA acetylsalicylic acid (aspirin)
American Society of Anesthesiologists

A.S.A. American Society of Anesthesiologists

A.S.A. 1 normal healthy patient

A.S.A. 2 patient with mild systemic disease

A.S.A. 3 patient with severe systemic disease

A.S.A. 4 patient with incapacitating systemic diease that is constant threat to life

ASAMI Association for the Study and Application of the Ilizarov Method

ASAP as soon as possible

ASB American Society of Biomechanics

ASBME Associated Students of Biomedical Engineering

ASBMR Austrian Society for Bone and Mineral Research (EFFO Member Society)

ASC arteriosclerosis
ascending

ASCAD arteriosclerotic coronary artery disease

ASCO American Society of Clinical Oncology

ASCUS atypical squamous cells of unknown significance

ASCVD arteriosclerotic cardiovascular disease

ASD atrial septal defect
autosensitization spongiotic dermatitis

ASDP American Society of Dermatopathology

ASES American Shoulder and Elbow Surgeons (also: AAOS Specialty Societies)

ASF African Swine Fever
anterior spinal fusion

ASH American Society of Hematology
asymmetrical septal hypertrophy

ASHD arteriosclerotic heart disease
atherosclerotic heart disease

ASHNR American Society of Head and Neck Radiology

ASI specific immunotherapy

ASIA American Spinal Injury Association (AAOS Related Organizations)

ASIC application specific integrated circuit

ASIS anterior superior iliac spine

ASM aggressive systemic mastocytosis
American Society for Microbiology

ASMI American Sports Medicine Institute

Asn asparagine

ASNR American Society of Neuroradiology

ASO Amplatzer septal occluder

A

ASO	antisense oligonucleotides
	antistreptolysin-O
	arteriosclerosis obliterans
ASOPA	American Society of Orthopaedic Physician's Assistants (also: AAOS Specialty Societies)
ASOS	Australian Society of Orthopaedic Surgeons
Asp	aspartic acid
ASPC	aspoxicillin
ASPNR	American Society of Pediatric Neuroradiology
ASPRS	American Society of Plastic and Reconstructive Surgeons
ASPVD	arteriosclerotic peripheral vascular disease
ASR	age standardized rate (incidence)
ASRT	American Society of Radiologic Technologists
Aß	amyloid beta-peptides
ASS	anterior superior spine
ASSH	American Society for Surgery of the Hand (also: AAOS Related Organizations)
assist	assistive
ASSR	American Society of Spine Radiology
ASSV	apple scar skin viroid
AST	all subjects treated
	alternate-site-testing
	antimicrobial susceptibility testing
	aspartate aminotransferase (formerly SGOT)
	Association of Surgical Technologists
	astigmatism
Astigm	astigmatism
ASTM	American Society for Testing and Materials
	American standard test method
as to	as tolerated
ASTRO	American Society for Therapeutic Radiology and Oncology
ASU	ambulatory surgery unit
ASVD	arteriosclerotic vascular disease
AT	achilles tendon
	anterior tibial
	athletic trainer
	atlas
at. Flutter	atrial flutter
ATF	amino-terminal fragment
	arrived to find
ATL	adult T-cell leukemia
	adult T-cell lymphoma
ATLL	adult T-cell leukemia
	adult T-cell lymphoma
ATLS	advanced trauma life support (training course)
ATN	acute tubular necrosis
ATNR	asymmetrical tonic neck reflex
AT/NC	atraumatic, normocephalic
ATP	attending physician
	autoimmune thrombocytopenic purpura
ATPS	ambient temperature and pressure saturated
atr	atrophy
ATR	Achilles tendon reflex
	alpha-thalassemia-mental retardation (syndrome)
	atracurium
	atrazine
	atrophy
ATRA	all-trans-retinoic acid (regimen used to treat acute promyelocytic leukemia)
Atr fib	atrial fibrillation
ATRIP	Africa Trade and Investment Program
ATRX	X-linked alpha-thalassemia-mental retardation (syndrome)
ATR-X	X-linked alpha-thalassemia-mental retardation (syndrome)

ATS Achard-Thiers syndrome
acid test solution
American Thoracic Society
American Trauma Society
American Trudeau Society
antirat thymocyte serum
antitetanus serum
antithymocyte serum
anxiety tension state
arteriosclerosis

ATSDR Agency for Toxic Substances and Disease Registry

att attending

ATT arginine tolerance test
aspirin tolerance time

ATV Abelson virus transformed
avian tumor virus

at vol atomic volume

at wt atomic weight

ATx adult thymectomy

atyp atypical

ATZ atypical transformation zone

Au Australia (antigen)
authorization
gold *(Lat: aurum)*

AU (auris unitas) both ears
according to custom *(Lat: ad usum)*
allergenic unit
Angstrom unit
antitoxin unit
arbitrary unit
Australia antigen
azauridine

A2U alpha 2u-globulin

AUA adenine-uracil-adenine codon for isoleucine
American Urological Association
asymptomatic urinary abnormalities

Au Ag Australia antigen

AUB abnormal uterine bleeding

AUC adenine-uracil-cytosine codon for isoleucine
area under the curve

aud, aud. auditory

AUD arthritis of unknown diagnosis

AUDIT alcohol use disorders identification test

aud-vis audiovisual

AUG acute ulcerative gingivitis
adenine-uracil-guanine codon for methionine

AUGH acute upper gastrointestinal hemorrhage

AuHAA Australia hepatitis-associated antigen

AUI Alcohol Use Inventory

AUL acute undifferentiated leukemia

AUMC area under the "moment" curve

AUO amyloid of unknown origin

AuP Australia antigen protein

AUPHA Association of University Programs in Health Administration

aur auric
auricle
auricular

Aur. Fib auricular fibrillation

aus auscultation

AuS Australia serum hepatitis

AUs alcohol users

AUS acute urethral syndrome

ausc auscultation

Ausc auscultation

AuSH Australia serum hepatitis

Auto-PEEP self-controlled positive end-expiratory pressure

AUU adenine-uracil-uracil codon for isoleucine

AuV Australia-Victoria strains of Newcastle disease virus

AUV anterior urethral valve
anterior uveitis

AUVIB	autotransfusion of UV-irradiated blood
aux	auxiliary
av	air velocity
	average
	avulsion
aV	abvolt
Av	average
	avoirdupois
AV	Adriamycin and vincristine
	air velocity
	allergic vasculitis
	anteroventral
	anteversion
	anticipatory vomiting
	antivirin
	aortic valve
	arteriovenous
	artificial ventilation
	assisted ventilation
	atrioventricular
	audio-visual
	augmented vector
	average
	aviation medicine
	avoirdupois
	avulsion
A/V	ampere/volt
	arteriovenous
A-V	arteriovenous
	atrioventricular
AVA	activity vector analysis
	antiviral antibody
	aortic valve area
	aortic valve atresia
	arteriovenous anastomosis
AV/AF	anteverted, anteflexed
AVB	atrioventricular block
AVC	aberrant ventricular conduction
	Academy of Veterinary Cardiology
	aortic valve closure
	Association of Vitamin Chemists
AVC (cont.)	associative visual cortex
	associative visual cortex
	atrioventricular cana
	automatic volume controll
AVCN	anteroventral cochlear nucleus
AVCS	atrioventricular conduction system
AVCx	atrioventricular circumflex branch
AVD	active vasodilator
	allograft vascular disease
	aortic valve defects
	aortic/acquired valvular disease
	apoptotic volume decrease
	apparent volume of distribution
	Army Veterinary Department
	arteriovenous delay
	atherosclerotic vascular disease
	atrioventricular dissociation/delay
	average vessel density
	avidin
AVD(O)	arteriovenous oxygen difference
AVDO2	arteriovenous oxygen saturation difference
AVDO2B	arteriovenous oxygen saturation difference, basal
avdp	avoirdupois
AVDP	average diastolic pressure
ave	average
AVE	aortic valve echocardiogram
aver	average
aVF	automated volt foot
	unipolar limb lead on the left leg in electrocardiography
AVF	antiviral factor
	arteriovenous fistula
avg	average
AVG	ambulatory visit group
	average
AVH	acute viral hepatitis
AVHD	acquired valvular heart disease
AVHS	acquired valvular heart syndrome
AVI	air velocity index

AVI (cont.) Association of Veterinary Inspectors
AVJ atrioventricular junction
atrioventricular junction rhythm
AVJRe atrioventricular junctional reentrant
aVL automated volt left
unipolar limb lead on the left arm in electrocardiography
AVLINE Audiovisuals On-Line (database)
AVM arteriovenous malformations
atrio-ventricular malformations
aviation medicine
AVMA American Veterinary Medical Association
AVN acute vasomotor nephropathy
atrioventricular nodal (conduction)
atrioventricular node
avascular necrosis (MRI evaluation)
AVND atrioventricular node dysfunction
AVNFH avascular necrosis of the femoral head
AVNFRP atrioventricular node functional refractory period
AVNR atrioventricular nodal reentry
AVNRT atrioventricular node reentry tachycardia
AVO aortic valve opening
aortic valve orifice
atrioventricular opening
A-VO2 arteriovenous oxygen
AVO2 arteriovenous oxygen ratio
AVP abnormal vasopressin
actinomycin-vincristine-Platinol
ambulatory venous pressure
antiviral protein
aqueous vasopressin
arginine–vasopressin
arteriovenous passage time
vasopressin
AVPU alert, verbal, painful, unresponsive (neurologic test)
aVR automated volt right
unipolar limb lead on the right arm in electrocardiography
AVR accelerated ventricular rhythm
antiviral regulator
aortic valve replacement
AVRI acute viral respiratory infection
AVRP atrioventricular refractory period
AVRR antiviral repressor regulator
AVRT atrioventricular reentrant tachycardia
atrioventricular reciprocating tachycardia
AVS aortic valve stenosis
arteriovenous shunt
auditory vocal sequencing
AVSD atrioventricular septal defect
AVSV aortic valve stroke volume
AVT Allen vision test
arginine vasotocin
Aviation Medicine Technician
Av3V anteroventral third ventricle
AVZ avascular zone
aw airway
water activity
AW able to work
above waist
abrupt withdrawal
alcohol withdrawal
alive and well
alveolar wall
anterior wall
atomic warfare
atomic weight
A+W alive and well
AWA as well as
AWAR anterior wall of aortic root
AWBM alveolar wall basement membrane
AW-GC apatite and wollastonite containing glass-ceramic
ax axillary
Ax. axilla, axillary

AX	axial
	axillary
AXR	abdominal x-ray
A.Z.	Ascheim-Zondek test
AZT	azidothymidine (zidovudine)
AZUR	6-azauridine

B

B	B-cells
	black
	born
	fever, sweats, or weight loss ("B" symptoms in Hodgkin lymphoma)
B.	bath
Ba	barium
BA	barium
	basic (for EMT-Basic level)
	blood alcohol
	bone age
	brachial artery
	bronchial asthma
BAB, Bab.	Babinski's sign
BAC	blood alcohol concentration
BACR	British Association for Cancer Research
bact	bacteriology
Bact	bacteriologist
	bacteriology
BaE, Ba.E	barium enema
BAER	brain stem auditory evoked response
BAIJP	Bovie-assisted uvulopalatoplasty
BAL	blood alcohol level
	bronchoalveolar lavage
BALF	bronchoalveolar lavage fluid
B-ALL	B-cell acute lymphoblastic leukemia
bals	balsam
BALT	bronchus-associated lymphoid tissue
BaM	barium meal
BAM	bamifylline
	basilar artery migraine
	bilateral augmentation mammoplasty
	brachial artery mean (pressure)
BAME	benzoylarginine methyl ester
BamHI	restriction enzyme from Bacillus amyloliquefaciens H
BAN	British Approved Name
	British Association of Neurologists
BANS	Back, posterior upper Arm, posterior Neck, Scalp
	prognostically high-risk sites for malignant melanoma
BAO	basal acid output
	brachial artery output
BAO-MAO	basal acid output to maximal acid output (ratio)
BAP	bacterial alkaline phosphatase
	Behavior Activity Profile
	beta-amyloid peptide
	blood-agar plate
	bovine albumin in phosphate buffer
	brachial artery pressure
BAPhysMed	British Association Physical Medicine
BAPI	barley alkaline protease inhibitor
BAPN	beta-aminoproprionitrile fumarate
BAPO	Belgian Association of Pediatric Orthopaedics
BAPP	beta amyloid precursor protein
BAPS	biomechanical ankle platform system
	bovine albumin phosphate saline
	British Association of Paediatric Surgeons
	British Association of Plastic Surgeons
BAPT	British Association of Physical Training

BAPTA 1,2-bis (aminophenoxy) ethane-N,N,N,N'-tetraacetic acid
BAPV bovine alimentary papilloma virus
BAQ brain-age quotient
bar barometric
BAR bariatrics
barometer
barometric
beta-adrenergic receptor
biofragmentable anastomosis ring
Barb barb, barbiturate, barbituric
BARB barbiturates
BARK beta-adrenergic receptor kinase
Barn benzamide
BARN bilateral acute retinal necrosis
BARS behaviorally anchored rating scale
BART blood-activated recalcification time
bas basilar
basophil, basophilic
Bas basophils
Bas. basal, basilar
BaS barium swallow
BAS balloon atrial septostomy
benzyl anti-serotonin
beta-adrenergic stimulation
boric acid solution
BASA Boston Assessment of Severe Aphasia
BASE B27-arthritis-sacroiliitis-extra-articular features (syndrome)
BASH body acceleration synchronous with heart rate
BASI barley alpha-amylase/subtilisin inhibitor
BASIC Beginner's All-Purpose Symbolic Introduction Code
baso basophil
BASO British Association of Surgical Oncologists
basos basophils (leukocytes)
BASPCAN British Association for the Study and Prevention of Child Abuse and Neglect
BAT basic aid training
best available technology
blunt abdominal trauma
brown adipose tissue
BAUS British Association of Urological Surgeons
BAV bicuspid aortic valve
BAVCP bilateral abductor vocal cord paralysis
BAVFO bradycardia after arteriovenous fistula occlusion
BAW bronchoalveolar washing
bb Bolton point
both bones
BB bad breath
bed bath
bed board
beta blockade, beta blocker
BioBreeding (rat)
blanket bath
blood bank
blood buffer
blow bottle
blue bloaters (emphysema)
borderline
both bones
breakthrough bleeding
breast biopsy
brush border
buffer base
bundle branch
isoenzyme of creatine kinase containing two B subunits
BBA born before arrival
BBB blood buffer base
blood-brain barrier
bundle branch block
BBBB bilateral bundle-branch block
BBBD blood brain barrier disruption

BBC Belgian Bone Club (EFFO Member Society)
bromobenzycyanide
BB/CC back board and cervical collar
BBD benign breast disease
BBE Bacteroides bile esculin (agar)
BBEP brush border endopeptidase
BBF bronchial blood flow
BB/FS breast biopsy/frozen section
BBI Biomedical Business International
Bowman-Birk soybean inhibitor
BBIW BioBreeding/Worcester (rat)
BBM brush border membrane
BBMV brush border membrane vesicle
BBN broad band noise
BBRS Burks' Behavior Rating Scale
BBS Barolet-Biedl syndrome
bashful bladder syndrome
benign breast syndrome
bilateral breath sounds
bombesin
borate-buffered saline
brown bowel syndrome
BBT basal body temperature
b/c benefit/cost (ratio)
BC Bachelor of Surgery *(Lat: Baccalaureus Chirurgiae)*
back care
bactericidal concentration
basal cell
basket cell
battle casualty
bicarbonate
biliary colic
bipolar cell
birth control
blastic crisis
blood count
blood culture
Blue Cross (plan)
board certified
bone conduction

BC (cont.) brachiocephalic
breast cancer
bronchial carcinoma
buccal cartilage
buccocervical
buffy coat
B+C biopsy and curettage
BCA balloon catheter angioplasty
basal cell atypia
bicinchoninic acid
blood color analyzer
Blue Cross Association
branchial cleft anomaly
breast cancer antigen
BCAA branched chain amino acid
BCAg basal-cell antigen
BCAT brachiocephalic arterial trunk
BCB blood-cerebrospinal fluid barrier
brilliant cresyl blue
BCBR bilateral carotid body resection
BCBSA Blue Cross and Blue Shield Association
BC/BS Blue cross/Blue shield
bcc body-centered-cubic
BCC basal cell carcinoma
benign cellular changes (pap smear)
biliary cholesterol concentration
birth control clinic
BCCG British Cooperative Clinical Group
BCCP biotin carboxyl carrier protein
BCD basal cell dysplasia
binary-coded decimal
bleomycin, cyclophosphamide, dactinomycin
BCDDP Breast Cancer Detection Demonstration Project
BCDF B-cell differentiation factor
BCDL Brachmann-Cornelia de Lange (syndrome)
BCDRS brief Carroll depression rating scale
BCDS bulimia cognitive distortions scale

BCDSP Boston Collaborative Drug Surveillance Program
BCE basal cell epithelioma
benign childhood epilepsy
bubble chamber equipment
BCEI breast cancer estrogen-inducible
BCF basophil chemotactic factor
bioconcentration factor
breast cyst fluid
BCFP breast cyst fluid protein
BCG bacille Calmette-Guérin (vaccine)
ballistocardiography, ballistocardiogram
bicolor guaiac test
bromcresol green
BCGF B-cell growth factor
BCh Bachelor of Surgery *(Lat: Baccalaureus Chirurgiae)*
BCH basal cell hyperplasia
BChD Bachelor of Dental Surgery
BCHE butyrylcholinesterase
BChir Bachelor of Surgery (Lat: Baccalaureus Chirurgiae)
Bchl, bChl bacterial chlorophyll
BCHS Bureau of Community Health Services
BCHT bicaval heart transplantation
BCI behavioral cues index
brain-computer interface
BCIA Biomedical Clinical Instrumentation Association
BCIP 5-bromo-4-chloro-3-inodolyl phosphate
BCKA branched-chain keto acid
BCKD branched-chain alpha-keto acid dehydrogenase
bcl-2 (B-cell lymphoma-2) a gene that inhibits apoptosis
overexpression may cause follicular lymphomas
BCL bandage contact lens
basic cycle length
BCL (cont.) B-cell leukemia/lymphoma
BCLPD B-cell chronic lymphoproliferative disorders
BCLs B cell lines
basic cycle lengths
bifocal contact lenses
BCLS basic cardiac life support
BCNU carmustine
BCP birth control pills
bcr breakpoint cluster region
BCS breast conservation surgery
BD band
barbital-dependent
barbiturate dependence
base deficit
base of prism down
basophilic degeneration
Batten disease
behavioral disorder
Behcet disease
belladonna
bicarbonate dialysis
bile duct
binocular deprivation
biotinylated dextran
birth date
black death
block design (test)
blood donor
blue diaper (syndrome)
board
border disease
borderline dull
bound
Bowen disease
brain damage
brain dead, brain death
Briquet disorder
bronchodilation, bronchodilator
buccodistal
bundle
buoyant density

BD (cont.)	Byler disease
	twice a day *(Lat: bis die)*
B-DD	B-domain-deleted
BDG	bidirectional Glenn shunt
BDI	blunt duodenal injury
BDI-1	monoclonal antibody against human bladder carcinoma
BDI-PC	Beck Depression Inventory for Primary Care
BE	barium enema
	below the elbow
	benzoylecgonine (cocaine)
	brisk and equal
BEA	2-bromoethylamine hydrobromide
BEC2	an anti-idiotypic monoclonal antibody that mimics the ganglioside GD3
BEE	basal energy expenditure
BELI	beta-endorphin-like immunoreactivity
BEMS	Bioelectromagnetics Society
BERG	balloon-assisted endoscopic retroperitoneal gasless (BERG lumbar interbody fusion)
BF	biofiltration
	black female
	blood flow
	bone fragment
bFGF	basic fibroblast growth factor
BFP	bilateral facial paralysis
	biological false positive
BG	bone graft
BGB	bisglucuronosyl bilirubin
BGS	balance, gate, station
BGTT	borderline glucose tolerance test
BHA	butylated hydroxyanisole
BH cells	baby hamster kidney cells
BHG	Belgian Hand Group
BHIA	British Healthcare Internet Association
BHP	benign hypertrophic prostate
BHS	beta hemolytic streptococcus
BHT	blunt head trauma
	butylated hydroxytoluene
BHV-1	Bovine Herpesvirus-1
BI	background interval
	bacterial index
	bactericidal index
	Barthel Index
	base-in (prism)
	basilar impression
	bilateral
	Billroth I (operation)
	biological indicator
	biotechnology informatics
	biphasic
	bodily injury
	bone impaction
	bone injury
	brain injury
	burn index
	both sides (e.g. bilateral)
	two components (e.g. biphasic)
Bic.	biceps
BID	brought in dead
bid, b.i.d.	twice a day (bis in die)
BID, BD	twice a day (bis in die)
BIH	bilateral inguinal hernia
BIJC	The British Isles Joint TNM Classification
BIL	bilateral
bilat.	bilateral
bili, BILI	bilirubin
BIN, b.i.n.	bin, twice a night
BIP	bronchiolitis obliterans with interstitial pneumonia
BIPAP	biphasic intermittent positive airway pressure
BIR	baculovirus IAP repeat
	British Institute of Radiology
BIRP	B1-independent rotation phase-cycled
	BIR-containing proteins
Bis-GMA	bisphenol-a-glycidyl methacrylate

BiVAS biventricular assist system
biw, BiW twice a week
BJ Bence Jones (proteinuria)
biceps jerk
bone and joint
BJE bones, joints, extremities
BJM bones, joints, muscles
BJP Bence Jones protein
BK back
below the knee
bk. back
BKA below knee amputation
BKP back pain
BL bilateral lower lung fields
blood loss
bl cult blood culture
Blad. bladder
bld. blood
BLE both lower extremities
BLEED bleeding (ongoing), low systolic blood pressure, elevated prothrombin time, erratic mental status, disease (unstable comorbid disease) (mnemonic for gastro-intestinal hemorrhage)
BLP beta-lipoprotein
BLPD B-cell lymphoproliferative disorder
BLQ both lower quadrants
BLS basic life support
BLS-D basic life support and defibrillation
Bl.T bleeding time
BM basal metabolism
black male
blood monitoring
body mass
bone marrow
bowel movement
BMA British Medical Association
butyl methacrylate
BMC bone mineral content
BMD 3-(s)-(benzyloxycarbonyl)methyl
Becker muscular dystrophies
BMD (cont.) Best's macular dystrophy
bone mineral density
BMES Biomedical Engineering Society
BMG benign monoclonal gammopathy
BMI body mass index
BMJ British Medical Journal
BMMEC bone marrow microvascular endothelial cells
BMN bone marrow necrosis
BMP bone morphogenetic protein
BMR basal metabolic rate
BMT bone marrow transplant (see HDC and HDC/BMT)
BMZ basement membrane zone
BN bound niacin
bulimia nervosa
BND barely noticeable difference
BNLI British National Lymphoma Investigation
BNO bladder neck obstruction
Bnp Bothrops neuwiedi pauloensis
BNP brain natriuretic peptide
BNP1350 7-[(2-trimethylsilyl)ethyl]-20(S)-camptothecin, a novel semi-synthetic, highly lipophilic, silicon-containing camptothecin + an inhibitor of topoisomerase I
bNP I+II bovine neurophysin-I and II
BNST bed nucleus of the stria terminalis
BNT bacterial nosocomial tracheitis
Bnu Bothrops neuwiedi urutu
BOA born on arrival
British Oncology Association
British Orthopaedic Association
BODMA British Oncology Data Managers Association (UK)
Body wt. body weight
BOE bilateral otitis externa
BOL buccal odontoblast layer
BOLD blood oxygenation level-dependent
BOM bilateral otitis media
BOMA otitis media, both ears, acute

BOO	bladder outlet obstruction
BOOP	bronchiolitis obliterans-organizing pneumonia
BOP	blood, ova, parasites
BOS	Bombay Orthopaedic Association
BOT	bottle
BOTA	Belgian Orthopaedic Trauma Association
BOW	bag of waters
BP	bipolar blood pressure body part British Pharmacopoeia bullous pemphigoid
B/P	blood pressure
BPC	blood pressure cuff
BPC	bronchoprovocation challenge
BPD	biparietal diameter borderline personality disorder bronchopulmonary dysplasia
BPH	benign prostatic hypertrophy
BPI	bactericidal permeability increasing protein Brief Pain Inventory
BPL	Bauchinia purpurea alba
bpm, BPM	beats per minute breaths per minute
BPP	blood pressure and pulse
BPPV	benign paroxysmal positional vertigo
BPR	brief psychiatric rating (scale)
B19-PRCA	pure red cell aplasia caused by parvovirus B19
BPS	Belgian Pain Society
BPTB	bone-patellar tendon-bone
BR	bacteriorhodopsin bathroom bed rest
Br.	breech presentation
brach.	brachial
brat	brain tumor gene
BRAT	a fusion protein between the membrane protein bacteriorhodopsin (BR) and the catalytic subunit of aspartyl transcarbamylase from Escherichia coli Baylor Rapid Autologous Transfusion system Behaviour Research and Therapy
BRB	bright red blood
BRBPR	bright red blood per rectum
BrBx.	breast biopsy
BRCA genes	"breast cancer genes", involved in a percentage of breast cancers (pron: bra,ka one ...)
BRD(C)	bovine respiratory disease (complex)
BRFSS	Behavioral Risk Factor Surveillance system
BRM	biological response modifier
broncho	bronchoscopy
BRP	bathroom privileges
BRW	breast meat weight
BRY	breast meat yield
BS	blood sugar body substance isolation bowel sounds breath sounds bronchial secretion
B.S.	breath sounds
BSA	body surface area bovine serum albumin bowel signs active
BSAEP	brain stem auditory evoked potentials
BSB	bedside bag
BSC	bedside commode
BSD	baby soft diet bedside drainage
BSE	bovine spongiform encephalopathy breast self examination

BSER brainstem evoked response audiometry
BSI bloodstream infections
BSL baseline
BSN bowel sounds normal
BSO bilateral salpingo-oophorectomy
BSP bromsulphalein (dye)
BSPh bachelor of science in pharmacy
BSQ behavior style questionnaire
BSR basal skin resistance
blood sedimentation rate
bowel sounds regular
brain stimulation reinforcement
Buschke selective reminding (test)
BSS Bachelor of Sanitary Science
balanced salt solution
Bernard-Soulier syndrome
black silk suture
British Scoliosis Society
buffered salt solution
buffered single substrate
BSSE bile salt-stimulated esterase
BSSG sitogluside
BSSH British Society for Surgery of the Hand
BSSL bile salt-stimulated lipase
BST bacteriuria screening test
blood serologic test
brief stimulus therapy
BSTFA bis-trimethylsilyltrifluoroacetamide
BSU Bartholin, Skene, urethral (glands)
basic structural unit
British standard unit
BSV binocular single vision
BT bedtime
bitemporal
bitrochanteric
bladder tumor
Blalock-Taussig (shunt)
bleeding time
blood type, blood typing
BT (cont.) blue tetrazolium
blue tongue
body temperature
borderline tuberculoid
botulinum toxin
bovine turbinate (cells)
brain tumor
breast tumor
base of tongue
BTA Blood Transfusion Association
BTB breakthrough bleeding
bromthymol blue
BTBL bromothymol blue lactose
BTC basal temperature chart
biliary tract complication
body temperature chart
Bt2cAMP N6,O2c- dibutyryladenosine 3c:5c-cyclic monophosphate, a dibutyryl derivative of cAMP
BTCG Brain Tumor Cooperative Group
BTD biliary tract disease
BTDS benzoylthiamine disulfide
BTE behind the ear (hearing aid)
bovine thymus extract
BTFS breast tumor frozen section
BTg bovine trypsinogen
BTG beta-thromboglobulin
BthU British thermal unit
BTL bilateral tubal ligation
basic trauma life support
BTM blood temperature monitor
benign tertian malaria
BTMSA bis-trimethylsilacetylene
BTP biliary tract pain
biological treatment planning
BTPABA N-benzoyl-L-tyrosyl-p-aminobenzoic acid
BTPS at body temperature and ambient pressure,and saturated with water vapor (gas)
BTr bovine trypsin
BTR Bezold-type reflex

BTR (cont.) biceps tendon reflex
biceps tendon reflex

BTS blood transfusion service
blue toe syndrome
bradycardia-tachycardia syndrome

BTSG Brain Tumor Study Group

bTSH bovine thyroid-stimulating hormone

BTU British thermal unit

BTV blue tongue virus

BTW back to work
by the way

BTx blood transfusion

BTX botulinum toxin
brevetoxin

BTZ benzothiazepine

Bu bushel
butyl

BU base of prism up
Bethesda unit
blood urea
Bodansky unit
bromouracil
burn unit
Buruli ulcer

BUA blood uric acid
broadband ultrasonic attenuation

BUAS Boston University Accutane Survey

Buc Bucc, buccal

BUDR bromodeoxyuridine

BUDS bilateral upper dorsal sympathectomy

BUE both upper extremities

BUF buffalo (rat)

BUG buccal ganglion

BUI brain uptake index

BULIT bulimia test

BuMed Bureau of Medicine and Surgery

BUMP behavioral regression or upset in hospitalized medical patients (scale)

BUN blood urea nitrogen

BUN/CR blood urea nitrogen/creatine ratio

BUO bleeding of undetermined origin,
bruising of undetermined origin

BUQ both upper quadrants

BUR bilateral ureteral occlusion

BUS busulfan
urethral, and Skene glands

But but, butyrate, butyric

BV bacitracin V
bacterial vaginosis
biological value
blood vessel
blood volume
bronchovesicular

BVA Blind Veterans Association
British Veterinary Association

BVAD biventricular assist device

BVAS Birmingham Vasculitis Activity Score (prognostic scoring systems)

BVC British Veterinary Codex

BVD bovine viral diarrhea

BVD-MD bovine viral diarrhea-mucosal disease

BVDT brief vestibular disorientation test

BVDU bromovinyldeoxyuridine

BVDV bovine virus diarrhea virus

BVE binocular visual efficiency
blood vessel endothelium
blood volume expander

BVGHV Belgian Society of Medicine and Surgery of the Foot

BVH biventricular hypertrophy

BVI blood vessel invasion

BVL bilateral vas ligation

BVM bag-valve-mask
bronchovascular markings
Bureau of Veterinary Medicine

BVMGT Bender Visual-Motor Gestalt Test

BVMOT Bender Visual-Motor Gestalt Test

BVMS Bachelor of Veterinary Medicine and Science

BVO branch vein occlusion

BVOT	Belgische Vereniging voor Orthopedie en Traumatologie
BVP	blood vessel prosthesis
BVP	blood volume pulse
	burst of ventricular pacing
BVR	baboon virus replication
	bureau of vocational rehabilitation
BVS	blanked ventricular sense
BVSc	Bachelor of Veterinary Science
BVU	bromoisovalerylurea
BVV	bovine vaginitis virus
BW	bacteriological warfare
	bed wetting
	below waist
	biological warfare
	biological weapon
	birth weight
	black woman
	bladder washout
	blood Wasserman (reaction)
	body water
	body weight
BWD	bacillary white diarrhea
BWFI	bacteriostatic water for injection
BWI	birth weight
BWS	battered woman (or wife) syndrome
BWS	Beckwith-Wiedemann syndrome
BWST	black widow spider toxin
BWSV	black widow spider venom
Bwt	body weight
BWYV	beet western yellow virus
bx, BX	bacitracin X
Bx, BX	biopsy
BXO	balanitis xerotica obliterans
ByCPR	bystander cardiac pulmonary resuscitation
BYDV	barley yellow dwarf virus
BYE	Barila-Yaguchi-Eveland (medium)
Bz	Bzl, benzoyl
BZ	benzodiazepine
BZD	benzodiazepine
BZQ	benzquinamide
BZRP	benzodiazepine receptor peripheral (type)
BZS	Bannayan-Zonana syndrome

C

c	clinical
	with *(Lat: cum)*
c.	with
C	Caucasian
	Celsius
	centigrade
	certainty factor
	cervical
	chlamydia
	clonidine
	complement
	concentration
	cortex
	cyanosis
	cysteine
	cytosine
	List
	standard clearance
	static respiratory compliance
C.	Celsius
	centigrade
	complement
c̄	with *(Lat: cum)*
CI-XII	1st to 12th cranial nerve
Ca	calcium
CA	cancer
	carbonic anhydrase
	carcinoma
	cardiac arrest
	catchment area
	Caucasian adult
	chromosomal aberration
	chronological age
	controlled atmospheres

C

CA (cont.)	cornu Ammonis (Ammon's horn)
	corpus allatum
	cytoxan plus adriamycin (treatment regimen)
CAA	cerebral amyloid angiopathy
	crystalline amino acids
	cytosine-adenine-adenine codon for glutamine
CAB	coronary artery bypass
CABG	coronary artery bypass graft (pron.: 'cabbage')
CAC	cytosine-adenine-cytosine codon for histidine
CACO3	calcium carbonate
CAD	coronary artery disease
CAE	carotid artery endarterectomy
CAF	caffeine
	Caucasian adult female
	cell adhesion factor
	chloramphenicol
	chronic atrial fibrillation
	citric acid fermentation
	cyclophosphamide, adriamycin, and 5-fluorouracil
CAG	cytosine-adenine-guanine codon for glutamine
CAH	chronic active hepatitis
CAHD	coronary atherosclerotic heart disease
CAI	carbonic anhydrase inhibitor
Cal	calorie(s)
CALGB	Cancer and Leukemia Group B (USA)
cALL	common ALL
CALLA	common acute lymphoblastic leukemia antigen
CAM	Caucasian adult male
	Complementary and Alternative Medicine
CAMIS	Computer Assisted Minimally Invasive Surgery (Cleveland Clinic Foundation)
CAMP	The Childhood Asthma Management Program
c-ANCA	cytoplasmic antineutrophil cytoplasmic antibodies
CAO	chronic airflow obstruction
CAOS	Computer Assisted Orthopaedic Systems (Hull University)
CAP	College of American Pathologists
	capsule
CAPD	continuous ambulatory peritoneal dialysis
CAPMR	Canadian Association of Physical Medicine + Rehabilitation
caps, Caps	capsules
Car	carbapenem
car.	carotid
Card Cath	cardiac catheterization
card.	cardiac
CAREMIS	Current Agricultural Management Information System
CAS	computer aided surgery (Journal)
CaSac	calcium saccharin
CASIB	computer-assisted frameless stereotactic interstitial brachytherapy
CAST-6	Children of Alcoholics Screening Test, 6-Item Version
CASTLE	carcinoma showing thymus-like differentiation
CAT	cataract
	chloramphenicol acetyltransferase
	coital alignment technique
	computed axial tomography
CATCH	critically attained threshold of cerebral hypoperfusion
cath	catheterization
	catheter
Cath	catheter
CAU	cytosine-adenine-uracil codon for histidine
CAV	cytoxan, adriamycin, and vincristine

CAVB chronic AV block
CAVH continuous arterio-venous haemofiltration
CAVHD continuous arterio-venous haemodialysis
CB cesarean birth
chest-back
chronic bronchitis
current complaint
CBC combinatorial chemistry
complete blood count
CB/CC centroblastic/centrocytic lymphoma
CBD common bile duct
corticobasal degeneration
CBDS corticobasal degeneration syndrome
CBF cerebral blood flow
core binding factor (16q22)
coronary blood flow
CBG capillary blood gas
cortisol binding globulin
CBGD cortical-basal ganglionic degeneration
CBI continuous bladder irrigation
CBP colon anastomosis bursting pressure
CBPP contagious bovine pleuropneumonia
CBQ California Behavior Questionnaire
cellobiose: quinone oxidoreductase
Childbearing Questionnaire
Children's Behavior Questionnaire
Conflict Behavior Questionnaire
CBR complete bed rest
CB3S Coxsackie B3 virus susceptibility
CBS cervicobrachial syndrome
chronic brain syndrome
clinical behavioral science
conjugated bile salts
culture-bound syndrome
cystathionine beta-synthase
CBT carotid body tumor
cognitive behavioral treatment/ therapy
computed body tomography
CBV capillary blood cell velocity
computed body tomography
central blood volume
cerebral blood volume
circulating blood volume
corrected blood volume
cortical blood volume
Coxsackie B virus
CBVD cerebrovascular disease
CBW chemical and biological warfare
CBX computer-based examination
CBZ carbamazepine
cc clean catch
concave
corrected
cubic centimeter
cc. cubic centimeter
Cc concave
CC Caucasian child
cc, cubic centimeter
chief complaint
closed cup
closing capacity
collagenous colitis
colony count
colorectal cancer
columnar cells
commission certified
common cold
complicating condition
compound cathartic
computer calculated
concordance
congenital cardiopathy
congenital cataract
consumptive coagulopathy
contrast cystogram
conversion complete

C

CC (cont.) coracoclavicular
cord compression
corpora cardiaca
corpus callosum
costochondral
Coulter counter
craniocervical
creatinine clearance
critical care
critical condition
Crohn colitis
Cronkhite-Canada (syndrome)
crus cerebri
Current Contents

C/C, C.C. chief complaint

C+C cold and clammy

C1 - C7 Cervical vertebrae

C1...C7 Cervical nerve 1 through 7, cervical vertebrae 1 through 7

C-C convexo-concavc

CCA cephalin cholesterol antigen
chick cell agglutination
chimpanzee coryza agent
choriocarcinoma
circulating cathodic antigen
circumflex coronary artery
common carotid artery
congenital contractural arachnodactyly
constitutional chromosome abnormality
Consultative Committee on Agriculture
cytosine-cytosine-adenine codon for proline

CCAT chick cell agglutination test
conglutinating complement absorption test

C-cath cardiac catheterization

CCB calcium channel blocker

CCBV central circulating blood volume

CCC care-cure coordination

CCC (cont.) cathodal closure contraction
chronic calculous cholecystitis
chronic catarrhal colitis
comprehensive care clinic
concurrent care concern
consecutive case conference
council on clinical classification
critical care complex
cylindrical confronting cistemae
cytosine-cytosine-cytosine codon for proline

CC+C colony count and culture

CCCAD The Canadian Consensus Conference on the Assessment of Dementia

CCCC centrifugal countercurrent chromatography

cccDNA covalently closed circular deoxyribonucleic acid

CCCE cross-cultural cognitive examination

CCCI cathodal closure clonus

CCCP carbonyl cyanide m-chloro-phenyl-hydrazone

CCCR closed chest cardiac resuscitation

CCCS Canadian Committee on Cancer Staging

CCCS condom catheter collecting system

CCCT closed craniocerebral trauma

CCCU comprehensive cardiac care unit

CCD calibration curve data
central core disease
charge-coupled device
childhood celiac disease
cleidocranial dysplasia
clinical cardiovascular disease
countercurrent distribution
cumulative cardiotoxic dose

CCDC Canadian Communicable Disease Center

CCDN Central Council for District Nursing

CcDNA closed circle deoxyribonucleic acid

CCE carboline carboxylic acid ester
chamois contagious ecthyma
clear-cell endothelioma
clubbing, cyanosis, edema
countercurrent electrophoresis
cyanosis, clubbing, edema

CCEHRP Committee to Coordinate Environmental Health and Related Programs

CCEI Crown-Crisp Experimental Index

CCF cancer coagulation factor
cardiolipin complement fixation
carotid-cavernous fistula
centrifuged culture fluid
cephalin-cholesterol flocculation
compound comminuted fracture
congestive cardiac failure
crystal-induced chemotactic factor

CCFA cefotoxin-cycloserine fructose agar

CCFAS compact colony-forming active substance

CCFE cyclophosphamide, cisplatin, fluorouracil, and extramustine

CCFMG Cooperating Committee on Foreign Medical Graduates

CCFPC Certificant member, College of Family Physicians of Canada

CCG Children's Cancer Group (USA)
cholecystogram, cholecystography
cholecystogram, cholecystography
cytosine-cytosine-guanine codon for proline

CCGC capillary column gas chromotography

CCH C-cell hyperplasia
cholinergic agonist carbachol
chronic chloride hemagglutination
chronic cholestatic hepatitis
circumscribed choroidal hemangiomas

CCHA Canadian Council on Hospital Accreditation

CCHD Chester County Health Department
cyanotic congenital heart disease

CCHE Central Council for Health Education

CCHFA Canadian Council on Health Facilities Accreditation

CCHMS Central Committee for Hospital Medical Services

CCHP Consumer Choice Health Plan

CCHS congenital central hypoventilation syndrome

CCI Cardiovascular Credentialing International
cyanotic congenital heart disease
chronic coronary insufficiency
common client interface
corrected count increment

CCID50 cell culture infectious dose 50 %

CCK cholecystokinin

CCK-8 cholecystokinin octapeptide

CCKLI cholecystokinin-like immunoreactivity

CCK-OP cholecystokinin octapeptide

CCK-PZ cholecystokinin-pancreozymin

CCKRB cholecystokinin receptor B

CCL carcinoma cell line
certified cell line
Charcot-Leyden crystal
continuing care level
critical carbohydrate level

CCLI composite clinical and laboratory index

CCM cerebrocostomandibular (syndrome)
chemical cleavage of mismatch
congestive cardiomyopathy
contextual choice model
craniocervical malformation
critical care medicine

CCMC Committee on the Costs of Medical Care

C

CCME Coordinating Council on Medical Education

CCMS cerebrocostomandibular syndrome
clean catch midstream (urine)
clinical care management system

CCMSU clean catch midstream urine

CCMT catechol methyltransferase

CCMU critical care medical unit

CCN caudal central nucleus
community care network
coronary care nursing
critical care nursing

CCNHP community college nursing home project

CCNU N-(2-chloroethyl)-N'-cyclo-hexyl-N-nitrosourea

CCO cytochrome C oxidase

CCOT cervical compression overloading test

CCPD continuous cycling peritoneal dialysis

CCR continuous complete remission

CCRG Children's Cancer Research Group (Oxford,UK)

CCS Canadian Cancer Society
serum corticosterone

CCSC Canadian Cardiovascular Society Classification

CCT central conduction time

CCU clean catch urine
coronary/cardiac care unit
cytosine-cytosine-uracil codon for proline

CCV critical closing volume

Ccy cystatin C

CCY casein hydrolysate-yeast extract-containing medium
cholecystectomy
coiled-coils gene

CD cadaver donor
Cadmium (Cd)
candela (cd)

CD (cont.) canine distemper
canine dose
carbohydrate dehydratase
carbon dioxide
cardiac disease
cardiac dullness
cardiac dysrhythmia
cardiovascular disease
Carrel-Dakin (fluid)
Castleman disease
caudad
caudal (cd)
cause of death
celiac disease
cell dissociation
cervico dorsal
cesarean delivery
chemical dependency
circular dichroism
cluster of differentiation (eg. CD4, CD8) - full list of CDs
coccygeal (cd)
color doppler
combination drug
common (bile) duct
communicable disease
compact disk
completely denaturated
conceptual design
conduct disorder
conduction disorder
condylion (cd)
conjugata diagonalis
consanguineous donor
consent decree
contact dermatitis
contagious disease
control diet
controlled drug
conventional dialysis
convulsive disorder
convulsive dose

CD (cont.)	corneal dystrophy Cotrel-Dubousset (rod) Crohn disease crossed diagonal curative dose cutdown cystic duct
CD50	fifty percent convulsant dose
CD138	plasma cell membrane receptor
CD138/B-B4	immunoperoxidase stain using an antibody against CD 138
CDA	chitin deacetylases congenital dyserythropoietic anemia
CDC	Centers for Disease Control
CDG	congenital disorders of glycosylation
CDGS	carbohydrate-deficient glycoprotein syndrome
CDH	congenital dislocation of hip congenital dysplasia of hip
CDI	clean, dry, intact
CDK	cyclin-dependent kinases
CDKI	cyclin-dependent kinases inhibitors
Cdiff	C-diff, Clostridium difficile
CDMS	clinically definite multiple sclerosis
cDNA	complementary DNA (a synthetic DNA copied from mRNA)
CDO	congenital duodenal obstruction
CDR	Clinical Dementia Rating complementarity-determining regions
CDS	cervico-dorsal syndrome
CDT	carbohydrate-deficient transferrin
CE	carboxylesterases chloracetate esterase european conformity angle (radiograph) center-edge angle
CEA	carcinoembryonic antigen
CEC	chloroethylclonidine
CEF	cytoxan plus epirubicin plus 5
Ceff	effective compliance; bedside method of monitoring the effectiveness of PEEP; equal with VT (tidal volume)/peak air pressure, should be greater than 50 cm3/cmH2O
CENELEC	European Committee for Electrotechnical Standardization
CERAD	Consortium to Establish a Registry for Alzheimer's Disease
c-erb	cellular erythroblastosis oncogene
Cerv.	cervix, cervical
Cervical dil.	cervical dilation
CEZ	cefazolin
CF	cardiac failure clofibrate compare, refer to complement fixation cystic fibrosis
CFAE	ceftiofur free acid equivalent
CFC	colony-forming cells
CFCOT	College Francais des Chirurgiens Orthopedistes et Traumatologues
CFDI	color flow duplex imaging
CFIDS	Chronic Fatigue and Immune Dysfunction Syndrome
CFM	continuous electronic fetal monitoring
CFNS	chills, fever, night sweats
CFP	call for papers
CFPC	College of Family Physicians of Canada
CFS	Chronic Fatigue (and Immune Dysfunction) Syndrome
CFS/ME	chronic fatigue syndrome (often called myalgic encephalomyelitis, especially in the UK)
CFTR	cystic fibrosis transmembrane regulator
CFU	colony forming units
CFUc	colony-forming unit cells

CFU-GEMM colony-forming units generating granulocytes, erythroblasts, macrophages, and megakaryiocytes
CFU-S spleen colony-forming units
cg centigram
CG chorionic gonadotropin
CgA chromogranin A
CGA compressed gas association
contact guard assist (physical therapy)
cytosine-guanine-adenine codon for arginine
CGC cytosine-guanine-cytosine codon for arginine
CGCGGATC Oct motif
CGD chronic granulomatous disease
CGG cytosine-guanine-guanine codon for arginine
CGH comparative genomic hybridization - cytogenetics method
CGL chronic granulocytic leukemia (previous name for CML)
CGN crescentic glomerulonephritis
CGS centimeter gram second
CGRP calcitonin gene-related peptide
CGU cytosine-guanine-uracil codon for arginine
cGy centi Gray (unit of radiation)
CH characteristic
chest
chief
chronic
crown-heel
CH50 total functional hemolytic complement
cHA coralline hydroxyapatite
CHA calcium hydroxyapatite
congenital hypoplastic anemia
cyclohexyladenosine
ch. br. syn. chronic brain syndrome
CHD congenital dislocation of the hip
CHD (cont.) congenital heart disease
coronary heart disease
ChE cholinesterases
Chem., chemo chemotherapy
CHF congestive heart failure
chronic heart failure
CHG change
CHI closed head injury
CHILD syndrome: congenital hemidysplasia with ichthyosiform erythrodermal and limb defects
ChIVPP chlorambucil, vinblastine, procarbazine, and prednisone
CHL classical Hodgkin lymphoma
CHO carbohydrate
Chol, CHOL serum cholesterol
Chr chronic
CHR chronic
chronological
CHS calvarial hyperostotic syndrome
Chediak-Higashi syndrome
customized headholder system
CHS1 Chediak Higashi syndrome gene, located on chromosome 1 (1q42-44)
CHT classical heart transplantation
CI cardiac index (cardiac output divided by the patient's body surface area); normal 2.8-4.2 L/min/m2
cardiac/coronary insufficiency
cerebral infarction
confidence interval
contraindications
C.I color index
CIA collagen-induced arthritis
CIBIC-Plus Clinician's Interview Based Impression of Change Plus Caregiver Input
CIC cardioinhibitor centre
certified infection control

CIC (cont.)	Chemical Institute of Canada: L'Institut de Chimie du Canada
	chronic inactive cirrhosis
	circulating immune complexes
	clean intermittent catheterization
	constant initial concentration
	coronary intensive care
	crisis intervention center/clinic
CICU	cardiac intensive care unit
CID	carpal instability dissociative
	collision-induced dissociation
CIDA	Canadian International Development Agency
CIDP	chronic inflammatory demyelinating polyneuropathy
cig	cigarette
cIg	cytoplasmic immunoglobulin
CIG	cigarette consumption
	cold insoluble globulin
	cryosurgical iceball gauge
cIgM	cytoplasmic immunoglobulin M
CIK	cytokine induced-killer cells
CIMF	chronic idiopathic myelofibrosis
CIMMYT	International Maize and Wheat Improvement Center
CIN	cervical intraepithelial neoplasia (grades I, II, III)
CIND	carpal instability non-dissociative
CIP	clinical investigation plan
	International Foot and Ankle Society
CIRC	circulation
	circumference
CIS	carcinoma in situ
CISD	critical incident stress debriefing team
cis-DDP	cis-diamminedichloroplatinum
CISH	chromosomal in situ hybridization
CJD	Creutzfeldt-Jakob disease
CJF	carotid-jugular fistula
CK	check
	creatine kinase
CK (cont.)	cytokeratin
CK 1-8	neutral to basic cytokeratin
CK 9-20	acidic cytokeratin
CK 18	cytokeratin found in hepatocyte, renal tubular cell, ductular epithelia, mesothelia, and respiratory epithelia
CKD	result checked
CKI	casein kinase
CK(-MB)	creatine kinase (MB)
CKMB	creatine kinase muscle band
CKS	classic Kaposi sarcoma
cl	centiliter
	clarified
	clean
	clear
	cleft
	clinic, clinical
	clonus
	clotting
	cloudy
Cl	chloride
	chlorine
	clavicle
	clear
	clinic
	Clostridium
	closure
	colistin
CL	capillary lumen
	cardiolipin
	cell line
	centralis lateralis
	chemiluminescence
	chest and left arm (lead in electrocardiography)
	cholelithiasis
	cholesterol-lecithin
	chronic leukemia
	cirrhosis of liver
	clavicle
	clean

C

CL (cont.)	clear liquid
	clearance
	cleft lip
	clinical laboratory
	clomipramine
	closed
	complex loading
	confidence limit or level
	constant domain of L chain
	contact lens
	corpus luteum
	corrected (echo long axis) length
	cricoid lamina
	criterion level
	critical list
	cycle length
	cytotoxic lymphocyte
	lung compliance
C-L	consultation-liaison (setting)
CLA	cerebellar ataxia
	Certified Laboratory Assistant
	cervicolinguoaxial
	contralateral local anesthesia
	cutaneous lymphocyte antigen
	cyclic lysine anhydride
	chloroacetyl
CLAH	congenital lipoid adrenal hyperplasia
Clam	cervical laminectomy
CLAS	congenital localized absence of skin
class	classification
clav, Clav.	clavicle
CLB	chlorambucil
	clobazam
	curvilinear body
CLBBB	complete left bundle branch block
CLBP	chronic low back pain
CLC	Charcot-Leyden crystal
	Clerc-Levy-Critesco (syndrome)
CLCD	cleidocranial dysostosis
CN	chloride channel
CLCP	chymotrypsin-like cationic protein
CL/CP	cleft lip/cleft palate
CLCS	colchicine sensitivity
CLD	chloride diarrhea
	chronic liver disease
	chronic lung disease
	congenital limb deficiency
	crystal ligand field
CLDH	choline dehydrogenase
CLDP	Commercial Law Development Program
cldy, Cldy	cloudy
CLE	centrilobular emphysema
	continuous lumbar epidural (anesthesia)
CLED	cystine-lactose-electrolyte-deficient (agar)
CLF	calcification of ligamentum flavum
	cardiolipin fluorescent (antibody)
	ceroid lipofuscinosis
	cholesterol-lecithin flocculation
CLH	chronic lobular hepatitis
	cleft limb-heart (syndrome)
	corpus luteum hormone
	cutaneous lymphoid hyperplasia
CLI	complement lysis inhibitor
	corpus luteum insufficiency
CLIA	Clinical Laboratory Improvement Act
CLIF	cloning inhibitory factor
	Crithidia luciliae immunofluorescence
clin	clinic, clinical
CLINPROT	Clinical Cancer Protocols
CLIP	capitolunate instability pattern
	corticotropin-like intermediate lobe peptide
CL-IVR	cycle length of the idioventricular rhythm
CLL	cholesterol-lowering lipid
	chronic lymphocytic leukemia
	cow lung lavage

CLL/SLL chronic lymphocytic leukemia/ small lymphocytic lymphoma
CLMA Clinical Laboratory Management Association
CLMF cytotoxic lymphocyte maturation factor
CLML Current List of Medical Literature
CLMV cauliflower mosaic virus
clo "clothing" - a unit of thermal insulation
CLO cod liver oil
CLOF clofibrate
Clon Clonorchis
CLON clonidine
Clostr Clostridium
ClP clinical pathology
CLP chymotrypsin-like protein
cleft lip with cleft palate
paced cycle length
CL(P) cleft lip without cleft palate
CL/P cleft lip with or without cleft palate
CLS café-au-lait spot
Clinical Laboratory Scientist
Coffin-Lowry syndrome
Cornelia de Lange syndrome
CLSE calf lung surfactant extract
CLSH corpus luteum stimulating hormone
CLSL chronic lymphosarcoma (cell) leukemia
CLSM confocal laser scanning microscopy
Cl.T clotting time
CLT Certified Laboratory Technician
chronic lymphocytic thyroiditis
Clinical Laboratory Technician
clot lysis time
clotting time
lung-thorax compliance
CLTB total body clearance
CLT(NCA) Laboratory Technician Certified by the National Certification Agency for Medical Laboratory Personnel
CLU clusterin
CLV cassava latent virus
constant linear velocity
CL VOID clean voided specimen (urine)
CLZ clozapine
cm, cm. centimeter - 0.01 meters
cm2 square centimeter
cm3 cubic centimeter
cM centi -morgan
Cm curium
maximum clearance
minimal concentration
CM California mastitis (test)
calmodulin
capreomycin
CarboMedics (heart valves)
carboxymethyl
cardiac murmur
cardiac muscle
cardiomyopathy
carpometacarpal
castrated male
Caucasian male
cause of death (form Latin causa mortis)
cavernous malformation
cell membrane
center of mass
centrum medianum
cerebral malaria
cerebral mantle
cervical mucosa or mucus
Chick-Martin (coefficient)
chloroquinemepacrine
chondromalacia
chopped meat (medium)
circular muscle
circulating monocyte
circumferential measurement

C

CM (cont.)	clindamycin
	clinical medicine
	clinical modification
	coccidioidal meningitis
	cochlear microphonic
	codling moth
	combined modality
	common migraine
	complete medium
	complications
	condition median
	congenital malformation
	congestive myocardiopathy
	continuous murmur
	contrast medium
	copulatory mechanism
	costal margin
	cow's milk
	cutaneous mastocytosis
	cytometry
	cytoplasmic membrane
	Master of Surgery (from Latin Chirurgiae Magister)
	narrow-diameter endosseous screw implant (form French crete manche)
C/M	counts per minute
C+M	cocaine and morphine
CMA	Canadian Medical Association
	Certified Medical Assistant
	chronic metabolic acidosis
	cow's milk allergy
	cultured macrophages
CMAP	compound muscle (or motor) action potential
CMAR	cell matrix adhesion regulator
Cmax	maximum concentration
CMB	carbolic methylene blue
CMB	Central Midwives' Board
	chloromercuribenzoate
CMBES	Canadian Medical and Biological Engineering Society
CMC	carboxymethylcellulose
	care management continuity
	carpometacarpal
	cell-mediated cytolysis or cytotoxicity
	chloramphenicol
	chronic mucocutaneous candidiasis
	critical micellar concentration
CMCC	chronic mucocutaneous candidiasis
CMCJ	carpometacarpal joint
CMCt	care management continuity across settings
CMD	campomelic dysplasia
	campomelic dwarfism
	cartilage matrix deficiency
	chief medical director
	childhood muscular dystrophy
	chronic myeloproliferative disease
	comparative mean dose
	congenital muscular dystrophy
	count median diameter
cmDNA	cytoplasmic membrane-associated deoxyribonucleic acid
CME	continuing medical education (American Medical Association On-Line CME Locator)
CMET	central mucoepidermoid tumor of the jaws
CMF	cyclophosphamide, methotrexate and 5-fluorouracil
	cytoxan, methotrexate and 5-fluorouracil
CMF/VP	cyclophosphamide, methotrexate, 5-fluorouracil, vincristine, and prednisone
CMH	Cochran-Mantel-Haenszel test
CMHC	community mental health centers
CMI	combined mechanical injury
CML	chronic myelogenous leukemia
CMM	cutaneous malignant melanoma
CMML	chronic myelomonocytic leukemia
CMO	centric relation occlusion

CMO (cont.) Chief Medical Officer (UK)
CMP cardiomyopathy
CMPF cyclohexylmethylphosphonofluoridate (organophosphate nerve agent)
CMQ Collège des médecins du Québec
CMR clinical materials requisition
CMS circulation, motion, sensation
CMT Charcot-Marie-Tooth (International)
combined modality therapy
CMT1A Charcot-Marie-Tooth disease type 1A
CMV cisplatin-methotrexate-vinblastine
control medical ventilation
cytomegalovirus
CMVIG cytomegalovirus immune globulin
CN cranial nerve
CN (2-12) cranial nerves (2 to 12)
CNB cannabinoids
CNL chronic neutrophilic leukemia
constant neutral loss (scanning)
CNPA chronic necrotizing pulmonary aspergillosis
CNR contrast-to-noise ratio
CNS central nervous system
cnst. constipation
CNTF ciliary neurotrophic factor
cNTS caudal region of nucleus tractus solitarius
CNU-TNM Comite Nacional Uruguayo TNM
CNV cranial nerve number 5
CNX cranial nerve number 10
Co cobalt
c/o complains of
complaints
CO carbon monoxide
cardiac output
check out
childhood-onset
C/O care of
complains of
CO2 carbon dioxide
COA California Orthopaedic Association
Canadian Orthopaedic Association (Canadian Medical Association Affiliates)
condition on admission
COAD chronic obstructive airways disease
COAG coagulation
COD cause of death
condition on discharge
Code full cardiac arrest
CO-GHD childhood-onset growth hormone deficiency
COGME Council on Graduate Medical Education
COLD chronic obstructive lung disease
comb. combine
combination
comm. communicable
COMP compound
comp. compound, compress
COMSS Council of Musculoskeletal Specialty Societies (also: AAOS Specialty Societies)
COMT catechol-O-methyltransferase
c-onc cellular oncogene
Conc concentrate
conc. concentrated
Con A concavalin A
Cong. fail. congestive failure
cons. consultation
Cons. consultant
CONs normal controls
cont continued
cont. continued
contractions
COOMR Center for Orthopaedic Oncology and Musculoskeletal Research
COP center of pressure
COPA Certified Orthotic and Prosthetic Advocates

COPD chronic obstructive pulmonary disease
COPE calendar of premenstrual experiences (scale)
chronic obstructive pulmonary emphysema
Cor heart
COR Center for Orthopaedic Research
CORF Carolina Orthopaedic Research Foundation
CORR Clinical Orthopaedics and Related Research (Journal)
COS Canadian Oncology Society
Clinical Orthopaedic Society (AAOS Related Organizations)
Colorado Orthopaedic Society
COSTA test compost stabilization test
COVD College of Optometrists in Vision Development
COX cytochrome C oxidase
COX-II cyclooxygenase-II
CP capsid protein
cerebral palsy
chest pain
choline phosphate
coat protein
CPAP continuous positive airway pressure
CPB cardiopulmonary bypass
competitive protein binding
CPC clinicopathological correlation
CPD cephalopelvic disproportion
chronic peritoneal dialysis
citrate-phosphate-dextrose
CP2D-A citrate-phosphate-double-dextrose adenine
CPE chronic pulmonary emphysema
complete physical examination
cytopathic effect
CPHL Central Public Health Laboratory
CPK creatine phosphokinase
CPM central pontine myelinolysis
clinical project manager
CPM (cont.) continuous passive motion machine (center for orthopaedics and sports medicine)
counts per minute
cyclophosphamide
CPMA California Podiatric Medical Association
CPMS chronic progressive multiple sclerosis
CPPB continuous positive pressure breathing
CPPD calcium pyrophosphate dihydrate
CPR cardiopulmonary resuscitation
checks with previous results
Contraceptive Prevalence Rate
C-reactive protein
CPS Children's Protective Services
CPT chest physical therapy
Current Procedural Terminology
CPV-2 parvovirus-2
CPX cardiopulmonary exercise testing
complete physical examination
CPZ cefoperazone
CPZ Chlorpromazine (Thorazine)
CQI continuous quality improvement
CR chest radiogram
clinical records
closed reduction
complete remission/complete response
conditioned reflex
crown-rump
CR (1, 2, 3) leukocyte complement receptors
CRA Clinical Research Associate
cran. cranial
Crani cranial (toward the head or proximal)
cranial (with reference to the cranium)
CRC Cancer Research Campaign (UK)
colorectal carcinoma
CR+C closed reduction and cast

CrCl, CRCL creatinine clearance
CRD chronic respiratory disease
Crea creatinine
CreA carbon catabolite repression in Aspergillus nidulans (the transcriptional repressor mediating)
creat. creatinine
CREST calcinosis, Raynaud's phenomenon, esophageal dysmotility, sclerodactyly, and telangiectasis
CRF case report form
case report forms
chronic renal failure
corticotropin-releasing factor or hormone
CRI chronic renal insufficiency
CRIS controlled-release infusion system
CRIT critical hematocrit
CRLs cervical root lesions
CRNA certified registered nurse anesthetist
CRO cathode ray oscilloscope
clinical research organizations
Contract Research Organization
CROM cervical range of motion
CROME congenital cataracts-epileptic fits-mental retardation (syndrome)
CROS contralateral routing of signals (hearing aid)
CrP creatine phosphate
CRP chronic relapsing pancreatitis
corneal-retinal potential
coronary rehabilitation program
C-reactive protein
cross-reacting protein
cyclic AMP receptor protein
CRPA C-reactive protein antiserum
CRPD chronic restrictive pulmonary disease
CRPF chloroquine-resistant Plasmodium falciparum
CRPF (cont.) closed reduction and percutaneous fixation
contralateral renal plasma flow
CRPS complex regional pain syndrome (type I and II)
CRRN certified rehabilitation registered nurse
CrRT cranial radiotherapy
CRS Carroll rating scale for depression
catheter-related sepsis
caudal regression syndrome
cervical spine radiography
Chinese restaurant syndrome
colon and rectum surgery
compliance of the respiratory system
congenital rubella syndrome
craniosynostosis
cryptidin-related sequence
CRSM cherry red spot myoclonus
CRSP comprehensive renal scintillation procedure
CRST calcinosis, Raynaud phenomenon, sclerodactyly, telangiectasia (syndrome)
crt hematocrit
CRT cadaveric renal transplant
capillary refill time
cardiac resuscitation team
cathode-ray tube
Certified Record Techniques
certified
choice reaction time
chromium release test
complex reaction time
computerized renal tomography
copper reduction test
corrected retention time
corrected
cortisone resistant thymocyte
cranial radiation therapy
CRTM cartilage matrix protein

CRTP Consciousness Research and Training Project
CRTT Certified Respiratory Therapy Technician
CRU cardiac rehabilitation unit
clinical research unit
CRV central retinal vein
CRVF congestive right ventricular failure
CRVO central retinal vein occlusion
CRYG gamma crystallin gene
CRYM crystallin, MU
cryo cryogenic
cryoglobulin
cryoprecipitate
cryosurgery
cryotherapy
Cryoppt cryoprecipitate
crys cryst, crystal, crystaline
cs chromosome
consciousness
cS centistoke
Cs case
cell surface
cesium
cyclosporine
CS calf serum
campomelic syndrome
carcinoid syndrome
cardiogenic shock
caries-susceptible
carotid sheath
carotid sinus
cat scratch
celiac sprue
central supply
central service
cerebral scintigraphy
cerebrospinal
cervical spine
cervical stimulation
cesarean section
chest strap

CS (cont.) chief of staff
cholesterol stone
chondroitin sulfate
chorionic somatomammotropin
chronic schizophrenia
cigarette smoker
citrate synthase
climacteric syndrome
clinic scheduling
clinical laboratory scientist
clinical stage
clinical status
Cockayne syndrome
complete stroke
compression syndrome
concentrated strength
conditioned stimulus
congenital syphilis
conjunctival secretion
conscious sedation
conscious, consciousness
conservative surgery
constant spring
contact sensitivity
continue same
contrast sensitivity (test)
control serum
convalescence, convalescent
coronary sclerosis
coronary sinus
corpus striatum
corticoid-sensitive
corticosteroid
crush syndrome
c-section, cesarean section
current smoker
current strength
Cushing syndrome
cycloserine
cyclosporine
C/S cesarean section
cycles per second

C+S	calvarium and scalp conjunctiva and sclera culture and sensitivity
C4S	chondroitin-4-sulfate
CsA	cyclosporine A
CSA	Canadian Standards Association canavaninosuccinic acid carbonyl salicylamide cell surface antigen chemical shift anisotropy chondroitin sulfate A chorionic somatomammotropin A colony-stimulating activity compressed spectral assay computerized spectral analysis Controlled Substances Act cross section area cyclosporine A
CSAA	Child Study Association of America
CSAD	corporate services administration department
CSAT	center for substance abuse treatment
CSAVP	cerebral subarachnoid venous pressure
csb	chromosome break
CSB	Canadian Society for Biomechanics (Société Canadienne de Biomécanique) congenital short bowel contaminated small bowel craniosynostosis, Boston type
CSBF	coronary sinus blood flow
CSBS	contaminated small bowel syndrome
CSC	blow on blow (administration of small amounts of drugs at short intervals) (Fr. coup sur coup) collagen sponge contraceptive corticostriatocerebellar cryogenic storage container
CSCC	cutaneous squamous cell carcinoma
CSCD	Center for Sickle Cell Disease
CSCI	corticosterone side-chain isomerase
CSCR	Central Society for Clinical Research
CSCV	critical serum chemistry value
CSD	carotid sinus denervation cat scratch disease combined system disease conditionally streptomycin dependent conduction system disease cortical spreading depression craniospinal defect critical stimulus duration
CSDB	cat scratch disease bacillus
CSDMS	Canadian Society of Diagnostic Medical Sonographers
CSE	clinical-symptom self-evaluation (questionnaire) cone-shaped epiphysis conventional spin-echo cross-sectional echocardiography
C sect	C-section, cesarean section
C-section	cesarean section
CSEP	cortical somatosensory evoked potential
CSER	cortical somatosensory evoked response
CSF	cancer family syndrome cerebrospinal fluid classical swine fever cold stability factor colony-stimulating factor contrast sensitivity function coronary sinus flow
CS-F	colony-stimulating factor
CSF-1	colony-stimulating factor 1 receptor
CSFH	cerebrospinal fluid hypotension

C

CSFP cerebrospinal fluid pressure
CSFR colony-stimulating factor receptor
CSFV cerebrospinal fluid volume
CSF-WR cerebrospinal fluid-Wassermann reaction
csg chromosome gap
CSG cholecystography, cholecystogram
CSGBI Cardiac Society of Great Britain and Ireland
CSGBM collagenase soluble glomerular basement membrane
CSH carotid sinus hypersensitivity
chronic subdural hematoma
combat support (army) hospital
cortical stromal hyperplasia
Canadian Study of Health and Aging
CSHE California Society for Hospital Engineering
CSHRH congenital self-healing reticulohistiocytosis
CSII continuous subcutaneous insulin infusion
CS IV clinical stage 4
CSK chronic superficial keratitis
CSM clinical supply management
CSMSD Czech Society for Metabolic Skeletal Diseases (EFFO Member Society)
CSOS Chinese Speaking Orthopaedic Society
CSOT Canadian Society of Orthopaedic Technologists
CSP cervical spine
cyclosporine
C-spine cervical spine
CSR central supply room
cervical spine radiography
CSRS Cervical Spine Research Society (also: AAOS Specialty Societies)
CSRT corrected sinus recovery time
CSS Churg-Strauss syndrome
Cst corticosterone
CSV Cordis Standard Valves
CSW Certified Social Worker
Children's Social Worker
ct. count
CT carpal tunnel
cerebral thrombosis
cervical traction
cervical-thoracic
chemotherapy
clinical trial
computerized tomography
cor triatriatum
cytotrophoblast
CTA clear to auscultation (about lungs)
CTAB clear to auscultation bilaterally (about lungs)
CTACK cutaneous T-cell attracting chemokine
CTB cholera toxin subunit B
confined to bed
CTC common toxicity criteria
CTD connective tissue disease
CTE coefficient of thermal expansion
CTEV congenital talipes equinovarus
CTF central tegmental field
CTGI continuous tracheal gas insufflation
CTL cervical, thoracic, lumbar
cytotoxic T lymphocytes
CTLA cytotoxic T-lymphocyte-associated antigen-4 (CD152)
CTNB CT-guided needle biopsy
CTO clinical trials office
CTR carpal tunnel release
coated tube radioimmunoassay
CTS carpal tunnel syndrome (carpal tunnel release: sample operative report)
CTSP called to see patient
CTV clinical target volume
CTX clinical trials exemption

cu cubic
CU cause unknown
clinical unit
CUA cytosine-uracil-adenine codon for leucine
CUC cytosine-uracil-cytosine codon for leucine
CUD cause undetermined
CUG cytosine-uracil-guanine codon for leucine
CUU cytosine-uracil-uracil codon for leucine
C-V cardiovascular
CV cardiac volume
cardiovascular
cervical vertebrae
color vision
cresyl violet (dye used in Gram staining)
curriculum vitae
CVA cerebrovascular accident (stroke)
costovertebral angle
CVAT CVA tenderness
CVC central venous catheters
CVD cardiovascular disease
cerebrovascular disease
CVG contrast ventriculography
CVI cerebrovascular insufficiency
chronic vascular insufficiency
CVL central venous line
CVMP Committee for Veterinary Medicinal Product
CVP central venous pressure (normal range: 0 to 9 cm of water)
cytoxan, vincristine, prednisone
CVS cardiovascular status
cardiovascular surgery
cardiovascular system
chorionic villous sampling
CVVH continuous veno-venous haemofiltration
CVVHD continuous veno-venous hemodialysis
CW chest wall
crutch walking
c/w compatible/consistent with
C/W continue with
CWHTO closing wedge high tibial osteotomy
CWI crutch walking instructions
CWP cell wall protein
childbirth without pain
coal workers' pneumoconiosis
Cx cervix
cultures
CX cervix
chest x-ray
consciousness
CxR, CXR chest x-ray
CYP cytochrome P450
Cys cysteine
cysto cystoscopic exam
Cysto cystoscopy
CZP clonazepam

D

d day(s)
per day
D aspartic acid
day
diopter (lens strength)
D1 – D12 dorsal vertebrae
thoracic vertebrae
D5 anti-microphthalmia transcription factor antibody (for diagnosis of clear cell sarcoma/malignant melanoma of soft parts)
DA degenerative arthritis
inbred strains of rats [DA(RT1a/AgB4)]
D/A date of accident

D/A (cont.)	date of admission
DAB	diaminobenzidine (chromogen for peroxidase-based detection systems)
	dorsal abductors
Dabs	absorbed radiation dose
	degassed by O2 absorption (lungs)
DABS	Derogatis Affects Balance Sheet
	diazobenzene sulfonate
DABS-AA	dimethylaminoazobenzene-sulfonyl-amino acid
DABS-Cl	dimethylaminoazobenzenesulfonyl chloride
DAF	decay-accelerating factor (CD55) - regulates C3
DAG	diacylglycerol
DAISY	the dairy information system (UK)
DAN	danazol
	diabetic autonomic neuropathy
	2,4-diaminonaphthalene
Dan-MONICA	Danish Monitoring trends in Cardiovascular diseases study
DAN-PSS	Danish prostate symptom score
DAO	dog aorta
DAP	Draw a Person Test
	distal airway pressure
	dystrophin associated protein
3,4-DAP	3,4-diaminopyridine
DAPC	dystrophin-associated protein complex
DAPK	death-associated protein kinase
DAP-Kinase	death-associated protein kinase
DAPT	diphtheria, acellular pertussis, and tetanus toxoids
DAR	double-antibody radioimmunoassay
DARF	dosage adjustment in renal failure
DAT	dementia of Alzheimer's type
	diet as tolerated
	direct antibody testing
DATT	defense attach
DAW	dispense as written
db, db.	decibel
DB	date of birth
	dapple apple viroid
	disability
DBE	deep breathing exercise
DBI	diazepam binding inhibitor
DBM	demineralized bone matrix
D/BMD	Duchenne and Becker muscular dystrophies
DBP	demineralized bone powder
	diastolic blood pressure
	dibutyl phthalate
DBPCFC	double-blind placebo controlled food challenge
DBSC	double-breath, single cycle
DBW	deficit birthweight
	desirable body weight
	diabetic black women
	dosing body weight
	dry body weight
dc, d/c	discontinue
DC	dendritic cells
	direct current
	disc, discharged, discontinue
	doctor of chiropractic
D/C	diarrhea/constipation
	discharge
	discontinue
D+C	dilatation and curettage
DCA	directional coronary atherectomy (for coronary ostial lesions)
DC+B	dilation, curettage and biopsy
DCBE	double-contrast barium enema
DCC	deleted in Colon Carcinoma gene (located on chromosome 18q21)
	dextran-coated charcoal
	direct current contershock
DCGF	dry corn gluten feed
DCh	dorsochiasmatic area
DCH	2,3-dicyanohydroquinone
	Day-case haemorrhoidectomy
	deep cerebral hemorrhages

DCH (cont.)	delayed cutaneous hypersensitivity
	diffuse chorioamnionic hemosiderosis
	diffuse choroidal hemangiomas
	double-crush hypothesis
DCIS	ductal carcinoma in situ - type of breast cancer
DCM	dilated cardiomyopathy
DCP	des-g-carboxy prothrombin, specific for HCC (hepatocellular carcinoma)
DCS	decompression sickness
DCT	distal convoluted tubule
3DCT	three dimensional (surface) CAT scan reconstruction images
dd	daily dose
dD	changes in vascular diameter
	dichotic listening test by Feldmann
Dd	diastolic diameters
	dictyostelium discoideum sorocarps
	dideoxy
DD	1, 4-bis(4'dihexylaminostyryl)-benzene
	Asp-Asp.
	constant darkness
	dangerous drug
	Darier's disease
	data definition
	day of delivery
	day-degrees
	death domain
	debridement and drilling procedure
	dedifferentiated
	deficiency disorders
	degenerated disc
	degenerative disease
	degree of deacetylation
	degree of dithiocarbamylation
	DeKalb Delta
	delivery day
	delusional disorder
	demineralized dentin
DD (cont.)	density dependence
	dependent drainage
	depersonalisation disorder
	depersonalisation-derealization
	depressive disorder
	depth dose [x-ray]
	designated driver
	desktop-display
	detrusor dyssynergia
	development(al) disorder
	developmental(al) disabilities
	developmental dyscalculia
	developmental dyslexis
	developmentally delayed
	dextran derivative
	di guglielmo's disease
	diadinoxanthin
	diallyl disulfide
	diaminedithiol
	diamond-shaped anastomosis duodenoplasty
	diaper dermatitis
	diarrheal disease
	diastolic depolarization
	diastolic dysfunction
	diastrophic dysplasia
	dibenzo-p-dioxin
	died of the disease
	dieldrin
	dielectro-deformation
	differential diagnosis
	differential display (analysis)
	differential mRNA display
	diffuse duodenitis
	diffusion-driven
	digestive disorder
	digital deficiencies
	dihydrodiol dehydrogenase
	D-dimers
	dipole-dipole
	disc diameter
	disc diffusion

D

DD (cont.) disc displacement
discharge diagnosis
discharged dead
dissociative (conversion) disorders
distance distribution
distortion of dots
district director
diverticular disease
DNA damage
DNA denaturation
DNA diploidy
dodecanedioic acid
dog danger
domain-deleted
dominance decay
donor-directed blood donation
dopamine-deficient
dorsal decubitus
dose-dependent
double depression
double diffusion
doubling dilutions
doubling doses
doxorubicin-docetaxel
Drew-Dickerson (sequence d[CGCGAATTCGCG])
dried-droplet
driving after drinking
drug delivery
drug dependence
dry dressing
Duchenne dystrophy
duodenal distension
duodenal diverticulum
duodenum
Duplex Doppler sonography
Dupuytren's disease
duration of diabetes
duration of disease
dynamic difference
dyscrasic diatheses
dysthymic disorder

DD-15 Lanthony Desaturated Panel D-15
dd-Ado 2', 5'-dideoxyadenosine
DDAVP desmopressin acetate
desmopressin test for urine osmolality
ddC zalcitabine
DDD degenerative disk disease
DDH developmental dysplasia of the hip (case report)
DD-Hep D-glycero-D-manno-heptose
ddI didanosine
DD-MVAC delipidated, deglycolipidated M. vaccae
DDP diamminedichloroplatinum
DDPAC dementia-parkinsonism-amyotrophy complex
DD-PCR differential-display polymerase chain reaction
DD-peptidase D-alanyl-D-alanine peptidase
DDPs designated driver programs
DDS Doctor of Dental Surgery
Dd-STATc dictyostelium STAT
DDT chlorphenotane
D/DW dextrose in distilled water
D5%DW dextrose 5% in distilled water
Ddx differential diagnosis
DDx differential diagnosis
DE delayed excitation
D+E dilatation and evacuation
DEA diethylamine
Drug Enforcement Agency
DEAE diethylaminoethyl
DEC deceased
decrease
decr. decreased
decub decubitus ulcer
DEF defecation
deferred
deficient
DEG degeneration
dehyd. dehydrated
Derm dermatology

Derm. dermatology
DES describe
desflurane
diethylstilbestrol
DET determine
DEV deviation
DEXA dual energy x-ray absorptiometry (accuDEXA™ bone densitometer by Schick Technologies)
Df dermatophagoides farinae
DF dibenzofuran
dietary fiber
dorsiflexion
DFA direct fluorescent antibody test
Dfb dermatophagoides farinae bodies
Dff dermatophagoides farinae faeces
DFF days to first flower
days of formalin fixation
dexfenfluramine
diastolic forward flow
diet free forever
dietary fat in feces
diflufenican
direct flow filtration
distal forearm fracture
DNA fragmentation factor
dried fat-free
DFI disease free interval
DFID British Department of International Development (Formerly ODA)
DFMO DL-alpha-difluoromethylornithine
DFS disease free survival - time without disease prior to relapse or last follow-up
DFSP dermatofibrosarcoma protuberans
DFT defibrillation threshold
DFX desferrioxamine
DGC differentiated type gastric carcinoma
dystrophin-glycoprotein complex
DGCR DiGeorge chromosomal region
DGGE denaturing gradient gel electrophoresis
DGI disseminated gonococcal infection
DGM duodenal gastric metaplasia
DGR duodenogastric reflux
DGS DiGeorge syndrome
DH dermatitis herpetiformis
D/H drug history
DHA docosahexanoic acid
DHEA dehydroepiandrosterone
DHEAS dehydroepiandrosterone sulfate
DHEA-ST dehydroepiandrosterone sulfotransferases
DHF dorsi-hyperflexion
DHHS Department of Health and Human Services
DHL diffuse histiocytic leukemia
DHS dynamic hip screw
DHx drug history
DI date of injury
deciliter
diabetes insipidus
D+I dry and intact (wound dressings)
diag diagnosis, diagnostic
DIAG. diagnosis
diam. diameter
DIB difficulty in breathing
DIBOA 2, 4-dihydroxy-1, 4-benzoxazin-3-one
DIC deviance information criterion
disseminated intravascular coagulation
Dict. dictation
DIF direct immunofluorescence
diff differential blood count
diff. differential
DIFF diff, differential blood count
dil. dilute
DIL dilated
dilute
dim. diminished
DIM diminished

MBOA	2, 4-dihydroxy-7-methoxy-1, 4-benzoxazin-3-one
Dind	indicative radiation dose
DIP	desquamative interstitial pneumonitis
	distal interphalangeal joints
	distal interphalangeal
DIPJ	distal interphalangeal joint
DIPP	diisopropyl phosphate
dIPSPs	depolarizing inhibitory postsynaptic potentials
dis.	disease
DIS	disabled
	disease
disch.	discharge
DISH	diffuse idiopathic skeletal hyperostosis
DISI	dorsal intercalate segment instability
DISL	dislocate
	dislocation
	dorsal intercalate segment instability
disp.	disposition
DISP	disposition
dist.	distilled
	distal
DIST	distal
	distended
DIT	diiodotyrosine
div.	divorced
DIV	divide/d
DIW	dextrose in water
DJD	degenerative joint disease
DKA	diabetic ketoacidosis
	did not keep appointment
DKB	deep knee bends
dl, dL	deciliter - 0.01 liters (100 ml)
DL	dual lumen
D/L	deciliter
DLA	dorsolateral area
DLC	diamond-like carbon (coatings)
DLCL	diffuse large cell lymphoma
DLCO	diffusing capacity of the lung for carbon monoxide
DLDH	dementia lacking distinctive histopathology
DLE	discoid lupus erythematosus
	disseminated lupus erythematosis
DLI	donor lymphocyte infusion
DLO	d-limonene 1,2-epoxide
	dorsolateral outflow
	octopamine-IR
D5LR	dextrose 5% with lactated ringers
DLS	date last seen
D-LST	drug lymphocyte stimulation test
DLT	dose limiting toxicity - determined by phase 1 studies
DM	dermatomyositis
	diabetes mellitus
	diastolic murmur
DM1	myotonic dystrophy gene
DM2	myotonic dystrophy gene 2 (linked to chromosome 3q)
DMA	dog mesenteric artery
DMAD	dimethylaminoadamantane
DMARD	disease modifying antirheumatic drugs
DMC	Data Monitoring Committee
DMD	dodecyloxycarbonyl-methyl-dioxane-diones
	daily maintenance dose
	delayed mental development
	depression and manic depression
	desmethyldiltiazem
	desmethyldoxepin
	diastolic myocardial dysfunction
	dietary management of diarrhea
	differential metabolic display
	differentially methylated domain
	digitoxigenin monodigitoxoside
	dimethadione
	dimethyldioxirane
	discontinuous molecular dynamics

DMD (cont.) disease modifying drug
disseminated malignant disease
disseminated mycobacterial disease
Doctor of Dental Medicine
dorsal medullary depressor area
Drug Misuse Databases
drusen-related macular degeneration
dry matter digestibility
Duchenne muscular dystrophy
Dynia-Majan-Drdlicka factor
dystonia musculorum deformans
dystrophin

DMG dimethylglycine

DMI Desipramine (Norpramin)
dry matter intake

DMN dorsal motor nucleus

DMP data management plan

DMPK dystrophia myotonica-protein kinase (gene on chromosome 19q)

DMR direct myocardial revascularization

3D-MRA three-dimensional magnetic resonance angiography

dms double minutes (chromosome-like structures)

DMS dimethylsulfone or methylsulfonylmethane (CH3SO2CH3)

DMSO dimethyl sulfamethoxazole (cryoprotective used to store cells from patients undergoing autologous transplantation)
dimethylsulfoxyde

DMT1 divalent metal transporter 1

DMV dog mesenteric vein
dorsal metatarsal veins

DN double negative

DNA deoxyribonucleic acid
did not attend (clinic)

DNC dominant-negative complementation

DND died a natural death

DNI do not intubate

DNI/DNR do not intubate, do not resuscitate

DNKA did not keep appointment

dnm daunosamine

dNM 1-deoxynojirimycin

DNM delayed nonmatching-to-sample
descending necrotizing mediastinitis
desmoplastic neurotropic melanoma
dominant negative mutant

DNR daunorubicin
do not resuscitate
dorsal nerve root

DNS did not show for appointment

D/NS dextrose in normal saline

D5%NS dextrose 5% in normal saline

DO disorder
doctor of osteopathy
dorsal outflow

DOA day of admission
dead on arrival
distal segment of ophthalmociliary artery

DOB date of birth

DOC deoxycholate
deoxycorticosterone
died of other causes

DOD date of death

DOD/OSD Department of Defense/Office of the Secretary of Defense

DOE date of examination
Department of Energy
dyspnea on exertion

DOES disorder of excessive somnolence (narcolepsy)

DOI date of injury

DOJ Department of Justice

DON demyelinating optic neuritis

Dors dorsal

DOS date of surgery
dead on scene

DOS (cont.)	Department of State
DOT	date of transfer
	Department of Transportation
D1OW	10% aqueous dextrose solution
DP	deep pulse
	diastolic pressure
	distal pulses
	dorsalis pedis pulse
	dorsalis pedis
DPC	desaturated phosphatidylcholine
	diethypyrocarbonate
	direct patient care
	disseminated peritoneal cancer
	distal palmar crease
	delayed primary closure
DPD	diffuse pulmonary disease
dpdt	time derivative of left ventricular pressure
DPDT-SP	D-Pro2-D-Trp7,9-SP
DPGN	diffuse proliferative glomerulonephritis
DPH	diphenylhydantoin
DPI	dry powder inhaler
DPKO	Department of Peacekeeping Operations
DPL	diagnostic peritoneal lavage
DPM	dipyridamole
	direct photometric method
	disintegrations per minute
	Doctor of Podiatric Medicine
	dog pancreas microsomal membranes
DPPC	dipalmitoyl phosphatidylcholine
DPT	diphtheria, pertussis, tetanus immunization
DPTA	diethylenetriaminepentaacetic acid
DPV	diameter of portal vein
dr	dram
DR	delivery room
	diabetic retinopathy
	diagnostic radiology
	dorsal root
DR (cont.)	dressing
	HLA DR antigen
D+R	dilation and radium implant
DRE	digital rectal examination
DREZ	dorsal root entry zone
DRG	diagnosis-related groups
	dorsal root ganglion
DRG/PPS	diagnosis-related-group/ prospective-payment system
DRN	disaster relief nurse
Drng	drainage
drsg, drsg.	dressing
Drsg	dressing
DRSP	drospirenone
drt	diffusional response time
DRt	dorsal reticular nucleus
DRT	daily rumination time
	delay-reduction theory
	Developmentally Regulated EPH-related Tyrosine kinase gene
	deviation ratio topography
	device readiness test
	device-related thrombosis
	dexamethasone-resistant thymocytes
	Diagnostic-Rhyme Test
	dichotic rhyme task
	Diet Readiness Test
	diffraction Radon transform
	diffuse rhythmic theta (waves)
	digestion-related thermogenesis
	discriminative reaction time
	discriminative response task
	disjunctive reaction time
	DNA-damage-repair/toleration activities
	dopamine replacement therapy
	dorsal root terminals
	dorsal roots
	Drug resistant typhoid fever
	dynamic regional thresholding
dRT-PCR	differential RT-PCR

DRUDP	Division of Reproductive and Urologic Drug Products
DRUJ	distal radioulnar joint
DRUL	distal radioulnar ligaments
DS	diagnostic sensitivity
	Durie-Salmon stage
D/S	discharge summary
DSA	defibrillation systems analyser
	digital substraction angiography
DSC	differential scanning calorimetry
DSCA	Defense Security Cooperation Agency
DSD	discharge summary dictated
	dry sterile dressing
DSE	disposable smoke evacuator
DSG	dressing
	dry sterile gauze
DSH	domestic shorthaired cat
DSHEA	Dietary Supplement Health and Education Act
DSK-TNM	Deutschsprachiges TNM-Komitee
DSM	Diagnostic and Statistical Manual
	Diagnostic and statistical manual of mental disorders
DSP	decreased sensory perception
D-spine	dorsal spine (thoracic spine)
DSR	Dahl salt-resistant rats
DSRF	drainage of subretinal fluid
	drosophila serum response factor
DSs	Dahl salt-sensitive
DSS	decision support system
	Dejerine-Sottas syndrome
	dengue shock syndrome
	Department of Social Services
	dextrane sulfate sodium
	digit symbol subtest
	distal splenorenal shunt
	disuccinimidyl suberate
	double simultaneous stimulation
DSSD	drug safety and surveillance management
DST	dexamethasone suppression test
DST (cont.)	distal straight tubule
DSV	Deep Submergence Vehicle
	dense-cored vesicles
	desulfoviridin
	diameter of splenic vein
	diastolic septal velocity
	diethylamine shift value
	diffuse sclerosing variant of papillary thyroid carcinomas
	digital subtraction venacavography
	digital subtraction venography
	Digitaria streak virus
	dithranol-2% salicylic acid-white soft vaseline
	DNA sequence variations
	dog saphenous vein
	Drosophila S virus
	Dual Switch Valves
DT	date and time
	delirium tremens
	date of treatment
	due to
	duration tetany
d/t	due to
DTP	diphtheria and tetanus toxoids with pertussis (killed, whole organism)
	distal tingling on percussion (over the site of a nerve, a.k.a. Tinel's sign or Hoffman-Tinel sign)
	distal tingling on percussion (Tinel's sign)
DTR	deep tendon reflex(es)
DTS	diametral tensile strength
DTSSP	3,3'-dithiobis-succinimidyl-propionate
DTT	dithiothreitol
DTZ	diltiazem
DU	decubitus ulcer
	diagnosis undetermined
	duodenal ulcer
DU-24	avian cell line

D

DUB dysfunctional uterine bleeding
DUI driving under influence
DUR duration (of action)
dus unknown gene tentatively designated "dus" for dut suppressor
Dus differential upstream sequence
DUs drug users
DUs duodenal ulcers
DUS distinctness, uniformity and stability (test for crops in UK)
divergent unilateral strabismus
Doppler ultrasound
Dusseldorf
DUS-3 avian rho0 cell line
dv double vibrations
D+V diarrhea and vomiting
3-DV three dimensional visualization
DVA developmental venous anomaly
distance visual acuity
duration of voluntary apnea
vindesine
DVB divinylbenzene
DVC divanillylcyclohexane
DVCC Disease Vector Control Center
DVD dissociated vertical deviation
DV+D Diploma in Venereology and Dermatology
dVDAVP 1 -deamine-4-valine-D-arginine vasopressin
DVE duck virus enteritis
DVH Diploma in Veterinary Hygiene
Division for the Visually Handicapped
dose volume histogram
DVI AV sequential (pacemaker)
deep venous insufficiency
diastolic velocity integral
digital vascular imaging
Doppler velocity index
digital vascular imaging system
DVIU direct-vision internal urethrotomy
DVL deep vastus lateralis
DVM digital voltmeter
Doctor of Veterinary Medicine
DVMS Doctor of Veterinary Medicine and Surgery
DVN dorsal vagal nucleus
DVP daunorubicin, vincristine and prednisolone
deep vascular plexus
defective viral particles
diastolic peak velocity prosthetic flow
diastolic ventricular pressure
digital video plotter
direct venipuncture
distal vein patch
distributed volume pair
divalproex sodium
divinylporphyrin
domestic violence programs
Doppler velocity profile
dorsal vein of the penis
draining vein pressure
ventriculo-peritonial derivations
digital vascular reactivity
Doctor of Veterinary Radiology
double valve replacement
double ventricular response
Doctor of Veterinary Science
Doctor of Veterinary Surgery
DVSc Doctor of Veterinary Science
DVT deep venous thrombosis
dw dwarf (mouse)
DW daily weight
deionized water
dextrose in water
distilled water
doing well
dry weight
D/W dextrose in water
discussed with
D5W 5% dextrose in water

D50W	50% dextrose in water
DWA	died from wounds by the action of the enemy
DWD	died with disease
DWDL	diffuse well-differentiated lymphocytic lymphoma
DWI	driving while impaired
	driving while intoxicated
DWM	Dandy-Walker malformation
DWR	delayed word recall
DWS	Dandy-Walker syndrome
	disaster warning system
dwt	pennyweight
DWT	dichotic word test
	discrete wave transform
DWW	diabetic white women
dx, Dx	diagnosis
DX	dextran
	diagnosis
	dicloxacillin
	discharged
	disease
DXA	dual energy X-ray absorptiometry
DXD	discontinued
DXM	dexamethasone
	dextromethorphan
DXP	digital x-ray prototype
DxPLAIN	Massachusetts General Hospital's expert diagnostic system
DXPNET	Digital X-Ray Prototype Network
DXR	deep x-ray
	doxorubicin
DXRT	deep x-ray therapy
DXT	deep x-ray therapy
	dextrose
dXTP	deoxyxanthine triphosphate
DXV	drosophila X virus
dy	dystrophia muscularis (mouse)
Dy	dysprosium
DY	dense parenchyma
dyn	dynamic
	dynamometer
dyn (cont.)	dyne
DYS	dysautonomia
dysp	dyspnea
dz	disease
	dozen
dZ	impedance change
DZ	diazepam
	dizygotic
	dizziness
DZM	dorsal zone of membranelle
DZP	diazepam

E

e	base of natural logarithms, approximately 2.7182818285
	egg transfer
	ejection
	electric charge
	electron
	elementary charge
	exchange
	without
e–	negative electron
e+	positron
E	air dose
	cortisone (compound E)
	each
	eating
	edema
	elastance
	electric charge
	electric field vector
	electrode potential
	electromotive force
	electron
	embyro
	emmetropia
	encephalitis
	endangered (animal)
	endogenous

E (cont.)	endoplasm
	enema
	energy
	Entamoeba
	enterococcus
	enzyme
	eosinophil
	epicondyle
	epinephrine
	error
	erythrocyte
	erythroid
	erythromycin
	Escherichia
	esophagus
	ester
	estradiol
	ethanol
	ethyl
	examination
	exhalation
	expectancy (wave)
	expected frequency in a cell of a contingency table
	experiment, experimenter
	expiration
	expired air
	exposure
	extract, extracted, extraction
	extraction fraction
	extralymphatic
	eye
	glutamic acid
	internal energy
	kinetic energy
	mathematical expectation
	redox potential
	involvement of a single extranodal site (in Hodgkin lymphoma)
	unit (Ger. Einheit)
Ē	average beta energy
4E	four-plus edema
E0	electric affinity
E0	standard electrode potential
E1	estrone
E2	17-estradiol
E3	estriol
E4	estetrol
E*	lesion on the erythrocyte cell membrane at the site of complement fixation
ea	each
Ea	kinetic energy of alpha particles
EA	early antigen (in EBV-IM)
	educational age
	egg albumin
	electric affinity
	electrical activity
	electroacupuncture
	electroanes thesia
	electrophysiological abnormality
	embryonic antibody
	endocardio graphic amplifier
	Endometriosis Association
	endurance athletes
	enteral alimentation
	entero anastomosis
	enzymatically active
	epiandrosterone
	erythrocyte antibody
	erythrocyte antiserum
	esophageal atresia
	estivo-autumnal
	ethacrynic acid
E/A	emergency admission
E+A	evaluate and advise
EAA	electroacupuncture analgesia
	Epilepsy Association of America
	essential amino acid
	extrinsic allergic alveolitis
	excitatory amino acid
EAAC	excitatory amino acid carrier
EAB	elective abortion
	Ethics Advisory Board

EABV effective arterial blood volume
EAC Ehrlich ascites carcinoma
electroacupuncture
epithelioma adenoides cysticum
erythema annulare centrifugum
erythrocyte, antibody, complement
external auditory canal
EACA epsilon-aminocaproic acid
EACD eczematous allergic contact dermatitis
EACH essential access community hospital
EACR European Association for Cancer Research
EACs endocrine-active chemicals
EAD early afterdepolarization
extracranial arterial disease
EA-D early antigen, diffuse
E-ADD epileptic attentional deficit disorder
E-ADM epiadriamycin
EADS early amnion deficit spectrum or syndrome
EAE experimental allergic encephalomyelitis
experimental autoimmune encephalitis
EAHP European Association for Hematopathology
EAN experimental allergic (autoimmune) neuritis
EANO European Association for NeuroOncology
EAS emergent abdominal sonography
EB epidermolysis bullosa
EBA epidermolysis bullosa acquisita
EBCT electron-beam computed tomography
EBER early EBV mRNA
EBL enzootic bovine leucosis
estimated blood loss
EBM evidence-based medicine
EBMT European Group for Blood and Marrow Transplantation
EBN Endemic Balkan nephropathy
EBNA Epstein-Barr nuclear antigen
EBV Epstein-Barr virus
EBV-IM Epstein-Barr virus infectious mononucleosis
EC Enzyme Commission of the International Union of Biochemistry
Eca Erwinia carotovora subsp. atroseptica (a phytopathogen)
Eca 109 human esophageal epithelial cancer cell line
ECA Echocontrast agents
ecternal/extracranial carotid artery
electrical control activity
endometrial cryoablation
enterobacterial common antigen
Epidemiological Catchment Area
external carotid artery
extra-cardiac structural or karyotypic anomalies
ECBO virus enteric cytopathogenic bovine orphan virus
ECC early childhood caries
emergency cardiac care
endocervical cell collector
extracorporeal circulation
ECCE extracapsular cataract extraction
ECF extended care facility
extracellular fluid
ECFV extracellular fluid volume
ECG electrocardiogram (also EKG)
ECH enoyl CoA hydratase
ECHO echocardiogram
enterocytopathogenic human orphan virus
ECM extracellular matrix
ECMO extracorporeal membrane oxygenation
E.coli Escherichia coli

ECoG Electrocorticograms
ECOMOG Economic Community of West African Monitoring Group
EcoRI restriction enzyme from Escherichia coli RY 13
ECOWAS Economic Community of West African States
ECRB extensor carpi radialis brevis
ECRL extensor carpi radialis longus
ECS endocervical scrape
ECT electroconvulsive therapy
ECTR endoscopic carpal tunnel release
ECU extensor carpi ulnaris
ECWSs endoluminal colonic wall stents
ED edema
emergency department
epidural
excision duodenoplasty
extradomain (the type III unit of fibronectin)
ED50 median effective dose
EDA Excess Defense Articles
EDAC early detection of alcohol consumption
EDC estimated or expected date of confinement
extensor digitorum communis
EDD esophageal detector device
estimated delivery date
EDDI Education for Development and Democracy Initiative
EDI electronic data interchange
EDIR emergency drug identification record
EDL extensor digitorum longus
EDM extensor digitis minimi
EDMR electrically detected magnetic resonance
EDOD estimated date of delivery
EDRF endothelium-derived relaxing factor
EDS Ehlers-Danlos syndrome
EDS (cont.) excessive daytime sleepiness
external defibrillation system
EDSTAC Endocrine-Disrupter Screening Testing Advisory Committee
EDTA ethylenediaminetetraacetic acid
EDV end diastolic velocity
EDX electrodiagnostic
EE energy expenditure
ethinyl estradiol
EEG electroencephalogram
EENT eye, ear, nose and throat
EES Ethicon Endo-Surgery
EEX electrodiagnosis
EEXOT Hellenic Orthopaedic Association
EF ectopic focus
edema factor
effects
ejection fraction
elastic fibril
electric field
elongation factor
embryo fibroblast
embryo-fetal
emergency facility
encephalitogenic factor
endothoracic fascia
endurance factor
eosinophilic fasciitis
epithelial focus
equivalent focus
erythroblastosis fetalis
erythrocyte fragmentation
exposure factor
extended field
extrafine
extrinsic factor
peptide elongation factor
EF-2 initiation factor in the translational step of viral replication
EFA essential fatty acids
EFAD essential fatty acid deficiency

EFFAS European Foot and Ankle National Societies
EFFO European Foundation for Osteoporosis and Bone Disease
EF-G elongation factor G
EFORT European Federation of National Associations of Orthopaedics and Traumatology
EFS event free survival - time from diagnosis to defined events (e.g. relapse or death)
EGA error grid analysis
estimated gestational age
EGC early gastric carcinoma
EGD esophagogastroduodenoscopy
EGDS esophagogastric devascularization with splenectomy
EGE eosinophilic gastroenteritis
EGF epidermal growth factor
EGFP enhanced green fluorescent protein
EHBA extrahepatic biliary atresia
EHBP extrahepatic biliary passages
EHEC enterohemorrhagic Escherichia Coli
EHL evaporative heat loss
extensor hallucis longus
EHS European Hip Society
EIC endometrial intraepithelial carcinogenesis
extensive intraductal component
EICESS European Intergroup Ewing's Sarcoma Study
EIN3 ethylene-insensitive3 (is a transcription factor that works in the ethylene signaling pathway in Arabidopsis)
EJ elbow jerk
EJC European Journal of Cancer
EJHS Electronic Journal of Hand Surgery
EJO Electronic Journal of Orthopaedics
EJS Electronic Journal of Surgery and Specialistic Medicine
EKG electrocardiogram (also ECG)
EL elbow
endoscopic ligation
ELAM-1 E-selectin adhesion molecule (on endothelial cells)
elev. elevated
ELF elective low forceps
ELISA enzyme-linked immunosorbent assay
Elix elixir
ELOS estimated lenght of stay
EM electron microscope, emmetropia
EMB eosin methylene blue agar
EmBx endometrial biopsy
EMC electromagnetic compatibility
EMCAP World Bank's Economic Management Capacity Project
EMD electromechanical dissociation
EMDR Eye Movement Desensitization and Reprocessing
EMEA European Agency for the Evaluation of Medicinal Products
EMG electromyogram, electromyography
EMH extramedullary hematopoiesis
EMM epithelial malignant mesotheliomas
EMP Embden-Meyerhof pathway
EMPD emergency medical priority dispatch
EMR electronic medical records
EMS electrical muscle stimulation
emergency medical service
endometrial scrape
EMST Emergency Management of Severe Trauma
EMT emergency medical technician
EMT-B Emergency Medical Technician basic
EMT-P Emergency medical technician paramedic
EMTALA Emergency Medical Treatment and Active Labor Act

EMUO	early morning urine osmolality (evaluating urine concentration)
EMV	eyes, motor, verbal response (Glasgow coma scale)
En.	enema
End	endothelial cells
ENG	electronystagmography
ENI	Bureau for Europe and the New Independent States
ENSG	European Neuroblastoma Study Group
ENT	ear, nose, and throat
EOA	Eastern Orthopaedic Association Egyptian Orthopaedic Association
Eoc.	eosinophiles
EOI	European Osteosarcoma Intergroup
EOM	extraocular movements
EOMI	extraocular movements intact
EOM(I)	extraocular muscles (intact)
EORS	European Orthopaedics Research Society
EORTC	European Organisation for Research and Treatment of Cancer
Eos	eosin, eosinophil(s)
EOS	eosinophil(s)
EP	ectopic pregnancy emergency physician endogenous pyrogens European Pharmacopoeia
EPA	Environmental Protection Agency controls the use of pesticides and monitors water pollution in general
EPB	extensor pollicis brevis
EPC	egg phosphatidylcholine
EPDM	ethylene propylene diene rubber
EPE	extraprostatic extension
EPEC	enteropathogenic Escherichia coli
Epi	epinephrine epithelial cells
EPI	epinephrine
Epis.	episiotomy
Epis. Med.	medial episiotomy
Epis. RML	right mediolateral episiotomy
Epis. LML	left mediolateral episiotomy
EPL	extensor pollicis longus
EPOC	excess post-oxygen consumption
EPOS	European Pediatric Orthopaedic Society
EPS	exophtalmos-producing substance extrapyramidal symptoms
EPSD	Early Periodic Screening Detection
EPSP	excitatory postsynaptic potential
EPSPS	5-enolpyruvylshikamate-3-phosphate synthetase
EPU	epidermal proliferative unit
EPV	Epstein-Barr virus
ER	emergency room endoplasmic reticulum external rotation
ERA	electrical response activity estradiol receptor assay evoked response audiometry
ERAD	endoplasmic-reticulum-associated degradation
ERCP	endoscopic retrograde cholangiopancreatography
ERE	external rotation in extension
ERF	external rotation in flexion
ERP	effective refractory period
ER/PR	estrogen/progesterone
ERT	empathy response task endurance run test enzyme replacement therapy estrogen replacement therapy external radiation therapy
Ery	erythrocytes
ES	electrical stimulation endoscopic sclerotherapy enzymatic spectrometric method enzyme-substrate complex
ESAF	Enhanced Structural Adjustment Facility
ESB	European Society of Biomechanics

ESBL	extended-spectrum beta-lactamase
ESD	esterase D
ESD Dus 2	a new rare allele for esterase D (ESD) described in a family from Dusseldorf
ESDS	European Spinal Deformities Society
ESF	Economic Support Fund
	European Science Foundation
ESFAS	European Society of Foot and Ankle Surgeons
ESI	electrospray ionization
	epidural steroid injection
	European Surgical Institute
ESO	European School of Oncology
EspA	E. coli secreted protein A
EspB	E. coli secreted protein B
EspD	E. coli secreted protein D
ESPD	electrosensitive protective device
	endogenous digoxin-like substance
ESPGHAN	European Society of Paediatric Gastroenterology, Hepatology, and Nutrition
ESR	electron spin resonance
	erythrocyte sedimentation rate
ESRD	end stage renal disease
ESRF	end stage renal failure
ESS	endometrial stromal sarcoma
	European Spine Society
ESSKA	European Society for Sports Medicine, Knee Surgery and Arthroscopy
EST	electroshock therapy
	estrogen sulfotransferases
	expressed sequence tag
ESTRO	European Society for Therapeutic Radiation and Oncology
ESWL	extracorporeal shock wave lithotripsy
et	and
ET	ejection time
ET (cont.)	endotracheal
	esotropia
	essential thrombocythemia
	eustachian tube(s)
	exercise training
ET-1	endothelin-1
ETA	estimated time of arrival
ETCO2	end tidal CO2
ETD	estimated time of departure
ETF	eustachian tube function
ETI	endotracheal intubation
Etio	etiology
etiol, etiol.	etiology
ETIOL.	etiology
EtO	ethylene oxyde
EtOH, ETOH	ethanol, alcohol
ETS	environmental tobacco smoke
ETT	endotracheal tube
	exercise tolerance test
ETX	ethosuximide
EU	European Union
EUA	examination under anesthesia
EUD	enzymatic ultrafiltrate digest
	equivalent uniform dose
	Eudragit
Eud-M	eudistomin M.
EU-NRLs	European Union National Reference Laboratories
EUP	eupneic
EUS	endoscopic ultrasound
EVA	economic value added
	electric vacuum aspiration
	ethylene-vinylacetate
eval	evaluate
EVAL	evaluation
eval.	evaluation
EVAL	ethylene-vinyl alcohol
EVH	enabled/VASP homology
	endoscopic vein harvest
	esophageal variceal hemorrhage
	eucapnic voluntary hyperventilation

EW	emergency ward
EWS	Ewing sarcoma gene (at 22q12)
ex.	exercise
	example
EX	exacerbate
	examination
	excision
	exercise
	extension
exam, Exam	examination
exc	excision
EXC	excellent
	except
	exchange
	excision
EXP	expand
	explain
expir	expiration
	expiratory
Exp. Lap	exploratory laparotomy
ext	external
ext.	extremities
	external
ExT	exfoliating toxin
EXT	extend
	external
	extremity
ext. gen.	external genitalia

F

f	normal
	steady
	unchanged
F	Fahrenheit degrees
	father
	female
	finger
	phenylalanine
F7	factor VII gene on chromosome 13q34-qter
FA	failed appointment
	Fanconi's anemia
	fluorapatite
	fluorescent antibody
	forearm
F.A.	first aid
FAA	Federal Aviation Agency
FAAN	Federal Airport Authority of Nigeria
FAAP	F-actin image analysis program
	Fellow of the American Academy of Pediatrics
	free amino acid pool
	functional activity of plasminogen activators in plasma
	N-formylaminoantipyrine
Faap(s)	fatty acid activation protein(s)
FAAU	functional activity of plasminogen activators in urine
FAB	French American and British classification scheme for leukemia
FABERE	external rotation and extension
FABP	fatty acid binding protein
FACC	Fellow of the American College of Cardiology
FACES-II	Family Adaptability and Cohesion Evaluation Scales, Version II
FACFAS	Fellow of the American College of Foot and Ankle Surgeons
FACOG	Fellow Of The American College Of Obstetrics And Gynecology
FACOI	Fellow of the American College of Osteopathic Internists
FACP	Fellow of the American College Of Physicians
FACS	Fellow of the American College Of Surgeons
	fluorescence-activated cell sorter
F-actin	filamentous actin
FACU	Federal Agricultural Coordinating Unit
FAD	flavin adenine dinucleotide

FADIR flexion, adduction and internal rotation
FADIRE flexion, adduction, internal rotation and extension
FAI Foot and Ankle International (Journal)
FALT follicle-associated lymphoid tissue
FAMS functional assessment of multiple sclerosis
FANA fluorescent antinuclear antibody test (see also ANA)
FAO United Nations Food and Agricultural Organization
FAOP Florida Association of Orthotists and Prosthetists
FAP familial adenomatous polyposis
FAQ frequently asked questions
FASIG Foot and Ankle Special Interest Group
FAS/ITP Foreign Agriculture Service/ International Trade Policy
FAWC Farm Animal Welfare Concil (UK)
f.b. foreign body
FB, F.B. foreign body
FBC full blood count
FBD Familial British dementia
feather and beak disease (a bird disease)
fibrin binding domain
fibrocystic breast disease
Flow-BOLD (blood oxygenation level-dependent) -Dependence
food-borne diseases
forearm bone density
functional bowel disorder/distress
functional breathing disorder
FB/Fb fingerbreadth
FBI Federal Bureau of Investigations
F-BKP femoral-below-knee-popliteal bypasses
FBM felbamate
FBP filtered back-projection
FBS fasting blood sugar
Finnish Bone Society (EFFO Member Society)
FC finger counting
free carnitine
FCA fracture, complete, angulated
FCAPM formal college approved postgraduate meeting
FCC Federal Communications Commission
fracture, complete/compound, comminuted
FCCC fracture, complete, comminuted, compound
FCCP Fellow of the American College Of Chest Physicians
FCD fracture, complete, deviated
FCE food conversion efficiency
FCI flow cytometric immunophenotyping
FCM flow cytometry
FCMC family-centered maternity care
FCOVD Fellow of the College of Optometrists in Vision Development
FCR flexor carpi radialis
FCS fetal calf serum
FCT Federal Capitol Territory
FCU flexor carpi ulnaris
FD familial dysautonomia
fire department
Forceps delivery
fully dilated
FDA Food and Drug Administration (US)
FDA-BAM Food + Drug Administration-Bacteriological Analytical Manual
FDC follicular dendritic cells
FDGB fall down - go boom
FDI first dorsal interosseus (muscle of the hand)
FDIM fluorescence digital imaging microscopy

E F

FDIO first dorsal interosseous (muscle)
FDMA first dorsal metacarpal artery
Fd-MIV Friend derived murine immunosuppressive virus
FDP fibrin degradation products
flexor digitorum profundus
fructose-1,6-diphosphate
FDS flexor digitorum superficialis
FDV four dimensional visualization
Fe iron
F+E flexion and extension
FEA focal epileptic activity
FEB fever
FECG fetal electrocardiogram
FECS Federation of European Cancer Societies
Fe def. iron deficiency
FEF forced expiratory flow
FEKG fetal electrocardiogram
FEL familial erythrophagocytic lymphohistiocytosis
FeLV feline leukemia virus
fem. femoral
fem. pop. femoral popliteal
FeNa fractional excretion of sodium: (UNa x PCr/PNa x UCr) x 100; <1 in prerenal azotemia and 1 in intrinsic renal azotemia
FEP free erythrocyte protoporphyrin
FER flexion, extension, rotation
FERC Federal Energy Regulatory Commission
fes feline sarcoma proto-oncogene
FES functional electric stimulation (Cleveland FES Center)
functional electrical stimulation
functional endoscopic sinus
FES-LCE functional electrical stimulation (FES)-induced leg cycle ergometer (LCE)
FESS functional endoscopic sinus surgery
FESSH Federation of the European Societies for Surgery of the Hand
fet. fetal
FEV forced expiratory volume
FEV1 forced expiratory volume in one second
Ff free fraction
FF forward flexion
f.f. force fluid
FFA for further appointment
FFD free from disability
FFM fat-free mass
Five-Factor Model of personality
FFP fresh frozen plasma
FFPET formalin fixed paraffin embedded tissues
FFR frequency following response
FFROM full, free range of motion
FFS failure-free survival
fee-for-service
Five-Factors Score (a prognostic scoring systems)
FFT forward flexion: fingertips to toes
FGF fibroblast growth factor
fh fundal height
FH family history
follicular hyperplasia
F.H., F/H family history
FHLH familial histiocytic lymphohistiocytosis
F(hor) horizontal ground reaction force
FHR fetal heart rate
FHR-UC fetal heart rate-uterine contraction
FHS fetal heart sounds
FHT fetal heart tones
FHx, FH(x) family history
F/I fever due to infection
Fib fibroblasts
FID flame ionization detectors (chromatography)
FIGO International Federation of Gynecology and Obstetrics

	(Federation Internationale de Gynecologie et d'Obstetrique)
FIM	functional independence measures
FIMS	Federation Internationale de Medecine Sportive (International Federation of Sports Medicine)
FIN	finasteride
FINCEN	Financial Center
FiO2	fraction of inspired oxygen
FISH	fluorescence in situ hybridization
FIT	Fracture Intervention Trial
FITC	fluorescein isothiocyanate
Five-DD	five dipolar dephasing
FIX	fixed arm support
FJRM	full joint range of motion
fl.	fluids
FL	flank
	flexion
	fluid
	follicular lymphoma
	fully lactating
flac.	flaccid
FLD	frontal lobe dementia
flex, flex.	flexion
	flexor
Flex, FLEX	flexion
Fli1	Friend leukemia integration 1 gene
FL-LC	follicular lymphoma large cell
FL-M	follicular lymphoma mixed small cleaved and large
FLMP	fuzzy logical model of perception
fl. oz.	fluid ounce
FL-SC	follicular lymphoma small cleaved
FLX	flexion
FM	finger movement
FMD	family medical doctor
	foot and mounth disease
FMF	Foreign Military Funding
FMH	fetal-maternal hemorrhage
FMP	first menstrual period
FMR-1	fragile X mental retardation 1 gene
FMRP	fragile X mental retardation protein(s)
FMS	fibromyalgia syndrome
FMSI	Federazione Medico Sportiva Italiana (Federation of Italian Sports Medicine) (ItalianMedSport)
FN	fibronectin
FNA	fine needle aspiration
FNAB	fine-needle aspiration biopsy
FNH	focal nodular hyperplasia
FNP	family nurse practitioner
FO	fecal output
FOBT	fecal occult blood testing
FOC	father of child
	flight of colors test
FOM	figure of Merit
	floor of mouth
	fosfomycin
FOM-1	anti-Forssman glycolipid antibody
FOM-8108	fungal strain isolated from a marine environment
FOP	fibrodysplasia ossificans progressiva
FORE	Foundation for Osteoporosis Research and Education
FOS	Finnish Osteoporosis Society (EFFO Member Society)
	full of stool/constipated
FOSA	Federation of Spine Associations (AAOS Specialty Societies)
FOSIT	Fosamax International Trial
FP	fluticasone propionate
FPA	fibrinopeptide A
FPAL	full term premature abortion living
FPB	fibrinopeptide B
	flexor pollicis brevis
FPD	fibrin(ogen) degradation products
FPIA	fluorescence polarization immunoassay
FPL	flexor pollicis longus
	functional profile length

FPM full passive movements
FPMA Florida Podiatric Medical Association
FPT farnesyl protein transferase
FR fracture
framework
frequency of respiration
full range
FR-I, II, III framework I, II, III
fract. fractional
FRBB fracture of both bones
FRC fibroblastic reticulum cells
functional residual capacity
FRCP Fellow of the Royal College of Physicians
FRCP(C) Fellow of the Royal College of Physicians of Canada
FRCSI Fellow of the Royal College of Surgeons in Ireland
FRET fluorescence resonance energy transfer
FRJM full range of joint movement
FROM full range of motion, full range of movement
FS finger stick
frozen section
fsa focal lymphocitic sialadenitis
fructose-six phosphate aldolase gene
FSA feline sarcoma A tumor-derived cell lines
fentanyl self-administration
fetal sialoglycoprotein
fetal sulfoglycoprotein antigen
fibroblast specific antigen
fibrosarcoma
fixed scheduled access
flexible spending account
fluorogenic matrix metalloproteinase substrate assay
focal suprabasal acantholysis
Food Safety Agency
FSA (cont.) food scrap ashes
Food Standards Agency (UK)
foot shock aggression
formaldehyde-treated albumin
fractal signature analysis
fractional shortening area
frozen section analysis
fructose-six phosphate aldolase
full-spectrum data analysis
FSa-II murine fibrosarcoma cell line
FSB Formosan Society of Biomechanics
FSC forward angle light scatter (flow cytometry term)
fracture, simple comminuted
FSCAI Fellow of the Society for Cardiac Angiography and Interventions
FSCC fracture, simple, complete, comminuted
FSCCL follicular small cleaved cell lymphomas
FSCPC fast-setting calcium phosphate cement
FSD functional sensory deficit
FSE fast-spin-echo
FSGS focal and segmental glomerulosclerosis
FSH follicle stimulating hormone
FSN Foreign Service National
FSOs family members and significant others
FSS frozen shoulder syndrome
ft Foot, feet (measure)
FT full-term
low-molecular polypeptide factors of thymus
FT4 free thyroxine
FTA-ABS fluorescent treponemal antibody absorption test
FTD failure to descend
frontotemporal dementia
FTI farnesyl transferase inhibitor
free thyroxin index

FT4I free thyroxin (T4) index
FTIR Fourier Transform Infrared
FT-IR Fourier Transform Infrared Spectroscopy
FTKA failed to keep appointment
FTND full term normal delivery
FTNM The French TNM Group
FTR fast-twitch red (skeletal muscle)
FTSG full thickness skin graft
FTT failure to thrive
FTW fast-twitch white (skeletal muscle)
fat weight
first time wheezing
FTY fat yield
FU, F/U, F-U follow-up
FU(5-) 5-fluorouracil (treatment regimen)
FUB functional uterine bleeding
FUBAR Fowled Up Beyond All Recognition
FUO fever of undetermined origin
fever of unknown origin
FVC forced vital capacity
FVII factor VII
FVIIa activated factor VII
FVIIAg factor VII antigen
FVIIc factor VII coagulant activity
FW fetal weight
FWB female worm burden
full weight bearing
Fx, FX fracture
FXBB fracture of both bones
FXS fragile X syndrome
FY fiscal year
FYI for your information

G

g gram
G gap (about cell cycle)
glycine
gram
gravida
G (cont.) guanine
histopathological grading
G0, G1, G2 gap 0 (about cell cycle), gap 1, gap 2
GA gastric analysis
general appearance
general anaesthetic/anesthesia
gestational age
granulocyte agglutination assay
GAA guanine-adenine-adenine codon for glutamic acid
GA/BW 16 gestational age/birthweight categories
GAC guanine-adenine-cytosine codon for aspartic acid
GAD generalized anxiety disorder
GADD45 growth arrest and DNA damage
GAERS genetic absence epilepsy rat from Strasbourg
GAF score global assessment of functioning
GAG guanine-adenine-guanine codon for glutamic acid
Gal gallon
GALOP Syndrome: Gait disorder, Autoantibody, Late-age Onset, Polyneuropathy
GAMC General Assistance Medical Care
GAO general accounting office
GAP GTPase-activating proteins
GAP-43 growth-associated protein-43
gastroc Gastrocnemius
GAU guanine-adenine-uracil codon for aspartic acid
GB gallbladder
GBD gallbladder disease
GBEF gallbladder ejection fraction
GBM glomerular basement membrane
GBS gallbladder series
Guillian-Barre syndrome
GC gas chromatography
general condition
germinal center

GC (cont.) gonococcal
gonococcus
gonorrhea

GCA giant cell arteritis
guanine-cytosine-adenine codon for alanine

GCC guanine-cytosine-cytosine codon for alanine

GCDFP-15 gross cystic disease fluid protein 15

GCG guanine-cytosine-guanine codon for alanine

GCI glial cytoplasmic inclusions

GC/MS gas chromatography/mass spectrometry

GCNST granular cell nerve sheath tumor

GCP Good Clinical Practice (guidelines)

GCRP good clinical research practice

GCS Glasgow Coma Scale

G-CSF granulocyte colony stimulating factor promotes production of white blood cells

GCT germ cell tumor

GCU guanine-cytosine-uracil codon for alanine

GD gastroparesis diabeticorum

G-DAP Geriatric Draw-A-Person

GDD Gly-Asp-Asp

GDM gestational diabetes mellitus

GDP Gross Domestic Product

GE gastroenteritis
gastroenterology
gastroesophageal
gradient echo (MRI)

G/E gastroenteritis

Ged end-diastolic conductances
left ventricle centers of gravity at end-diastole

GED gas electron diffraction
gastric emptying duration
gastric epithelial dysplasia
general emergency department
general equivalency diploma

GED (cont.) generalised exfoliative dermatitis
generalized epileptiform discharges
Gln-enriched diet
glutamic acid diethyl ester
Graves' eye disease
GTPase effector domain
guanidinoethyldisulphide

GED-ELISA gel electrophoresis-derived enzyme-linked immunosorbent assay

GEDs Glycosphingolipid-enriched domains

gen, genl. general

GERD gastroesophageal reflux disease

Ges end-systolic conductances

gest. gestation

GETT general by endotracheal tube

GFAP glial fibrillary acidic protein

GFP green fluorescent protein

GFR glomerular filtration rate

GFW Guizhi-Fuling-Wan (prescription of Traditional Chinese Medicine for liver disease)

GG gamma globulin

GGA guanine-guanine-adenine codon for glycine

GGC guanine-guanine-cytosine codon for glycine

GGF glial growth factor
grifolafrondosa

GGG guanine-guanine-guanine codon for glycine

g, gm gram

GGT gamma-glutamyltransferase
gamma-glutamyltranspeptidase

GGU guanine-guanine-uracil codon for glycine

GH general health
growth hormone (somatotropin)

G.H. growth hormone

GHBP growth hormone binding protein

GHD growth hormone deficiency

GHRF growth hormone releasing factor
GHSG
German Hodgkin Lymphoma Study Group
GHT geniculo-hypothalamic tract
growth hormone therapy
GI [gaster (Greek)] gastrointestinal
gonion
G.I. gastrointestinal
GIC glass ionomer cement
GICD Groupe Internationale Cotrel Dubousset
GIF granulocyte immunofluorescence assay
GIFT gamete intrafallopian transfer
GIH gastrointestinal hormone
GIN glucose/nitrogen ratio
GINS glucose in normal saline (solution)
GIP gastric inhibitory peptide
giant cell interstitial pneumonia
glucose-dependent insulinotropic peptide
gonorrheal invasive peritonitis
GIT gastrointestinal tract
GIS Global Information System
GLC gas-liquid chromatography
Gln glutamine
GLP good laboratory practice
Glu glucose
glutamic acid
GLU glutamic acid
gluc glucose
GLUC glucosidase
GLUD glutamate dehydrogenase
GLUDP glutamate dehydrogenase pseudogene
GLUL glutamate (ammonia) ligase
GLUR glutamate receptor
GLUT glucose transporter
GLV gibbon ape leukemia virus
Gross leukemia virus
GLVR gibbon ape leukemia virus receptor
Gly glycine
GLY gly, glycine
glyc glyceride
gm gram
g-m gram-meter
gm.% grams per 100 c.c.
Gm an allotype marker on the heavy chains of immunoglobins
GM gastric mucosa
Geiger-Muller (counter)
general medicine
genetic manipulation
geometric mean
giant melanosome
gram
grand mal (epilepsy)
grand multiparity
grandmother
granulocyte-macrophage
gray matter
gross motor
growth medium
GM- gram-negative
GM+ gram-positive
G-M Geiger-Muller (counter)
G/M granulocyte/macrophage
GMA glyceral methacrylate
grand mal attack
gross motor activity
GMB gastric mucosal barrier
granulomembranous body
GMBF gastric mucosa blood flow
GMC general medical clinic
general medical council
giant migratory contraction
grivet monkey cell
gm/cc grams per cubic centimeter
GMCD grand mal convulsive disorder
GM-CFU granulocyte and macrophage colony forming unit
GM-CSF granulocyte and macrophage colony stimulating factor

GMD geometric mean diameter
glycopeptide moiety modified derivative
GME graduate medical education
GMENAC Graduate Medical Education National Advisory Committee
gm, GM gram
GMH germinal matrix hemorrhage
GMK green monkey kidney (cells)
GML gut mucosa lymphocyte
g/ml grams per milliliter
gm/l grams per liter
gm-m gram-meter
GMN gradient moment nulling
gm. neg. gram negative
g-mol gram-molecule
GMP glucose monophosphate
good manufacturing practice
granule membrane protein
guanosine monophosphate
3':5'-GMP guanosine 3':5'-cyclic phosphate
GMPR guanine monophosphate reductase
GMPs GDP-mannose pyrophosphorylases
GMR gallops, murmurs, rubs
gradient motion rephasing
GMRH germinal matrix related hemorrhage
GMRI gated magnetic resonance imaging
GMS General Medical Service
geriatric mental state
Gilbert-Meulengracht syndrome
glyceryl monostearate
Gomori methenamine silver stain
goniodysgenesis-menta1 retardation-short stature (syndrome)
GM+S general medicine and surgery
GMSC General Medical Services Committee
GMT geometric mean titer
gingival margin trimmer
GMV gram molecular volume
GMW gram molecular weight
Gn gnathion
gonadotropin
GN gaze nystagmus
glomerulonephritis
glucose nitrogen (ratio)
gnotobiote
graduate nurse
gram-negative
guanine nucleotide
GNA general nursing assistance
GNAT guanine nucleotide-binding protein, alpha-transducing
GNAZ guanosine nucleotide-binding alpha Z pol, peptide
GNB ganglioneuroblastoma
gram-negative bacillus
guanine nucleotide-binding (protein)
GNBM gram-negative bacillary meningitis
GNBT guanine nucleotide-binding protein, beta transducing
GNC general nursing care
General Nursing Council
geriatric nurse clinician
Gram-negative diplococci
GNID gram-negative intracellular diplococci
GNP geriatric nurse practitioner
gerontologic nurse practitioner
Gross National Product
GNR gram-negative rods
GnRF gonadotropin-releasing factor
GnRH gonadotropin-releasing hormone
GnRHR gonadotropin-releasing hormone receptor
GNTP Graduate Nurse Transition Program
Go gonion
GO gastro-(o)esophageal
geroderma osteodysplastica
glucose oxidase
gonorrhea

G+O gas and oxygen
GOA generalized osteoarthritis
gone on arrival
GOAT Galveston Orientation and Amnesia Test
GOBAB gamma-hydroxy-beta-aminobutyric acid
GOE gas, oxygen, and ether
GOG Gynecologic Oncology Group
GOH gemderma osteodysplastica hereditaria
GOK God only knows (the diagnosis)
GOMER Get Out of My Examination Room
Grand Old Man of the Emergency Room
GON gonococcal ophthalmia neonatorum
Government of Nigeria
GOND glaucomatous optic nerve damage
GOQ glucose oxidation quotient
GOR gastroesophageal reflux
general operating room
GOS Glasgow outcome score
GOT aspartate aminotransferase
glucose oxidase test
glutamate oxaloacetate transaminase
goal of treatment
GOTM glutamic-oxaloacetic transaminase, mitochondrial
GOX glyphosate oxydoreductase
gp gene product
gp46 viral protein specific to HIV virus
Gp parallel conductance
GP gangliocytic paraganglioma
gastric pneumatosis
gastroplasty
general paralysis
general paresis
general physic
general practice
general practitioner
GP (cont.) genetic prediabetes
geometric progression
globus pallidus
glucose phosphate
glutathione peroxidase
glycerophosphate
glycogen phosphorylase
glycopeptide
glycophorin
glycoprotein
Goodpasture syndrome
gram positive
gross product
group
guinea pig
gutta percha
G/P gravida/para
G-1-P glucose-1-phosphate
G3P G-3-P, glyceraldehyde-3-phosphate
glycerol-3-phosphate
G3PD glucose-3-phosphate dehydrogenase
G6P G-6-P, glucose-6-phosphate
G6Pase G-6-Pase glucose-6-phosphatase
G6PD glucose-6-phosphate dehydrogenase
Gpa the phosphorylated high-activity form of glycogen phosphorylase (GP)
GPA glucose pentaacetate
Goodpasture antigen
grade point average
Group Practice Association
growth-promoting activity
guinea pig albumin
3-GPA 3-guanidinopropionic acid
GPA(3) 3-guanidinopropionic acid
GPAIS guinea pig anti-insulin serum
G6Pase G-6-Pase glucose-6-phosphatase

G

GPb the dephosphorylated low-activity form of glycogen phosphorylase (GP)
GPB glossopharyngeal breathing
glycophorin B
GPC gastric parietal cell
gel permeation chromatography
giant papillary conjunctivitis
glycophorin C
glycerophosphorylcholine
granular progenitor cell
guinea pig complement
GPCI geographic practice cost index
G3PD glucose-3-phosphate dehydrogenase
G6PD G-6-PD, glucose-6-phosphate dehydrogenase
GPD glucose-6-phosphate dehydrogenase
glycerol-phosphate dehydrogenase
GPI glycophosphatidilinositol (anchor surface protein deficient in PNH)
glycosylphosphatidylinositol
GPOH Gesellschaft fur Padiatrische Onkologie und Hamatologie (German Paed. Onc Group)
GPP good pharmacy practices
GPR good partial remission
GPT glutamic pyruvic transaminase
GPx glucathione peroxydase
gr grain
1 grain = 65mg (Therefore Vgr = 325mg)
GR gastric resection
great
greater
gross
grossly
group
glutathione reductase
Gra granulocytes
GRAIL Gene Recognition and Analysis Internet Link
Grav. pregnancy
GRAV Grav., gravida, a pregnant woman
GRE gradient echo
GRF guanine releasing factor
GRH growth hormone-releasing hormone (somatocrinin)
GRID gay-related immunodeficiency
GRM gallop, rub, murmur
GS glycogen synthase
GSC gas-solid chromatography
GSH reduced glutathione
GSM grams per square meter
GSS Gerstmann-Sträussler syndrome
glucose-saline solution
Gruppo di Studio della Scoliosi e delle Patologie Vertebrali
GSSG oxidized glutathione
GST-P glutathione S-transferase P form
GSW gun shot wound
gt drop, drops
gt. drop
GT gait training
GTD gestational trophoblastic disease
gtt drops (Lat: guttae)
GTT glucose tolerance test
Gtt drops
Gt.tr. gait training
Gtts drops per minute
gtts. drops
G-tube gastrostomy tube
G-type gastric type
GU (genitalis) genitourinary
gastric ulcer
GUA guanine-uracil-adenine codon for valine
GUC guanine-uracil-cytosine codon for valine
GUG guanine-uracil-guanine codon for valine

Guppying the complete exterior and interior alteration that most World War II boats experienced after the war
GUS genitourinary system
GUU guanine-uracil-uracil codon for valine
GvHD graft versus host disease
GVHR graft vs. host reaction
GW gigaohm (one billion ohms)
G/W glucose and water
GXT graded exercise test
graded exercise tolerance (Stress test)
Gy grays (units of radiation)
Gyn gynecology
GYN gyn, gynecology

H

h hour(s)
H histidine
hypodermic
hydrogen
HA headache
hemolytic anemia
high anxiety
hospital admission
hydroxylapatite
H/A headache
HAA hepatitis associated antibodies
HA/AI hydroxyapatite coated porous alumni (ceramic)
HAART highly active antiretroviral therapy
HAC hydroxylapatite ceramic
HACCP Hazard Analysis and Critical Control Point
HAD high-alcohol-drinking
HADD highest average daily dose
HADS Hospital Anxiety and Depression Scale
HaeIII restriction enzyme from Haemophilus aegyptius
HAF hyperalimentation fluid
HAL hypocellular acute leukemia
HAM human alveolar macrophage
HASCVD hypertensive arteriosclerotic cardiovascular disease
HAT Halsted aphasia test
harmonic attenuation table
head, arm, trunk
heparin-assosiated thrombocytopenia
hepatic artery thrombosis
heterophil antibody titer
high albumin transport
histone acetyltransferase
hospital arrival time
hypoxanthine, aminopterin and thymidine
hypoxanthine, azaserine and thymidine
HAV hepatitis A virus
HAZMAT hazardous materials
Hb hemoglobin
HB heart block
HbA1c hemoglobin A1c - used for monitoring blood glucose
HBD has been drinking
hydroxybutyrate dehydrogenase
HBF hepatic blood flow
HBIG hepatitis B immune globuline
Hbp high blood pressure
HBP high blood pressure
HBPV Hemophillus influenzae type B polysaccharide vaccine
HBSAG hepatitis B surface antigen
HBSE Human Behavior + Social Environment
HBV hepatitis B virus
HC Hassal's corpuscles
head circumference
H+C hot and cold

HCA hepatic cell adenomas
homocysteic acid
Murex Hybrid Capture CMV DNA assay
HCC hepatocellular carcinoma
HCFA Health Care Financing Administration (US)
HCG human chorionic gonadotropin
HCGs hyperchromatic crowded groups
HCl hydrochloric acid
hydrochloride
HCII heparin cofactor II
HCL hairy cell leukemia
HCM health care maintenance
hypertrophic cardiomyopathy
HCO3 bicarbonate
HCPS hantavirus cardiopulmonary syndrome
hct, Hct, Hct. hematocrit (also packed cell volume, see PCV)
HCT hematocrit (also packed cell volume, see PCV)
helical computed tomographic
HCTZ hydrochlorothiazide
HCV hepatitis C virus
hog cholera virus
HCVD hypertensive cardiovascular disease
h.d. at bedtime
Hd head
HD hearing distance
heart disease
helper-dependent (e.g. adenoviral vectors)
hemodialysis
herniated disks
high dose
Hodgkin's disease (lymphoma)
hospital day
HDC high-dose chemotherapy (often used as HDC/BMT)/PSCT or/PSCR, "used with HDC, means with peripheral" stem cell transplant or rescue
HDCT high-dose chemotherapy
HDCV human diploid cell vaccine
HDF human diploid fibroblast
HDL high density lipoprotein
HDN hemolytic disease of the newborn
HDPE high-density polyethylene
HDS herniated disc syndrome
HDU hemodialysis (high dependency) unit
HE Hektoen enteric agar
hereditary eliptocytosis
H+E hematoxylin and eosin stain
hemorrhage and exudate
hematocrit and hemoglobin
HEADS home, education + employment, activities, drugs, and sexuality (special history taking technique for adolescents)
HEC Hemorrhagic Escherichia Coli
HECOS Health and Economic Consequences of Smoking
HEDIC Healthcare Electronic Data Interchange Corporation
HEENT head, ears, eyes, nose, and throat
HELLP hemolysis, elevated liver enzymes, low platelets syndrome
Hem hematology
HEMA 2-hydroxyethylmethacrylate
HEMA-MMA hydroxyethyl methacrylate-methyl methacrylate
Hem Pro hematology profile
HEP home exercise program
HEPA high-efficiency particulate air/adsorption
Hep. Lock heparin lock
HER2 human EGF-like receptor no. 2; short for HER2, ECD (extra cellular domain) (also called Her2/neu)
hern. hernia
12-HETE 12-hydroxyeicosatetraenoic acid

HETE's	HydroxyEicosaTetraEnoic acids
HEV(s)	high endothelial venule(s)
HF	hay fever
	heart failure
HFC	high frequency cells
H. flu	Haemophilus influenzae
HFOV	high-frequency oscillatory ventilation
HFRT	hyperfractionated radiotherapy
HFV	hippocampal formation volume
Hg	Mercury
HG	herpes gestationis
	Hog Cholera
hgb	Hb, HGB, hemoglobin
Hgb	hemoglobin
HGE	human granulocytic ehrlichiosis
HGH	human gastric mucin
	human growth hormone
HGO	hepatic glucose output
HGPRT	hypoxanthine guanine phosphoribosyl transferase
HGSIL	high-grade squamous intraepithelial lesion
HH	hard of hearing
	hiatal hernia
H/H	henderson-hasselbach equation
	hemoglobin/hematocrit
Hha	Halobacterium halobium
HHC	hereditary hemochromatosis
HHI	heat-humidity index
HHNK	hyperglycemic hyperosmolar non-ketotic
HHV	human herpes virus
HHV-8	human herpes virus 8
Hi	hemiglobin (methemoglobin)
HI	head injury
	hemagglutination inhibition
	hepatic insufficiency
HIAA (5-)	5-hydroxyindoleacetic acid
Hib	Hemophillus influenzae type B conjugate vaccine
HiB	high brooding temperature
HIB	Haemophilus influenzae type B
HIBCC	Health Industry Bar Code Council
HiCN	hemiglobincyanide
HIDA	Health Industry Distributors Association
	hepatic iminodiacetic acid (imaging or scanning)
	tetrahydroindazolone carboxylic acid
HIDA (scan)	hepatobiliary scan
HIE	hypoxic ischemic encephalopathy
HIER	heat induced epitope retrieval
HIFU	high intensity focused ultrasound
HIM	Health Information Management
HIMA	Health Industry Manufacturers Association
HindIII	restriction enzyme from Haemophilus influenzae Rd
HIPAA	Health Insurance Portability and Accountability Act
HIPSOC	Hip Society (also: AAOS Related Organizations)
His	histidine
hist.	history
	histology
HIT	heparin induced thrombocytopenia
	Holtzman Inkblot Technique
HIV	human immunodeficiency virus
HIV/AIDS	Human Immuno-Deficiency Virus/ Acquired Immune Deficiency Syndrome
H-J	hepatojugular
HJR	hepatojugular reflux
HK	high molecular weight kininogen
HK (3-)	3-hydroxykynurenine
HKAFO	hip-knee-ankle-foot orthosis
HKCOS	Hong Kong College of Orthopaedic Surgeons
HKOA	Hong Kong Orthopaedic Association
HL	hearing loss
	heart and lungs

HLA heart, lungs, abdomen
histocompatibility locus antigen
human leukocyte antigen
HL-A Human Leukocyte Associated antigens (HL-A matching for BMT)
HLA-DR D-related human leukocyte antigen
HLFs human lung fibroblasts
HLH histiocytic lymphohistiocytosis
HLK heart, liver, kidney
HLV herpes like virus
HM hand motion
heart murmur
HMD hyaline membrane disease
HME heat and humidity exchanger
HMG human menopausal gonadotropin
HMGI high mobility group I
HMGR 3-Hydroxy-3-methylglutaryl-coenzyme A reductase
HMO health maintenance organization
HMP hexose monophosphate (oxidative shunt)
hot moist packs
HMPAO hexamethyl propyleneamine oxime
HMSN hereditary motor and sensory neuropathies
HMWK high-molecular weight kininogen
HNP herniated nucleus pulposus
HNPCC hereditary nonpolyposis colon cancer syndrome
HNPP hereditary neuropathy with liability to pressure palsies
HNV has not voided
HO heterotopic ossification
history of
house officer
h/o history of
H/O history of
h20, H2O water
h202, H2O2 hydrogen peroxide
HOA hypertrophic osteoarthropathy
HOB head of bed
HOCM hypertrophic obstructive cardiomyopathy (pron.: 'hocum')
HoFH homozygous familial hypercholesterolaemia
HOH hard of hearing
HOMC hypertrophic obstructive cardiomyopathy
HON Health On the Net Foundation
HONC hyperosmolar nonketotic coma
Hop H. pylori outer membrane protein
hor horizontal
hOR human oestrogen receptor
human oxidoreductase
Hor-1 fucan sulfate isolated from the hot water extract of an edible brown alga, Sargassum horneri
HOR Health outcomes research
high outlet resistance
higher-order repeat
homing receptor
homologue of rap
hordein genes
horizontal movable arm support
hydroxysteroid oxidoreductase
hyperosmolarity-responsive
rehydrated Hemoccult
HOR (17beta-) 17beta-hydroxysteroid oxidoreductase
horiz. horizontal
Hor v 9 group IX pollen allergen from barley (Hordeum vulgare)
HOS Hawaii Orthopaedic Society
Hemoccult sensa
Hox homeobox gene
HP haloperidol
haptoglobin
helicobacter pylori
hemipelvectomy
hot pack
hot-plate
H+P history and physical (examination)

HPA hypothalamo-pituitary-adrenocortical
HPC hematopoietic progenitor cells
HPC-PEP peplomycin emulsion in hydroxypropylcellulosum
HPE history and physical examination
HPETE hydroperoxyeicosatetraenoic acid
h.p.f. high power field
HPF high power field
HPFH hereditary persistence of fetal hemoglobin
HPI history of present illness
hPL human placental lactogen
HPL Human Performance Laboratory
HPLC high pressure (or performance) liquid chromatography
HPMC hydroxypropyl methylcellulose
HPNS high pressure neurologic syndrome
HPP hereditary pyropoikilocytosis
HPSA health professional shortage area
HPT hyperparathyroidism
HPTR hypoxanthine phosphoribosyltransferase
HPV human papilloma virus
HQoL health-related quality of life
Hr hour
HR heart rate
high risk
hospital record
HRDO Human Resources Development Office
HRF homologous restriction factor (regulates C9)
HRIG human rabies immunoglobin
HRMS Human Resources Management Systems
HRP horseradish peroxidase
HRQL health-related quality of life
HRQOL health-related quality of life
HRRR heart regular rate and rhythm
HRS Hodgkin and Reed-Sternberg cells
H.R.S.T. heat, reddening, swelling, tenderness
HRT hormone replacement therapy
hs, h.s., Hs hora somni – hour of sleep, at bedtime
HS heart sounds
hereditary spherocytosis
herpes simplex
H2S hydrogen sulfide
HSA human serum albumine
hs-CRP high-sensitivity C-reactive protein
HSDA test high solids anaerobic digestion test
HSEL Hemeselect
HSG hysterosalpingography
HS-GC head space gas chromatography
HSIL high squamous intraepithelial lesion
HSM hepatosplenomegaly
holosystolic murmur
HSP Henoch-Schönlein purpura
HS purpura Henoch-Schönlein purpura
HSR homogeneous staining regions
HSS Hospital for Special Surgery
HSV herpes simplex virus
ht height
HT heart
hospital treatment
hypertension
hyperthyroidism
HT-BCLs homozygous typing B cell lines
HTLV-I human T-cell lymphotropic virus types I
HTLV-III human lymphotropic virus, type III (AIDS agent, HIV)
HTMT heptane carboxamide (an H1 receptor antagonist)
HTN hypertension
HTS high throughput screening
HUS head ultrasound
hemolytic uremic syndrome
HUVEC human umbilical vein endothelial cells

HV	half-value
	healthy volunteers
	hepatic vein
	herpes virus
	home visit
	hospital visit
	hyperventilation
HVA	homovanillic acid
HVD	hypertensive vascular disease
HVL	half-value layer
HVO	Health Volunteers Overseas
HW	healing well
	hemodynamically weighted
HWA	horticulture waste ashes
HWI	hazardous waste incinerator
	Hazardous Waste Index
	head-out water immersion
	Heart weight index
	Heart work index
	heartworm infection
	height-width index
	hemodynamically weighted imaging
	Hepatic weight index
	high water intake
	hip-waist index
	hot-water irrigation (was introduced as a treatment of epistaxis more than 100 years ago)
HWL	healthy way of life
	Heat-Withdrawal Latency
	height-width-length
	hindpaw withdrawal latency
	hybrid white leghorn
HWL-12	2-phenyl-3-(3',5'-dimorpholinomethyl-4'-hydroxy)-benzoyl-indole
HWP	hot wet pack
HWT	H-wave therapy
Hx	history
	hospitalization
HY	Hoehn and Yahr (scale)
hyp.	hypodermic
HYP	hyperpneic
Hyperal.	hyperalimenation
hypo	hypodermically
Hz	Hertz (cycles per second)
HZT	high zone tolerance
HZV	herpes zoster virus

I

I	isoleucine
	radioactive iodine
IA	incurred accidentally
	intra-arterial
	invasive aspergillosis
IABP	intraaortic balloon pump
IAC	infinite amplitude clipping
	internal acoustic canal
IACR	International Agency on Cancer Research
IADH	inappropriate secretion of antidiuretic hormone
IADHS	inappropriate secretion of antidiuretic hormone syndrome
IAHL	infection-associated hemophagocytic lymphohistiocytosis
IAHS	infection-associated hemophagocytic syndrome
IAP	inhibitor of apoptosis
IAPM	International Association of Medical Prosthesis Manufacturers
IARC	International Agency for Research on Cancer
IAS	Indian Arthroscopy Society
IASLC	International Association for the Study of Lung Cancer
IASP	International Association for the Study of Pain
IATMR	tetramethylrhodamine-iodoacetamide

IBA incinerator bottom ashes

IBC idiopathic bone cavity
idiotype binding capacity
immunoglobulin bearing cells
incidence of bacteria-carrier
indirect bilirubin concentrations
inflammatory breast cancer
Injury Behavior Checklist
Inoue balloon catheter
Institutional Biosafety Committee
insulin binding capacity
integrated backscatter coefficient
Integrated Broadband Communication
International BioClinical
International Bioethics Committee (of UNESCO)
International Biophysics Corporation
International Business Communications
interval breast cancer (breast cancer diagnosed within 1 year of a negative annual screening examination)
intraductile breast cancer
invasive bladder cancer
invasive breast cancers
iodine binding capacity
ionophore of bivalent cations
iron binding capacity
isobutyl cyanoacrylate
isobutylchloroformate

IBD inflammatory bowel disease

IBF individual bioequivalence

IBG iliac bone graft

IBIDS Syndrome: ichthyosis, brittle hair, impaired intelligence, decreased fertilityshort stature

IBMTR International Bone Marrow Transplant Registry

IBP Ibuprofen

IBS irritable bowel syndrome

IBSE International Federated Body on Scoliosis Etiology

IBW ideal body weight

i.c. intracutaneous(ly)

IC between meals
incident command
inspiratory capacity
intensive care
intracerebral

I/C instructor coordinator

ICA immunohistochemical assay
internal carotid artery

ICAM intercellular adhesion molecules

ICAM-1 intercellular adhesion molecule 1 (endothelial cell adhesion molecule)

ICAO International Civil Aviation Organization

ICARE International Cancer Alliance for Research and Education (ICARE)

ICASS Internal Cooperative Agreement Support and Services

ICBG iliac crest bone graft

ICC inferior colliculus
intensive coronary care

ICCG International Collaborative Cancer Group

ICCPO Icelandic Childhood Cancer Parent Organisation
International Confederation of Childhood Cancer Parent Organizations

ICCU intensive coronary care unit

ICD implantable-cardioverter defibrillator
International Statistical Classification of Disease, published by WHO
isocitrate dehydrogenase

ICD-9 International Classification of Diseases, 9th Revision

ICD-9-CM International Classification of Diseases, 9th Revision, clinical modification
ICD-10 International Classification of Diseases, 10th Revision, maintained by WHO
ICDA international classification of diseases, adapted
ICD-O International Classification of Diseases for Oncology (coding system)
ICD-O M morphologic rubric of ICD-O
ICD-O T topographic rubric of ICD-O
ICEID 2000 The International Conference on Emerging Infectious Diseases 2000
ICER incremental cost-effectiveness ratio
ICF informed consent form
intensive care facility
intermediate care facility
intracellular fluid
ICFX intracapsular fracture
ICH human infantile cortical hyperostosis
International Conference on Harmonization (GCP)
intracerebral hemorrhage
ICM intercostal margin
ICN intensive care nursery
ICOE International Center for Orthopaedic Education (US)
ICP intracranial pressure
ICPA International Chiropractic Pediatric Association
ICRF Imperial Cancer Research Fund (UK)
ICRS International Cartilage Repair Society
ICS intercostal space
International Continence Society
ICSF International College of Surgery of the Foot
ICSI intracytoplasmic sperm injection
ICT insulin coma therapy
intermittent cervical traction
ICU intensive care unit
i.d. during the day
ID during the day
identification
ill defined
ineffective dose
infectious disease
internal diameter
intradermal
I+D incision and drainage
IDA iron deficiency anemia
IDC infiltrating ductal carcinoma
interdigitating cells
IDD insulin dependent diabetes
internal disc disruption
IDDM insulin-dependent diabetes mellitus, type I
IDDS importable drug delivery system
IDET intradiscal electrothermal therapy
IDK internal derangement of the knee
IDU injection drug users
IDW ideal body weight
IE inner ear
I+E internal and external
I/E inspiratory, expiratory
IEC independant ethics committee
Information, Education, and Communication
IEEE Institute of Electrical and Electronics Engineers
IESS Intergroup Ewing's Sarcoma Study (USA)
IF index finger
IFA indirect immunofluorescent IgG antibody
IFC International Finance Corporation
IFCCs intraperitoneal free cancer cells
IFE immunofixation electrophoresis
IFER International Federation of the Eye Banks

IFG impaired fasting glucose
IFMBE International Federation for Medical and Biological Engineering
IFN interferon
IFOSA International Federation of Spine Associations
IFPOS International Federation of Pediatric Orthopaedic Societies
IFR inspiratory flow rate
IFSC International Federation of Surgical Colleges (WHO non-governmental organizations)
IFSSH International Federation of Societies for Surgery of the Hand
IG immature granulocyte
Ig immunoglobulin
IgA, IGA immunoglobulin A
IgD, IGD immunoglobulin D
IgE, IGE immunoglobulin E
IGF insulin-like growth factor (somatomedin)
insulin-like growth factor
IGFBP insulin-like growth factor binding protein
IGFBP-5 insulin-like growth factor-binding protein-5
IgG, IGG immunoglobulin G
IGHD IB isolated growth hormone deficiency type IB
IgM, IGM immunoglobulin M
IgSF Ig superfamily
IGT impaired glucose tolerance
IGV immunoglobulin variable region gene
IH infectious hepatitis
interval history
IHA inhibition of hemagglutination
IHC immunohistochemistry
Internet Healthcare Coalition
IHD ischemic heart disease
IHHNV infectious hypodermal and hematopoietic necrosis virus
IHR intrinsic heart rate
IHS International Hip Society
IHSS idiopathic hypertrophic subaortic stenosis
IHT intermittent hypoxic training
IID insulin dependent diabetes
IIF indirect immunofluorescence
IIS Intergalactic Institute of Shoulderology
IITS International Intradiscal Therapy Society
IL ilio-lumbar
interleukine
IL2 Interleukin2
IL-1 Rrp IL-1 receptor related protein
ILC interstitial laser coagulation
ILCOR Interrnational Liaison Committee on Resuscitation
Ile isoleucine
ILL intermediate lymphocytic lymphoma
ILO International Labor Office
ILP isolated limb perfusion
ILSG International Lymphoma Study Group
I.M. intramuscular
IM infectious mononucleosis
intermediate (for EMT-intermediate level)
internal medicine
intramedullary
intramuscular
IMBC indirect maximum breathing capacity
Im-DCH-beta-Gal O-[4-(1-imidazolyl)butyl]-2,3-dicyano-1,4-hydroquinonyl beta-D-galactopyranoside
IME independent medical examiner
IMF International Monetary Fund
International Myeloma Foundation

IMHO	in my humble opinion
IMI	Imipramine (Tofranil)
	intramuscular injection
	inferior myocardial infarction
IML	intracranial mass lesion
IMLAS	International Musculoskeletal Laser Society
IM-like	infectious mononucleosis-like
IMM	immediate
	immobilize
	immunize
	interdigestive migratory motor complex
IMO	in my opinion
imp	impression
	important
	improved
Imp	impression
IMP	immuno magnetic particles
	important
	impression
	improved
	inosine 5'-monophosphate
	inpatient multidimensional psych scale
IMPOX	immunoperoxidase
IMRI	Interventional Magnetic Resonance Imaging
IM-ROD	intramedullary rod
IMRT	intensity-modulated radiotherapy
IMS	immunomagnetic separation
IMV	intermitt. mandatory ventilation
In.	inches
INC	incomplete
	inconclusive
	increase
Inc. AB	incomplete abortion
INCB	International Narcotics Control Board of United Nations
incr.	increased (ing)
Incr	increase
IND	independent
IND (cont.)	indication
	Indomethacin
	investigational new drug (see FDA)
Inev. AB	inevitable abortion
inf	infusion
	inferior
Inf.	infusion
INF	infant
	infarction
	infected
	inferior
	infusion
INFA	International Neurofibromatosis Association
INH	isoniazid
Inhal	inhalation
INI	initial(ly)
inj	inject(ion)
	injured
INJ	inject
	injection
	injury
INK	inhibitors of CDK4 and CDK6
	injury not known
INL	International Narcotics and Law Enforcement Affairs Bureau (DOS)
iNO	inhaled nitric oxide
INR	intermittent
	International Normalized Ratio (standard of care for the management of anticoagulation)
	interval
INS	Immigration and Naturalization Service
	insulin
	insurance
InsP(3)	inositol 1,4,5-trisphosphate
inspir	inspiration
	inspiratory
INSS	International Neuroblastoma Staging System
int, int.	internal

Int. internal
INTHC intrathecally
Intra inside (e.g. intracavitary)
during (e.g. intraoperative = during surgery)
IO inferior oblique
intestinal obstruction
intraosseous
I+O intake and output (as for fluids)
IOA Indian Orthopaedic Association
IOFB intraocular foreign body
IOL intraocular lens
IOM interosseous membrane
IOP intraocular pressure
IORT intraoperative radiotherapy
IOU intensive therapy observation unit
IP inpatient
interphalangeal
intraperitoneal
IP3 inositol-1,4,5,-triphsophate
Ipa invasion plasmid antigens proteins
pasiniazid
IPA 5-(N-methyl-N-isopropyl) amiloride
idiopathic premature adrenarche
invasive pulmonary aspergillosis
IPA immunoprecipitation assay
Independent Practice Associations
indices of platelet activation
indole-3-pyruvic acid
indole-3-propionic acid
inferior phrenic artery
infiltrating pancreatic ductal adenocarcinoma
Information Processing Ability
inherited paternal HLA antigens
integrated pulse amperometry
interference pattern analysis
International Paediatric Association
International Pharmaceutical Abstracts
intimate partner abuse
IPA (cont.) intralobar pulmonary arteries
intraperitoneal
intrapulmonary arteries
iodo-l-phenylalanine
ipamorelin
irrigation pipe-associated
isopropyl alcohol
isopropylamine
Isopropylantipyrine
IPA-EST indophenyl acetate esterase
IPC in-process control
IPC(foot) intermittent pneumatic foot compression
IPE iris pigment epithelium
IPHC International Prostate Health Council
intraperitoneal hyperthermic perfusion chemotherapy
isoproterenol hydrochloride
IPI international prognostic index
IPJ interphalangeal joint
IPK isolated perfused rat kidney
IPOP immediate postsurgical prosthetics
IPPA inspection, palpation, percussion, auscultation
IPPB intermittent positive pressure breathing
IPPO intermittent positive-pressure inflation with oxygen
IPPR intermittent positive pressure respiration
IPPS Independent Power Producers
IPPV intermittent positive pressure ventilation
IPRAF International Plastic, Reconstructive and Aesthetic Foundation
IPRAS International Confederation for Plastic, Reconstructive and Aesthetic Surgery
IPS initial patient survey

IPSID immunoproliferative small intestinal disease
IPSM Institute for Preventative Sports Medicine
IPSP inhibitory postsynaptic potential
The Italian Prognostic System Project
IPSS International Prostate Symptom Score
IPTG isoproylthiogalactoside
IPV inactivated poliovirus vaccine
IPx impaired glucose tolerance
phosphoinositide
IPX immunoperoxidase
I.Q. intelligence quotient
IQ intelligence quotient
IQC instrument quality control
Ir iridium
IR immunoreactive
incident report
infrared
internal rotation
intracellular receptor
IRB institutional review board
IRBBB incomplete right bundle-branch block
IRDS infant respiratory distress syndrome
IRE internal rotation in extension
IRF internal rotation in flexion
IRI immunoreactive insulin
IRMA intraretinal microvascular abnormalities
irreg, irreg. irregular
irrig irrigation
IRrs Inspiratory Rrs
IRS Internal Revenue Service
IRSSD International Research Society for Spinal Deformities
IS in situ
intercostal space
ISA intrinsic sympathomimetic activity
ISAC International Society for Analytical Cytology
ISAG International Society for Animal Genetics
ISAK International Society for the Advancement of Kinathropometry
ISAKOS International Society of Arthroscopy, Knee Surgery, and Orthopaedic Sports Medicine (also: AAOS Specialty Societies)
ISAZ International Society for Anthrozoology
ISB International Society of Biomechanics
ISBS International Society of Biomechanics in Sports
ISC instrument standardization and calibration
irreversibly sickled cells
ISCAS International Society for Computer Aided Surgery
ISDRF International Spinal Development + Research Foundation
ISEP International Society of Educators in Physiotherapy
ISG immune serum globulin
International Shoulder Group
ISH in situ hybridization
isolated systolic hypertension
ISHLT the International Society for Heart and Lung Transplantation
ISI international sensitivity index
ISIS International Spinal Injection Society
ISL interscapular line
ISM indolent systemic mastocytosis
ISMISS International Society for Minimal Intervention in Spinal Surgery
ISO isoflurane
ISOST Internet Society of Orthopaedic Surgery and Traumatology
ISP intraocular silicone prosthesis

ISPO International Society for Prosthetics and Orthotics
ISR induced systemic resistance
ISS Integrated Summary of Safety
International Society of Surgery
ISSC investigative site support center
ISSI Interview Schedule of Social Integration
IST insulin shock therapy
IT idiopathic thrombocythemia
individual therapy
inhalation therapy
intensive therapy
intermediate trophoblast
interthecal
IT15 interesting transcript 15 in Hungtington disease
ITB iliotibial band
ITC interagency testing committee
ITP idiopathic thrombocytopenic purpura
ion transport peptide
ITs immunotoxins
ITT internal tibial torsion
interstitial tumor therapy
ITU Intensive Therapy Unit
I-type intestinal type
IU immunizing unit
international units
intrauterine
I.U. international unit
IUC intrauterine catheter
IUCD intrauterine contraceptive device
IUD intrauterine contraceptive device
intrauterine device
IUFD intrauterine fetal death
IUGR intrauterine growth retardation
IUP intrauterine pregnancy
IUT intrauterine transfusion
IUTP intrauterine term pregnancy
Iv intravenous, intravenous line
I.V. IV, intravenous
IV in vitro
in vivo
intervertebral
intravascular
intravenous
IVC inferior vena cava
intravenous cholangiography
isovolumic contraction
IVCD intraventricular conduction defect
IVD intervertebral disc
IVDA intravenous drug abuse
intravenous drug addict
IVDU intravenous drug use/user
IVEC in vitro expression cloning
IVF intravenous fluids
in vitro fertilization
IVH intrafascial vaginal hysterectomy
intravenous hyperalimentation
intraventricular hemorrhage
IVI intravenous injection
IVIG intravenous immunoglobulin
IVJC intervertebral joint complex
IVP intravenous pyelogram
intravenous push
ivpb intravenous piggyback infusion
IVPB intravenous piggyback infusion
IV-QAR in vitro quantitative autoradiography
IVR idioventricular rhythm
iliac vascular resistance
immersive virtual reality
in vitro released
in vivo recovery
inhibitor of virus replication
interactive voice response
intermediate view reprojection
intervascular ridging
interventional radiology
interventional vascular radiology
intestinal vascular resistance
intramolecular vibrational energy redistribution

IVR (cont.)	intrarenal vascular resistance
	intravaginal ring
	intravenous regimen
	intraventricular reentry
	inverted repeats
	in-vitro-retinae
	isovolumetric regulation
	isovolumic relaxation
	ivermectin
IVRA	intravenous regional anesthesia
IVR-OD	inverted repeat outer domain
IVSD	interventricular septal defect
IVU	intravenous urogram
	intravenous urography
IVUS	intravascular ultrasonography
IvVD	intravenous administration of high and intermittent doses of calcitriol
IW	infarction weight
IWMF	International Waldenstrom's Macroglubulinemia Foundation

J

J	joint
JAAD	Journal of the American Academy of Dermatology
JAAOS	Journal of the American Academy of Orthopaedic Surgeons
JAB	Journal of Applied Biomechanics
JACS	Journal of the American College of Surgeons
Jak(s)	Janus kinase(s)
JAMA	Journal of the American Medical Association
JAOA	Journal of the American Osteopathic Association
JBJS	Journal of Bone and Joint Surgery (UK)
	Journal of Bone and Joint Surgery (US)
JBMR	Journal of Back and Musculoskeletal Rehabilitation
JCAHO	Joint Commission on Accreditation of Healthcare Organizations
JCD	Jakob-Creutzfeldt disease
JCO	Journal of Clinical Oncology
JCOA	Japanese Clinical Orthopedic Association (Japanese only)
JCT	junction
JHS	Journal of Hand Surgery (US)
JJ	jaw jerk
JJC	The Japanese Joint Committee
JNC	Joint National Committee
JND	just noticeable difference
JNMS	Journal of Musculoskeletal System
JOA	Japanese Orthopaedic Association (UMIN: Japanese only)
JOCD	juvenile osteochrondritis dissecans
JOD, JODM	juvenile onset diabetes mellitus
JOD(M)	juvenile onset diabetes mellitus
JOS	Internet Journal of Orthopaedic Surgery and related subjects
JOSPT	Journal of Orthopaedic and Sports Physical Therapy
JOT	Journal of Orthopaedic Trauma
JP	Jackson-Pratt (drains)
JPC	junctional premature contraction
JPO	Journal of Prosthetics and Orthotics
JRA	juvenile rheumatoid arthritis
JSCAS	Japan Society for Computer Aided Surgery (only Japanese)
JSN	joint space narrowing
JSOA	Journal of the Southern Orthopaedic Association
JSR	Journal of Sport Rehabilitation
JSS	Junior Secondary School
jt, jt.	joint
JT	joint
J-tube	jejunostomy tube
JUV	juvenile
JV	jugular vein

JV (cont.) jugulovenous
JVC jugular venous catheter
JVD jugular-venous distension
JVP jugular venous pressure
jugular venous pulse

K

K kidney
lysine
potassium
K+ potassium
KA ketoacidosis
KASS Kaneda anterior spinal/scoliosis system
kb kilobases (1kb = 1000 nucleic acid bases)
KB knee bearing amputation
kcal kilocalorie (food calorie)
Kcal. kilocalorie
calorie
KCl potassium chloride
KCS keratoconjunctivitis sicca
KD knee disarticulation
KEE Klebsiella spp., E.coli, and Enterobacter soo., the lactose fermentation bacteria that are most commonly isloated from urine
KETO ketoconazole
KFD Kikuchi-Fujimoto disease
KFH Kaiser Foundation Hospital
killifish
King Fahad Hospital, Riyadh, Saudi Arabia
KFT kidney function test
kg, kg. kilogram
Kg. kilogram
KGS(17-) 17-ketogenic steroids
KH Krebs-Hensleit buffer
KHK coronary heart disease (German abbreviation)
Ketohexokinase
Kupat Holim Klalit (a health insurance institution)
Ki-67 proliferation index
KI Karolinska Institut (Musculoskeletal Diseases)
potassium iodide
KIA Kliger iron agar
KIB836 Monroe county EMS call letters/ numbers
KID Syndrome: keratitis, ichthyosis, and deafness
KJ, K-J knee-jerk
KK knee kick
KLS kidney, liver, spleen
KO keep open
KOH potassium hydroxide
KOR keep open rate
KPS Karnofsky performance status
KR keratinocytes
KS Kaposi sarcoma
kidney stone
Knee Society (AAOS Specialty Societies)
KS(17-) 17-ketosteroids
K-SADS schedule for affective disorders and schizophrenia for school-age children
KSHV Kaposi sarcoma herpes virus
KUB kidneys, ureters, bladder (x-ray)
KVO keep veins open
K-wire Kirschner wire

L

l liter
L Lactobacillus
lambda
latex

L (cont.) Latin
left
Legionella
Leishmania
length
lente insulin
lethal
leucine
levo-
lidocaine
ligament
light
lingual
Listeria
liter
liver
low
lower
lumbar
luminance
lymph
lymphatic invasion
lymphocyte
outer membrane layer of cell wall of gram-negative bacteria (layer)
pound
syphilis *(Lat: lues)*

L1 - L5 Lumbar vertebrae 1 - 5 (spine e.g. L1 = 1st lumbar vertebra)

L_1 ... L_5 lumbar vertebrae 1 - 5 (spine e.g. L1 = 1st lumbar vertebra)

L2 second lumbar vertebra

L3 third lumbar vertebra

L6 (vertebra) lumbarization of S1 or sacralization of L5

LA left atrium
linoleic acid
local anesthesia

L+A light and accommodation

LAAD lymphadeno(nodal)-dysplasia

Lab, lab. laboratory

LABC locally advanced breast cancer

lac, lac. laceration

Lac laceration

LAC long arm cast

lact. lactic

LAD left anterior descending (coronary artery)
left axis deviation
leukocyte adhesion deficiency
ligament augmentation device
linoleic acid-deficient
low-alcohol-drinking
lymphadenomegaly/lymphadenopathy

LAD I lymphangiodysplasias

LAD II lymphadeno(nodal)dysplasia

LADD laparoscopic appendectomy and duodenocolonic dissociation

Ladd's syndrome, intestinal obstruction from peritoneal bands

LADDs lifetime average daily doses

LADDs liquid automatic dishwashing detergents

LAE left atrial enlargement
long above elbow (cast)

LAFB left anterior fascicular block

LAH left atrial hypertrophy

LAHB left anterior hemiblock

LAM laminectomy

LAM-1 L-selectin adhesion molecule (on leukocytes)

LANC long arm navicular cast

LA-NSCLC locally-advanced non-small-cell lung cancer

LAO left anterior oblique

lap laparoscopy

LAP left atrial pressure
leukocyte alkaline phosphatase

lap chole laparoscopic cholecystectomy

lapt laparotomy

LAR linoleic acid-rich

LASIK laser in-situ keratomileusis

lat, lat. lateral

LAT lateral (view in x-rays)
lat. flap latissimus dorsi flap reconstruction
LATS long-acting thyroid stimulator
LAVH laparoscopic assisted vaginal hysterectomy
lax laxative
lb, lb. pound(s)
LB large bowel
Lewy body
Lyme borreliosis
LBB low back bending
LBBB left bundle branch block
LBCD left border of cardiac dullness
LBD Lewy body dementia
LBL lecture-based learning
lymphoblastic lymphoma
LBM lean body mass
LBO large bowel obstruction
lower body obesity
LBP lower back pain
low blood pressure
LBT low back tenderness
LBW low birth weight
LC Langerhans' cells
lateral compression
lymphocyte corona
LC50 lethal concentration 50%
LCA lateral costal artery (branch of internal mammary artery)
left coronary artery
leukocyte common antigen
LCCY laparoscopic cholecystectomy
LCDCP limited/low-contact dynamic compression plate
LCE leg cycle ergometer
LCEA latency corrected ensemble average
lung carcinoma expressed antigens
LCH Langerhans cell histiocytocis
LCI Leydig cell insufficiency
LCIS lobular carcinoma in situ (breast carcinoma)
LCL lateral collateral ligament
LCM left costal margin
LCNEC large cell neuroendocrine carcinoma
LCR ligase chain reaction
LCSW licensed clinical social worker
LCTA lungs clear to auscultation
LCX left circumflex coronary artery
LD Leao's spreading depression
lidocaine
low dose
luminance-defined
L.D. lethal dose
L+D labor and delivery
L/D level-dose (ratios)
LD100 lethal dose 100 %
LDC leprosy-derived corynebacteria
LDCHL lymphocyte-depleted classical Hodgkin lymphoma
LDF laser Doppler flowmetry
LDGS life-death growth standard
LDH lactate dehydrogenase
LDL low-density lipoprotein
LDL chol. low-density lipoprotein cholesterol
LDM lipoatrophic diabetes mellitus
LDP lumbo-dorsal pain
LDRP Labor Delivery Recovery Postpartum
LDW low-dose warfarin
LE left eye
lower extremity
lupus erythematosis
L.E. lower extremities
LEE locus of enterocyte effacement
LEL lowest effect level
LES lower esophageal sphincter
Leu leucine
leuc. leukocytes
LF left foot
linear fracture
low flap
low forceps
low frequency

LFA left forearm
left frontoanterior
lymphocyte function-associated antigen
LFA-1 leukocyte function-associated antigen-1
lymphocyte function-associated antigen 1
LFB Luxol fast blue
LFD low fat diet
low forceps delivery
LFLA antilactoferrin latex bead agglutination test
LFS light fragment sleep
LFT left frontotransverse
liver function tests
lg large
leg
LGA large for gestational age
LG-ABN licking/grooming and arched-back nursing
LGB lateral geniculate body
LGI (see GI) lower gastrointestinal tract
LGV lymphogranuloma venereum
LH luteinizing hormone
luteotropic hormone
L+H lungs and heart
lymphocytic and/or histiocytic Reed-Sternberg cell variants
LHG left hand grip
LHRH luteinizing hormone-releasing hormone
LHS left hand side
LHT left hypertrophia
LIc lacunar ictus
LIC left iliac crest
LICS left intercostal space
lido lidocaine
Lig, lig. ligament
LIH left inguinal hernia
LIMA left internal mammary artery
LINCL late infantile form of neuronal ceroid-lipofuscinosis
LIP lymphoid interstitial pneumonitis
liq, liq. liquid
LIQ left inner quadrant
LIR left iliac region
LIS laboratory information system
LK left kidney
LKS liver, kidney, spleen
LL late-lactating
left lateral
left leg
left lower
left lung
lower lid
LLB left lateral bending
long leg brace
LLC long leg cast
LLCC long leg cylinder cast
LLD leg length discrepancy
LLE left lower extremity
LLF left lateral flexion
left little finger
LLG left lateral gaze
LLL left lower leg
left lower lid
left lower lobe (lung)
LLN lower limit of normal
LLQ left lower quadrant (abdomen)
LLR left lumbar region
long-latency response
LLS long leg splint
LLWC long leg walking cast
LLX left lower extremity
LM lentigo maligna
L/m one liter per minute
LMA left mentoanterior
LMD left midline deviation
local medical doctor
LMDS L. monocytogenes detection system
LML left mediolateral
LMM lentigo maligna melanoma

LMN lower motor neuron (signs)
LMO local medical officer
LMP last menstrual period
left mentoposterior
LMPM L. monocytogenes plating medium
LMR Lambertville/Maybee/Raisinville
LMT left mentotransverse
LMWH low molecular weight heparin
LN lupus nephritis
lymph node
LNMP last normal menstrual period
LO lysyl oxidase
LOA left occipitoanterior
lob lobular
LOC level of care
level of consciousness (in Glasgow Coma Scale)
loss of consciousness
L.O.C. laxative of choice
LOD limit of detection
loss on drying
LOH loss of heterozygosity
Lol leucinol
loline alkaloid
LOL left occipitolateral
limitation of liability
limits of linearity
lingual odontoblast layer
load on the lumbar vertebrae
lysyl oxidase-like protein
LOL I, II isolectin I, II from the seeds of Lathyrus ochrus
Lol p I lolium perenne group I allergen
LOM left otitis media
limitation of movement
loss of movement
LOP left occipital posterior
LOQ left outer quadrant
limit of quantification
LOR low outlet resistance
LOS length of stay
LOS (cont.) lipooligosaccaride (endotoxin virulence factor of N. gonorrhoeae)
load on the sacrum
loss of sight
LOT left occiput transverse
ligament of Treitz
LP light perception
lumbar puncture
lymphocyte predominant (Hodgkin lymphoma)
LPA left pulmonary artery
lpcAB lipopolysaccharide (LPS) core AB cluster genes
lpcC lipopolysaccharide (LPS) core C gene
LPCC liver primary cell cultures
LPD late Parkinson's disease
luteal phase defect
lpf low power field
LPFB left posterior fascicular block
LPHB left posterior hemiblock
LPHL lymphocyte predominant Hodgkin lymphoma
LPL lipoprotein lipase
LPLK lichen planus-like keratosis
LPN licensed practical nurse
LPS lipopolysaccharides
LQ lower quadrant
LQTS long QT syndrome
LR labor room
lactated Ringer's solution
lateral rectus
light reflex
LRCHL lymphocyte-rich classical Hodgkin lymphoma
LREC Local Research Ethics Committee (UK)
LRF Leukaemia Research Fund (UK)
LRFA Lymphoma Research Foundation of America
LRQ lower right quadrant

K L

LRT	lower respiratory tract
LRTI	ligament reconstruction tendon interposition (procedure)
	lower respiratory tract infection
Ls.	loose
LS	left side
	liver and spleen
	lumbar spine
	lumbosacral
L/S	lecithin/shingomyelin ratio
L+S	liver and spleen
LSA	lateral sacrum anterior
	left sacrum anterior
LSB	left sternal border
LSCS	lower segment Cesarean section
LSD	lysergic acid diethylamide
LSF	lateral spread of freeze (of a cryosurgical iceball)
LSIL	low grade squamous intraepithelial lesion
LSK	liver, spleen, kidney
LSM	long slender microvilli
LSMFT	liposclerosing myxofibrous tumor
LSN	lateral spinal nucleus
LSO	left salpingo-oophorectomy
LSP	left sacrum posterior
	lumbar spine
LSS	lumbar spinal stenosis
LST	left sacrum transverse
Lt.	left
	light
LT	lunotriquetral
LTB4	leukotriene B4
LTC	long term care
LTCF	long term care facility
LTCS	low transverse Cesarean section
ltd.	limited
LTg	low iodine thyroglobulin
	lysosomal thyroglobulin
LTG	lamotrigine
	late transplant generation
	lateral tegmental tract
LTG (cont.)	lean tissue growth
	leukocyte thermostable alpha-glycoprotein
	liquid form triglycerides
	liver triglycerides
	long term goal
	long-term gentamicin
	long-term group
	Lotus tetragonolobus
	low temperature group
	low tension glaucoma
	low transcript gene
	low transport group
	LysoTracker Green DND-26
LTGBMS	long-term glioblastoma multiforme survivor
LTG/NP	Lie Transformation Group Theory of Neuropsychology
LTK	laser thermokeratoplasty
LTP	long-term potentiation
LTR	long terminal repeats
	lower trunk rotation
LTRPC	long TRPC
LTSC	long-time (72-96 hours) stimulated cultures
LUA	left upper arm
LUE	left upper extremity
LUL	left upper lobe (lung)
LULA	laparoscopy under local anesthesia
LUOQ	left upper outer quadrant
LUP	specimen lipemic, unable to perform
LUQ	left upper quadrant (abdomen)
LV	left ventricle
LVAS	left ventricular assist system
LVEDP	left ventricular end-diastolic pressure
LVEDVI	left ventricular end-diastolic volume index
LVEF	left ventricular ejection fraction
LVESVI	left ventricular end-systolic volume index

LVF left ventricular failure
LVH left ventricular hypertrophy
LVSEM low-voltage scanning electron microscopy
LVSF left ventricular shortening fraction
LVSR low viscosity silicone rubber
LW Large White (pig)
L+W living and well
LWCT Lee-White clotting time (coagulation time)
LX lower extremity
LXRs liver X receptors
LYMP lymphocyte
Lymphs lymphocytes
LyP lymphomatoid papulosis
Lys lysine
LYS life years saved
lytes, Lytes electrolytes
LZT low zone tolerance

M

m male
married
mass
meter
minimum
molar
multiple tumors
murmur

M distant metastasis
male
married
mass
medulla
metal
meter
methionine
molar
monocytes
mother

M (cont.) mortality

M0 metastases absent
M1 metastases present
M30 antibody against epitope 387-396 AA of cytokeratin
MA marketing authorization
Master of Arts
mechanism of action
medial amygdala
medical advisor
medical authorization
mental age
moderately advanced
muscle activity
MAA minimum audible angle
MAbs maternal derived antibodies
MAC macerated
maximum allowable concentration
membrane attack complex
minimum alveolar concentration
Mycobacterium avium complex
MACE major adverse clinical event
MACOP-B methotrexate, doxorubicin, cyclophosphamide, vincristine, prednisone, bleomycin
macro. macrocytic
macroscopic
MAE major arrhythmic events
median absolute error
medical air evacuation
medication administration errors
microwave-assisted extraction
motion aftereffect
moves all extremities
murine aortic endothelial cells
myoclonic absence epilepsy
myoclonic-astatic epilepsy
MAG myelin-associated glycoprotein
MAHA microangiopathic hemolytic anemia

MAIGA	monoclonal antibody immobilization of granulocyte antigens
MAJ	major
	majority
MAL	malignant
	middle axillary line
MALT	mucosa associated lymphoid tissue
mammo	mammogram
MANe	Argosy's Manhattan II, experimentally modified
MANE	The Morrow Assessment of Nausea and Emesis
MANOVA	multivariate analysis of variance
MAO	maximal acid output
	monoamine oxidase
MAOI	monoamine oxidase inhibitor
MAP	mean arterial pressure
MAPSS	multi angle polarised scatter separation
MAPT	Master of Physical Therapy
mar	married
Mar	Medication Administration Record
MAR	matrix attachment region
MARCM	mosaic analysis with a repressible cell marker
MART-1	melanoma antigen recognized by T cells
MAS	manifest anxiety scale
	meconium aspiration syndrome
	meconium aspiration
	membrane anaerobic system
MASS	massage
	massive
MAST	medical antishock trousers
	military antishock trousers
MAT	maternal
	multifocal atrial tachycardia
max.	maxillary
	maximum
MAX	maxilla
	maximal
MAX (cont.)	maximum
	muscle
MB	muscle balance
m-BACOD	methotrexate, bleomycin, doxorubicin, cyclophosphamide, vincristine, dexamethasone
MBC	maximum breathing capacity
	minimum bactericidal concentration
MB ChB	Degrees of Bachelor of Medicine and Bachelor of Surgery (UK)
mbcr	minor breakpoint cluster region
MBH	maximum benefit from hospitalization
MBP	major basic protein
	myelin basic protein
MBPC	knee arthroplasty with metal-backed patellar components
MBs	Mallory bodies
	medulloblastomas
	melanoblastoma
	molecular beacons
	mushroom bodies
MBS	Marie-Bamberger syndrome
	modified barium swallow test
	myosin-binding subunit
MC	mast cells
	metastatic carcinoma
	mixed cellularity (classical Hodgkin lymphoma)
MCA	medical control authority
	Medicines Control Agency
	multiple correspondence analysis
McAb	monoclonal antibodies
MCAO	middle cerebral artery occlusion
MCD	multivessel coronary disease
mCE	monomeric carboxylesterases
MCF	monocyte chemotactic factor
mcg	μg, microgram
MCh	Master of Surgery
MCH	mean corpuscular hemoglobin

MCHC mean corpuscular hemoglobin concentration
MCHL mixed cellularity classical Hodgkin lymphoma
mCi millicurie
MCI mandibular cortical index
mass casualty incident
MCI-154 a cardiac Ca2+ sensitizer
MCI-186 a newly-developed free radical scavenger
MCI-2016 bifemelane hydrochloride
MCI-225 a new selective noradrenaline reuptake inhibitor with 5-HT3 receptor blocking action
MCL mantle cell lymphoma
mast cell leukemia
midclavicular line
MCP metacarpophalangeal joint
MCP-1 monocyte chemoattractant protein
MCS mast cell sarcoma
master cell stock
motor conduction studies
multiple chemical sensitivity
MCTD mixed connective tissue disease
MCU medical care utilization
MCV mean corpuscular/cell volume (a parameter of red blood cells)
MD medialis dorsalis
Medical Doctor
muscular dystrophy
motion-defined
MDA 4,4'-methylenedianiline
maternal derived antibodies
Medical Devices Agency (UK)
Meniere's disease
mouse diaphragm assay
MDC minimum detectable concentration
MDD Medical Devices Directorate (UK)
maximum daily dose
manic-depressive disorder
MDDe major depressive disorders, endogenous
MDDE 1,1-dichloro-2,2-bis(4-methoxyphenyl)ethene
MDGCR minimal DiGeorge critical region
MDH malate dehydrogenase
MDI metered-dose inhaler
MDII multiple daily insulin injections
MDM-2 mouse double minute protein
Mdnt. midnight
MDPB Medical direction and practice board
MDR mitochondrial diazepam binding inhibitor (DBI) receptor
multi drug resistant
MDS myelodysplastic syndrome
MDS/MPS myelodysplastic/myelproliferative syndromes
MDV Marek disease virus
multiple dose vial
ME medical examiner
middle ear
MEA multiple endocrine adenomatosis
MEC medical emergency clinic
medical ethical committee
mitoxantrone, etoposide and Ara-C regimen
Med. medicine
MED minimum effective dose
medial
MEDFLAG Military Medical Exercise
MEDLARS medical literature analysis and retrieval system
Meds, meds medication
MEE middle ear effusion
MEF maximal expiratory flow
MEFR maximal expiratory flow rate
MEH medical eye history
MEIA microparticle enzyme immunoassay
MEKO methyl ethyl ketone
MEL melanoma
melatonin
MEN multiple endocrine neoplasia

MEN I	multiple endocrine neoplasia (1.pituitary; 2.parathyroids; 3.pancreas)
MEN II	multiple endocrine neoplasia (1.thyroid; 2.parathyroids; 3.adrenals)
MEP	motor evoked potentials
mEq	milliequivalent
mEq/L	milliequivalents per liter
MES	microembolic signals
MESA	myoepithelial sialoadenitis
Met	methionine
MET	methamphetamine
mets	metastases
MF	marrow fibrosis middle finger myelofibrosis
M+F	mother and father
MFD	medical first responder midforceps delivery minimum fatal dose
MF/MM	myelofibrosis/myeloid metaplasia
MFS	manual function score
MFT	muscle function test
MFU	medical follow up
MFV	maximum flow velocities
MFW	multiple fragment wounds
mg	milligram - 0.001 gram
Mg	Magnesium
MG	muscle group myasthenia gravis
MGB	malachite green brucellae medium medial geniculate body Michaelis-Gutmann body micropouch gastric bypass minor groove binder monoglucuronosyl bilirubin myoglobin
MgCl2	magnesium chloride
MGCT	malignant granular cell tumor
MgD	magnesium-deficient
MGd	medial geniculate body dorsal
MGD	mammary gland density mean glandular dose meibomian gland disease mixed gonadal dysgenesis modulation gap detection molybdopterin guanine dinucleotide monogalactosyl diacylglycerol monolayer growth defect Mouse Genome Database multiglandular disease
MGD1	Mytilus galloprovincialis defensin 1
MGD-1	Mediterranean mussel defensin
MGD-Fe	N-methyl-D-glucamine dithiocarbamate/ferrous sulfate mixture
MGF	maternal grandfather
MGG	May-Grünwald-Giemsa stain
MGGM	maternal great grandfather
MGM	maternal grandmother
m.g.r.	murmurs, gallops, or rubs
MGUS	monoclonal gammopathy of undetermined significance
MGv	medial geniculate body ventral
M/H	medical history
MH	maleic hydrazide malignant histiocytosis malignant hyperthermia Mannheimia (Pasteurella) haemolytica Mantel-Haenszel (test) marital history Mayfield skull pin head holder medical history mental health metal halide mild hypoxia morbus Hodgkin Mueller-Hinton (medium) multiheaded multiply handicapped municipal hospital

MHA May-Hegglin anomaly
Mental Health Association
microangiopathic hemolytic anemia
microhemagglutination
MHAC Mental Health Act Commission (UK)
MHAM Mueller-Hinton agar medium
mutiple hamartoma
MHAQ Modified Health Assessment Questionnaire
MHA-TP microhemagglutination Treponema pallidum
MHb methemoglobin
myohemoglobin
MHB maximum hospital benefit
Mueller Hinton Base
MHBSS modified Hank balanced salt solution
MHC major histocompatibility complex (see HLA)
MHC Mental Health Care
MHCA Managed Health Care Associates
MHCI major histocompatibility complex
MHCS mental hygiene consultation service
MHCU Mental Health Care Unit
MHD magneto hydrodynamics (nuclear)
maintenance hemodialysis
mean hemolytic dose
Mental Health Department
minimum hemolytic dilution
minimum hemolytic dose
Mulberry heart disease
MHDP methylene hydroxydiphosphonate
MHDPS Mental Health Demographic Profile System
MHG Metropolitan Health Group
mHg millimeter of mercury
MHI malignant histiocytosis of intestine
mental health index
mental health information
MHI (cont.) mental health inventory
minimal head injury
MHIQ McMaster Health Index Questionnaire
MHL medial hypothalamic lesion
MHLC multidimensional health locus of control
MH-like BCL malignant histiocytosis-like B-cell lymphoma
MHLS metabolic heat load stimulator
MHLW Ministry of Health, Labor and Welfare
MHN massive hepatic necrosis
Mohshardness Number
morbus hemolyticus neonatorum
MHO microsomal heme oxygenase
MHP 1-mercury 2-hydroxypropane
hemiplegic migraine
Maternal Health Program
Medical Center Health Plan
Metropolitan Health Plan
monosymptomatic hypochondriacal psychosis
MHPG 3-methoxy-4-hydrophenylglycol
MHR maximal heart rate
mi microphtalmia gene
MI mental foramen
mental illness
mitral insufficiency
myocardial infarction
MIA medically indigent adults
missing in action
multi-institutional arrangements
MIB1 antibody against Ki-67 (a proliferating marker)
mIBG Radioactive Iodine Metaidobenzoguanidine (mIBG scans or mIBG therapy)
MIBI (99mTc-MIBI or setamibi) Technetium-99m 2-methoxyisobutylisonitrile

M N

MIBI (cont.) methoxyisobutylisonitrile (as in 99mTc-MIBI or setamibi = Technetium-99m 2-methoxy-isobutylisonitrile)
MIC minimal inhibitory concentration
MICE Medical Insurance Claim Examiner
micro microcytic
microscopic
MICU mobile intensive care unit
MID maximum inhibitory dilution
mesioincisodistal
minimum infective dose
minimum inhibitory dose
minimum irradiation dose
multi-infarct dementia
multiple ion detection
MIDCAB minimally invasive directed coronary bypass
MIDD renal monoclonal immunoglobulin deposition disease
MIF maximal inspiratory flow
MIFR maximal inspiratory flow rate
MIH maturation-inducing hormone
medication-induced headache
molt-inhibiting hormone
mullerian inhibiting hormone
myointimal hyperplasia
min, min. minimum
minutes
MIN mammary intraepithelial neoplasia
minimal
minor
MIP maximum intensity projection
MIRL membrane inhibitor of reactive lysis (CD59)
MIS maximal isometric strength
melanoma in situ
minimal incision surgery
minimally invasive surgery
MISS minimally invasive spinal surgery
MIT monoiodotyrosine
Mitf microphtalmia transcription factor
Mitr.I mitral insufficiency
Miv matured in vitro
mitral valve
MiV Miltenberger class V-like molecule (a human glycophorin variant)
MIV impurities and volatile matter
major injury vector
major interspecific variant
maternal intravenous administration
mature intermediate villi
maximal isocapnic ventilation
maximization of interclass variance
maximum increase value
mean integrated voltage
mean number of infective vector
minimal inhibitory volumes
minimum immobilizing viscosity
mitoxantrone, ifosfamide, and etoposide (chemotherapy)
mivacurium
Mivazerol
mosquito iridescent virus
multivalent influenza vaccine
Miv-CC Microhodotermes viator corpus cardiacum peptide
MK marked
megakaryocyte
MKS meter kilogram second
MKV measles, killed vaccine
ml, mL milliliter 0.001 liter
ML maximum to left
midline
MLAT Mutual Legal Assistance Treaty
MLC minimum lethal concentration
mixed lympohocyte culture
MLD mean lung dose
minimum lethal dose
minimum lumen diameter
MLE mariner-like elements
midline episiotomy
MLF medial longitudinal fasciculus

MLMP mucinous tumor of low malignant potential
MLO mediolateral oblique
MLR mixed lymphocyte reaction
MLU mean length of utterance (a standard by which speech development is measured)
MLV murine leukemia virus
ML-VRI mandibular lingual vertical releasing incisions
mm, mm. millimeter - 0.001 meters
methylmalonyl
mucous membrane
multiple myeloma
muscles
mM millimole
MM macromolecul
Maelzels metronome
major medical
malignant melanoma
malignant mesothelioma
manubrium to malleus
Marshall Marchetti
Master of Management
medial malleolus
mediastinal mass
megamitochondria
meningococcal meningitis
menstrually related migraine
metastatic melanoma
methadone maintenance
millimolar/millimole
minimal medium
mismatched
morbidity and mortality
mucous membrane
multiple myeloma
murmur
muscle mass
muscles
muscularis mucosae
myeloid metaplasia

MM (cont.) myelomeningocele
M+M morbidity and mortality
MMA marketing authorization application
mastitis, metritis, agalactia
medical management analysis
medical materials account
methyl methacrylate
methylmalonic acid
middle meningeal artery
minor morphologic aberration
mono-methyladenosine
multiple module access
MMAAP monomethylaminoantipyrine
MMEF maximal mid expiratory flow
MMEFR maximum mid expiratory flow rate
MMF maximal midexpiratory flow
MMFR maximal midexpiratory flow rate
MMG mammogram
mechanomyography
mm Hg millimeters of Mercury
MMI maximum medical improvement
methimazole
MMM mixed malignant mesothelioma
mucus membranes moist
MMMT malignant mixed mesodermal tumor
mmol millimole
MMP matrix metalloproteinase
MMPI Minnesota multiphasic personality inventory
MMR measles, mumps, rubella (live attenuated vaccine)
MMS Mini-Mental State
Mohs micrographic surgery
MMSE mini-mental state examination
MMST muscle strength
MMT manual muscle test
MMTS maximum mean total score
methylmethanethiosulfonate
MMVA methylmevinolinic acid
Mn. manganese

Mn. (cont.)	midnight
M.N.	mononuclear lymphocytes
MN	malignant neoplasm
MND	dementia with motor neuron disease
MNJ	1-deoxymannojirimycin
	myoneural junction (disease)
mo	month(s)
MO	metal oxide
moA	8-methoxy-2'-deoxyadenosine
MoA	mechanism of action
MOA	10-methyleneoctadecanoic acid
	fatty acid cis 9
	malignant oligoastrocytomas
	Marasmius oreades agglutinin
	mean orthostatic acceleration
	medial orbital
	medical office audit
	memorandum of agreement
	mesoxalic acid
	method of adjustment
	methoxyacrylate
	middle segment of ophthalmociliary artery
	migraine without aura
	mineral oil adjuvant
	mitral orifice area
	mixed oligoastrocytomas
	moderate osteoarthritic
	motion onset asynchrony
	Motor Age Score
	multiplicity of attachment (of a virion)
	myxothiazol
	The Rorschach Mutuality of Autonomy Scale
MoA-I	mouse apo A-I
MoAs	monoclonal antibodies
MOC	maintenance of certification
mod	moderate
MOD	medical officer of day
	moderate
MODEMS	Musculoskeletal Outcomes Data Evaluation and Management System
MODS	multiorgan dysfunction syndrome
MODY	maturity onset diabetes of the young
MOF	multiple organ failure
MOI	mechanism of injury
MOL	more or less
mol wt	molecular weight
MOM	milk of magnesia
mono	monocytes
MOP	methoxypsoralen
8-MOP	8-methoxypsoralen
MOPP	mechlorethamine, vincristine (Oncovin), procarbazine, and prednisone (combination of drugs used for treatment of Hodgkin's disease)
MOS	mitral opening snap
MOSF	multiple organ system failure
mOsm	milliosmole
MP	melphalan and prednisone
	menstrual period
	metacarpal phalangeal (also MCP)
	metatarsalphalangeal joint
MP(6-)	6-mercaptopurine (anti cancer drug)
MPA	malpractice attorney
	medroxyprogesterone acetate
	microscopic polyangiitis
MPC	maximum permissible concentration
	methoxypropyl cyanoacrylate
	mucopurulent cervicitis
MPCM	maculopapular cutaneous mastocytosis
MPD	(chronic) myeloproliferative disorder
	maximum permissible dose
	myeloproliferative disorders
MPEG	Moving Picture Experts Group

MPF maturation-promoting factor
MPGN membranoproliferative glomerulonephritis
MPH midparental height
MPK Minipig Kidney cell line
MPL Maclura pomifera
mouse potency level
MPO Medical and Pediatric Oncology (journal)
myeloperoxidase
MPOA medial preoptic area
MPP multipurpose phantoms
MPS mononuclear phagocyte system
myeloproliferative syndromes
M-PST monoamine-sulfating form of sulfotransferases
mPT mutant pertussis toxin
MPT mean peripheral temperature
mechanical pain threshold
mechanical pressure therapy
Methylphenidate treatment
modified physiotherapy
MPTP synthetic narcotic related to meperidine that selectively destroys dopaminergic neurons of the substantia nigra (considered a "designer drug")
MPV mean platelet volume
MPXI neutrophil myeloperoxidase activity
MR maximum to right
medial rectus
mental retardation
mitral regurgitation
mutual recognition
MRA magnetic resonance angiography
mycoplasma removal agent
MRC Medical Research Council (UK)
MRCAS (Center for) Medical Robotics and Computer Assisted Surgery
MRCGP membership examination of the Royal College of General Practitioners
MRD Medical Records Department
MRDD max. recommended daily dose
MREC Multi-center Research Ethics Committee (UK)
MRG murmurs, rubs or gallops
MRI magnetic resonance imaging
MRKH Mayer-Rokitansky-Kuster-Hauser syndrome
MRL maximum residual limits
MRM magnetic resonance neurography
Modified Radical Mastectomy
MRN magnetic resonance neurography
mRNA messenger RNA
MRP multidrug resistance protein
mRRp mouse ribosome receptor protein
MRSA Methicillin resistant Staphylococcus aureus
MRSE methicillin-resistant staphylococcus epidermis
MRT magnetic resonance tomography
mean residence time
MRV magnetic resonance venography
ms mitral stenosis
MS mass spectrometry
medical student
mental status
minor surgery
mitral stenosis
morphine sulfate
multiple sclerosis
multiple sleep latency test
murmurs
MSAFP maternal serum α-fetoprotein
msc meiotic sister-chromatid recombination
milliseconds
mSC membrane secretory component
motor layers superior colliculus
MSc muscimol

MSC glomerular mesangium cell
macrocystic serous cystadenoma (of the pancreas)
macrodactyly simplex congenita
magnitude squared coherence
magnocellular neurosecretory cell
major septic complications
major symptom complex
malignant spindle-shaped cells
mammosomatotroph cells
mantle storage cells
marrow stromal cells
Master of Science
Materials Services Center
maternal serum cortisol
maxillary sinus carcinoma
Meadowlands Sports Complex
meat starter culture
mechanosensitive ion channels
medial septum cholinergic (neurons)
medial septum complex
mediastinoscopy
Medical Sciences Campus
Medical Service Corps
medical smart card
Mercurascan
mesangial cells
mesencephalon
mesenchymal stem cells
mesothelial cells
methylselenocysteine
middle subcutaneous (adipose tissue)
midpalatal suture cartilage
mid-systolic click
migrating spike complexes
milk somatic cell
miniature squamous cells
minimal sporocidal concentrations
minimum significant change

MSC (cont.) minimum spirocheticidal concentration
modified sampling connections
modified semi-circular (spot electrode array)
modified synaptonemal complexes region
molecular shape comparison
Moloney sarcoma cell
monocyte synergistic cytotoxicity
monosynaptic connection
morphine sulphate Contin
motile sperm count
motor-sensory cortex
mouse spinal cord
mouse splenocytes
MS Contin tablets
mucosal starter culture
Multimedia Super Corridor
multiple synchronous cancer
multiplicative scatter correction
multipotential subserosal cells
multipurpose silastic catheters
muscle satellite cells
muscle score
musculoskeletal
myelin-forming Schwann cells
myeloid suppressor cells

MSC80 mouse Schwann cell line

MSC-LSMS mid-systolic click-late systolic murmur syndrome

MSCT Multi-Slice CT (scan)

mSCs miniature synaptic currents

MSDS material safety data sheet

MSE mental status examination

MSF Médecins Sans Frontières

MSG monosodium glutamate, a food additive causing neuronal necrosis in micein high doses

MSH melanocyte-stimulating hormone

MSL midsternal line

MSLT multiple sleep latency test

MSM methylsulfonylmethane or dimethylsulfone (CH3SO2CH3)
MSO4 morphine sulfate
MSOA Missouri State Orthopaedic Association
MSP methylation-specific polymerase chain reaction
motor, sensory, pulse
mss massage
MSSA methicillin-sensitive staphylococcus aureus
MSSE medicine + science in sports + exercise
MSSU mid stream specimen urine
MST mean survival time
median survival times
mini stress test
morphine sulfate tablets
MS-TBI multi-syringe time-based injection
MSTI multiple soft tissue injuries
M.S.U. midstream urine
monitored stroke unit
MSU midstream specimen of urine
monosodium urate
MSV master seed virus
MSW Mallory-Weiss syndrome
Master in Social Work
municipal solid waste
MT manual traction
maximal therapy
metacarpophalangeal (joint)
more than
muscles and tendons
muscle test
M.T. muscles and tendons
MTAL medullary thick ascending limb
MTB maternal blood type
MTBI mild traumatic brain injury
MTD maximum tolerated dose - phase 1 studies
MTO methyltrioxorhenium
MTOC microtubule organizing centers
MTP metatarsal-phalangeal
MTR magnetization transfer ratio
masses, tenderness, rebound
MTRG masses, tenderness, rebound, guarding
MTS Musculoskeletal Tumor Society (AAOS Specialty Societies)
MTSS medial tibial stress syndrome
MTX methotrexate (anti cancer drug)
M-type mixed gastric and intestinal type
MUA manipulation under anaesthesia
medically underserved area
MUAP's motor unit action potentials
MUAR multilevel upper airways reconstruction
MUC maximum use concentration
MUC2 goblet cell mucin
MUC5AC gastric-foveolar mucin
MUC6 pyloric-gland mucin
MUD matched unrelated donor - for bone marrow transplant
MUG 4-methylumbellyferyl-*-D-glucuronide
MUGA multigated acquisition (scanning)
MUO myocardiopathy of unknown origin
MUP maximum urethral pressure
mouse urinary protein
MUS muscle
MUSOC Musculoskeletal Ultrasound Society
mV mean velocity
millivolt
MV medial vestibular nucleus
mitral valve
mva min of visual angle
MVA malignant ventricular arrhythmias
manual vacuum aspiration
marginal vascular arcade (about intestines)
market value added
massive volume administration
maximal voluntary activation

MVA (cont.)	Maximum Volunteer Activity (software)
	mechanical ventricular assistance
	medioventral area
	medullary ventral areas (about medulla oblongata)
	megabalanus volcano
	mesopic visual acuity
	methanococcus vannielii
	mevalonic acid
	mevalonic aciduria
	mevinolinic acid
	microvascular anastomosis
	microvascular angina
	microvascular architecture
	microvillous atrophy
	minimum visible angle
	mitral valve area
	modified vaccinia virus Ankara
	Montserrat volcanic ash
	mosaic variegated aneuploidy
	motor vehicle accident
	multiple vessel angioplasty
	multivariate analysis
	multivesicular aggregates
	myelo-vertebral abnormalities
MVA-1	agglutinin isolated from the hemolymph of the acorn barnacle, Megabalanus volcano
MVA-2	agglutinin isolated from the hemolymph of the acorn barnacle, Megabalanus volcano
M-VAC	methotrexate, vinblastine, doxorubicin, cisplatin
MVc	caudal part of the medial vestibular nucleus
MVC	maximum voluntary contraction
	methotrexate, vinblastine and cisplatin
	microvascular cells
	microvessel count
MVC (cont.)	microvillar cells (in the olfactory epithelium)
	minute virus of canines
	motor vehicle collision/crash
MVD	mitral valve defects
MVI	multiple vitamin injection
MVMT	movement
MVP	mitral valve prolaps
MVR	mitral valve replacement
MVV	maximum volume ventilation
	maximum voluntary ventilation
MW	Megawatt
	molecular weight
MWA	migraine with aura
MWLT	multiple wake latency test
Mx	metastases unknown
MX	metastasis cannot be, or has not been, assessed
MYH11	smooth muscle myosin heavy chain (gene 16p13)
myop.	myopia
MZ	marginal zone
MZL	mantle zone lymphoma
MZPC	mezlocillin

N

n.	nerv
N	asparagine
	nerve
	nitrogen
	normal (concentration of solution)
	regional lymph node metastasis
N2	nitrogen
Na	sodium
NA	no abnormalities
	not admitted
	not applicable
	not available
N/A	not applicable
NAA	no apparent abnormalities

NAACCR North American Association of Central Cancer Registries
NAAOP National Association for the Advancement of Orthotics + Prosthetics
NABCO National Alliance of Breast Cancer Organizations
NABS normoactive bowel sounds
Nac nucleus accumbens
NaC Na channels
NAC N-acetyl-L-cysteine
nascent polypeptide associated complex
nitrogen assimilation control protein
non-amyloid component (of Alzheimer'salpha-synuclein disease amyloid)
NaCl sodium chloride
NACP non-amyloid-beta-component precursor (a.k.a. synuclein)
NAD nicotinamide adenine dinucleotide
no active disease
no acute disease
no acute distress
no apparent distress
nothing abnormal detected
NADP nicotinamide-adenine dinucleotide phosphate
NADW National Arthritis Data Workgroup
NAHCO3 sodium bicarbonate
Na-HOR sodium hornan
NAI no acute infection
nonaccidental injury
NANA N-acetylneuraminic acid
NAON National Association of Orthopaedic Nurses
NAOT National Association of Orthopaedic Technologists
NAPRA National Association of Pharmacy Regulatory Authorities
NAR nagase analbuminemic rats
NAR (cont.) narcotic
no action required
NARD National Association of Retail Druggists
Netherlands Centre for Monitoring of Adverse Reactions to Drugs
no apparent respiratory distress
nominal absorbed radiation dose
NAS National Academy of Sciences
no added salt
NASH nonalcoholic steatohepatitis
NASPEM North American Society for Pediatric Exercise Medicine
NASS North American Spine Society (also: AAOS Related Organizations)
NAT nucleic acid amplification testing
NATA National Athletic Trainers Association
NaTT sodium tetrathionate
nb note well *(Lat: nota bene)*
NB nail bed
neuro Behçet
neuroblastoma
neurometric battery
newborn
nitrous oxide-barbiturate
normoblast
note well *(Lat: nota bene)*
nutrient broth
NBI no bone injury
NBM nothing by mouth
NBN newborn nursery
NBP non-invasive blood pressure
NBs neuroblasts
nuclear bodies
N-bromosuccinimide
Nijmegen breakage syndrome
nucleotide-binding site
NBS normal breath sounds
NBSS The Canadian National Breast Screening Study

NC	nasal cannula no change no complaint non-contributory normocephalic nuclear cytoplasmic (ratio)
N/C	nucleocytoplasmic area ratio
NC/AT	normocephalic/atraumatic
NCBI	National Center for Biotechnology Information (US)
NCC	National Competition Council (AU) National Consumer Council (UK) National Coordinating Center
NCCF	National Childhood Cancer Foundation (USA)
NCCI	National Consultative Committee on Immunization nervi corpori cardiaci interni noncardiac cerebral ischemia
NCCLS	National Committee for Clinical Laboratory Standards
NCD	not considered disabling
NCEP	National Cholesterol Education Program
NCHS	National Center for Health Statistics
NCI	National Cancer Institute (USA)
N-CLB	n-desmethyl-clobazam
NCNS	no complications, no sequelae
NCO	no complaints offered
NCPP	National Collaborative Perinatal Project
NCR	no cardiac resuscitation
NCRA	National Cancer Registrars Association (USA)
NCR paper	no carbon required paper
NCS	nerve conduction studies
NCV	neocarzinostatin nerve conduction velocities non-cholera vibrios nuclear coefficient of variance
ND	non distended
ND (cont.)	nondisabling not detected not diagnosed not done
NDA	new drug application
NDF	neutral detergent fiber
NDI	nephrogenic diabetes insipidus
NDPs	nucleoside diphosphates
NDSAC	National Drug Scheduling Advisory Committee (Canada)
NE	nerve ending neurologic examination norepinephrine
NEC	necrotizing enterocolitis Nursing Education Coalition
NECCR	North of England Children's Cancer Research Unit
NED	no effort detected no evidence of disease
NEFA	non-esterified fatty acids
neg	negative
NEJM	New England Journal of Medicine
NEO	neostigmine
NEP	neutral endopeptidase
NER	no evidence of recurrence
NERD	no evidence of recurrent disease
NETA	norethisterone acetate
Neur.	neurology
Neuro	neurology neurological
NF	neurofibrillary (changes in Alzheimer's disease)
NF-1	neurofibromatosis type 1 gene (17q11.2) neurofibromin (a GTPase-activating protein)
NF-2	neurofibromatosis type 2 gene (22q12)
NFP	neurofilament protein
NFR	not for resuscitation
NFRA	National Fibromyalgia Research Association (US)

NFs neurofilaments
NFT neurofibrillary tangles
ng nanogram (millimicron) - 0.000000001 gram
NG nasogastric
N-G nasogastric
NGO Non-Governmental Organization
NGT nasogastric tube
NGU nongonococcal urethritis
NH natural health
neurologic history
neuropsychiatric hospital
nursing home
NHANES National Health and Nutrition Examination Survey
NHANES II Second National Health and Nutrition Examination Survey
NHE Naples-High Excitability rats
NHIS National Health Interview Survey
NHL non-Hodgkin's lymphoma
NHP natural head position
NHS National Health Service
NHSCR National Health Service Central Registry (UK)
NI no insurance
NIA National Institute on Aging
NIAMS National Institute of Arthritis and Musculoskeletal and Skin Diseases (US)
NIC neonatal intensive care
NICU neonatal intensive care unit
neurointensive care unit
NIDA National Institute on Drug Abuse
NIDDM non insulin-dependent diabetes mellitus, type II
NIDRR National Institute on Disability and Rehabilitation Research
NIF negative inspiratory force
NIH National Institute of Health (US)
NIHSS National Institutes of Health Stroke Scale
NII neuronal intranuclear inclusion
NIL nothing
NIMH National Institute of Mental Health
NIP no infection present
no inflammation present
NIPB non-invasive blood pressure
NIR near infrared
NIRS near infrared spectroscopy
NIRVANA NIR Vascular Advanced North American
NISMAT Nicholas Institute of Sports Medicine and Athletic Trauma
NIV non-invasive ventilation
NK natural killer cells (large lymphocytes, part of the immune system)
not known
N/K not known
NKA no known allergies
NKCA National Kidney Cancer Association (USA)
NKD no known disease
NKDA no known drug allergies
NKH nonketotic hyperglycinaemia
NKHS non-ketotic hyperosmolar syndrome
NKI a subset of natural killer (NK) cells
neurokinin I receptor
The Netherlands Cancer Institute (Nederlands Kanker Instituut)
NKI 42255 anti-insect agent (2-(1-imidazolyl)-1-(4-methoxyphenyl)-2-methyl-1-propanone)
NL normal limits
normal
NLE naples low-excitability
NLG natural latex gloves
nerve conduction velocities
Nictitans lacrimal gland
noreleagnine
NLM National Library of Medicine (part of NIH)

M N

NL/NP	non-lactating/non-pregnant
NLP	no light perception
	normal light perception
NL/P	nonlactating/pregnant
NLPHL	nodular lymphocyte predominant Hodgkin lymphoma
NLS	nuclear localization signal
NLT	not lower than
NM	neuromuscular
	nodular melanoma
	not measured
	not mentioned
N+M	nerves and muscles
NMA	neurogenic muscular atrophy
NMBA	neuromuscular blocking agent
NMDA	N-methyl-D-aspartate
NMdNM	N-methyl-1-deoxynojirimycin
NMDP	National Marrow Donor Program
NMJ	neuromuscular junction
NMKI	Nordic Committee for Food Analysis
NMR	nuclear magnetic resonance (scan)
NMR (31P-)	phosphorous-31 nuclear magnetic resonance spectroscopy
NMS	neuroleptic malignant syndrome
nmSC	nonmyelinating Schwann cells
NMSC	non melanoma skin cancer
	nonmyelin-forming Schwann cells
NMSS	National Multiple Sclerosis Society
NMT	not more than
NMZL	nodal marginal zone b-cell lymphoma
NN	neonatal
	nerves
	nurse notes
NNFF	National Neurofibromatosis Foundation (USA)
NNP	4-hydroxy-3.5-dinitrophenyl
	diabetic non-neuropathic
	neonatal nurse practitioners
	nerve net pulses
	N-nitroso-2-nitrophenacetin
NNP (cont.)	N-nitrosopiperidine
	N-nitrosopropranolol
	N-nitrosopyrrolidine
	non-histone nuclear proteins
	non-neoplastic pneumopathy
	nonneoplastic polyps
	non-pregnant normotensive women
	normal non-pregnant
	nose/nasopharynx
	sodium nitroprusside
NNP-1	novel nuclear protein (HGMW-approved symbol D21S2056E)
NNPs	nerve net pulses
NNR	not necessary to return
NNT	number needed to treat
no	number
NO	nitric oxide
NO2	nitrogen dioxide
NOAEL	no observable adverse effect level
NOC	night
noct	at night *(Lat: nocte)*
NOD	non-obese diabetic
NOEL	no observable effect level
NOF	National Osteoporosis Foundation
	neck of femur
NOHA	Nominal Ocular Hazard Area
NOK	next of kin
NONAS	number of non-aligned proximal tooth surfaces
non-IgSF	non-Ig superfamily
NONMEM	nonlinear mixed effect model
NOP	no ocular pain
	not otherwise provided for
NORD	National Organization for Rare Disorders (USA)
NOS	nitric oxide synthase
	no organisms seen
	not on staff
	not otherwise specified
NotI	restriction enzyme from Nocardia otitidis-cavarium

NOV Nederlandse Orthopaedisch Vereniging (Dutch Orthopaedic Association)
NOW navel orangeworm
NP nasopharyngeal
nasopharynx
neuritic plaques
neuropathology
neuropsychiatric
not palpable
nonpreferring (alcohol)
nurse practitioner
N.P. neuropsychiatry
NPBE non-protein-bound estradiol
NPC nasopharyngeal carcinoma
NPC no previous complaint
NPCMD p-nitrophenoxycarbonyl methyl disulfide
NPD no pathologic diagnosis
NPDL nodular poorly differentiated lymphocytes
NPH neutral protamine Hagedorn - an intermediate acting insulin
no previous history
normal pressure hydrocephalus
NPI National Program of Immunization
NPI-NH neuropsychiatric inventory/nursing home
NPN nonprotein nitrogen (BUN and creatinine)
nPNA normalized protein nitrogen appearance rates
NPO nil per os, nothing by mouth
NPO MN nothing by mouth after midnight
NPP National Population Policy
NPT normal pressure and temperature
NPV negative predictive value
NQMI non-Q-wave myocardial infarction
NQWMI non-Q-wave myocardial infarction
NR nasal airflow resistance
nerve root
non-rebreather oxygen mask
NR (cont.) not recommended
not remarkable
nrb nuclear RNA-binding protein
NrB normal brooding temperature
NRb nasal airflow resistance in the basal state
NRB Naples random-bred rats
nasal root breadth
neuroblastoma
neutral red bioassay
nitrate-reducing bacteria
Non-institutional Review Board (EU)
non-rebreather mask
nonrejoining break
norbromide
normalized relative backscatter
nucleotide releasing bacterial Lumac
squats without rebound (non-rebound)
NRBC nucleated red blood cells
NRC National Research Council
NRCS Natural Resources Conservation Service
NRCT National Registry of Childhood Tumors (UK) held by the CCRG at Oxford
NRI nerve root involvement or irritation
NRL natural rubber latex
NRM non-rebreather mask
no regular medications
normal range of motion
NRN no return necessary
NROM normal range of motion
NRS nucleotide releasing somatic Lumac
NRT nicotine replacement therapy
NRTI nucleoside analogue reverse transcriptase inhibitors
Ns. nerves
NS nephrotic syndrome
nerves

M N

NS (cont.) neurosurgery
nodular sclerosis (classical Hodgkin lymphoma)
no show
nonspecific
nonserrated cells (type of basal epidermal cells)
normal saline (solution)
not specific
nucleotide sugar

N.S. nervous system

N/S normal saline

NSA no significant abnormalities

NS5A. nonstructural protein 5A

NSAD no sign of significant disease

NSAID non-steroidal anti-inflammatory drugs

NSC neurosecretory cells
no significant change

NSCIA National Spinal Cord Injury Association

NSCLC non-small cell lung cancer

NSD N-acetylneuraminic acid (NANA) storage disorders
Nairobi sheep disease
nasal septal deformity
neurosecretory dysfunction
neurosensory deficit
night shift dose
nigrostriatal degeneration
nitrofurazone soluble dressing
nominal standard dose
non surgical doctors
nonsegmental defect
non-soap detergent
non-specific damage
non-specific defense
non-specific dermatitis
non-specific duodenitis
non-sudden death
nonsuicidal depressed
nonsyndromic prelingual deafness

NSD (cont.) normal sodium dialysate
normal spontaneous delivery
normal-coordinate structural decomposition
normalized slope descriptors
normalized spin density
normalized standard deviation
normal-salt diet
normotensive sedentary
no significant defect
no significant differences
no sleep deprivation
number of step-down

nsd-1 nonsusceptibility to DNV-1 (a recessive gene in the silkworm, Bombyx mori)

NSD-1015 3,4-hydroxybenzyl-hydrazine dihydrochloride

NSD 2023 gamma-morpholino-butyrophenone (a monoamine oxidase inhibitor)

NSD 3004 2-amino-4-phenylsulphonylbenzenesulphonamide

NSDD-38 National Security Decision Directive-38

NSE neuron-specific enolase - a neural marker
non-specific esterase

NSF no significant findings

NSG nursing

NSH National Health Service (UK)

NSHD nodular sclerosing Hodgkin's disease

NSHL nodular sclerosis classical Hodgkin lymphoma

NSI no sign of infection, inflammation

NSM neurosecretory material

NSMI National Sports Medicine Institute of the United Kingdom

NSR non significant result
normal sinus rhythm

NSS normal saline solution
normal size and shape
NST non-stress test
NSVD normal spontaneous vaginal delivery
NSx neonatally splenectomized (animals)
NSX N4-acetylsulfisoxazole
nt nucleotide
NT nasotracheal
nerve treatment
neuropil threads
normal range
normal temperature
no test
not tender
not tested
N/T numbness and tingling
N+T nose and throat
NTCP normal tissue complication probability
NTD neural tube defect
nothing to do
NTG nitroglycerine
NTLI neurotensin-like immunoreactivity
NTM nontuberculous mycobacteria
NTP National Toxicology Program
nitroprusside infusion
nonthrombocytopenic preterm
normal temperature and pressure
NTPs nucleotide triphosphates
NTS nucleus tractus solitarius
NTT nasotracheal tube
nonthrombocytopenic term
N-type null type
NUFIP nuclear FMRP-interacting protein
nullip never gave birth
NV nausea vomiting
neurovascular
N/V, N+V nausea and vomiting
NVD nausea, vomiting, diarrhea
N/V/D/C nausea/vomiting/diarrhea/constipation
NVI iris neovascularization
N+W normal and well
NWB non-weight bearing
NWDA National Wholesale Druggists' Association
NWOTA North West Orthopaedic Trainees Association
NXG necrobiotic xanthogranuloma
NYD not yet diagnosed
NYHA New York Heart Association

O

o none
without
O objective
oral
O2 oxygen
O2 cap. oxygen capacity
O2 sat. oxygen saturation
O2Sat oxygen saturation
OA occiput anterior
occiput posterior
oligoastrocytomas
osteoarthritis
O.+A. odontectomy and alveolectomy
OAF osteoclast-activating factor
OAP osteoarthropathy
OAR Office of Air and Radiation
organ at risk
Ottawa Ankle Rules
OARG Osteoporosis and Arthritis Research Group
OARS Osteoarthritis Research Society
OATA Ohio Athletic Trainers Association
OATS osteochondral autograft transfer system
OAVD optimal AVD
OAW occipital acoustic window

OB	obstetrics
	occult blood
	obstetrics
Ob-GYN	obstetrics and gynecology
OBJ	object
	objective
OBL	oblique
OB/OJ ratio	overbite (OB) and horizontal overjet (OJ) ratio
OBP	ova, blood and parasites
Obs	observation
OBS	observer
	obstetrics
	organic brain syndrome
OC	obsessive/compulsive
	office call
	on call
	oral contraceptive
	oryzacystatin
occ	occasionally
OCC	occasionally
	occiput
	occupation
OCC.	occipital
OCD	obsessive-compulsive disorder
	osteochrondritis dissecans
oCE	oligomeric carboxylesterases
OCE	comprehensive exam
	observable cholinomimetic effects
	odd-carbon fatty acid enriched
	oral conjugated estrogens
	osteocartilaginous exostoses
OCEs	Oct-containing composite elements
OCF	occipital-frontal circumference
OCG	oral cholecystogram
OCME	Office of chief medical examiner
OCP	oral contraceptive pills
OCR	oculocephalic reflex
OCS	open canalicular system (about platelets)
OCT	oral contraceptive therapy
OD	oculus dexter
	occupational disease
	officer of the day
	once daily
	optic density
	outer diameter
	overdose
	right eye *(Lat: oculus dexter)*
ODA	on day of admission
ODC	ornithine decarboxylase
ODN	oligodeoxynucleotide
ODS	Oswestry Disability Score
OE	on examination
	orthopedic examination
	otitis externa
O/E	on examination
O+E	observation and examination
OECI	Organization of European Cancer Institutes
OES	old english sheepdog
OF	open fracture
OFFA	Orthopaedic Foundation for Animals
Oflx	ofloxacin
OGE	U.S. Office of Government Ethics
OGTT	oral glucose tolerance test
OH	occupational history
OHCS(17-)	17-hydroxycorticosteroids
OHD	organic heart disease
OHS	open heart surgery
OHSD (17-)	17 beta-hydroxysteroid oxidoreductase
OHT	Open Health Terminology
OI	opportunistic infections
	osteogenesis imperfecta
OIA	optical immunoassay
OIB	2-oxo-3-[4-(1-oxo-2-isoindolinyl)phenyl]-butanamide
	obturator internus bursa
	ortho-iodobenzoate
	osmiophilic inclusion bodies
	osseointegrated implant bridge

OIF Osteogenesis Imperfecta Foundation
Oint ointment
OJ isoleucyl-tRNA synthetase
obstructive jaundice
orange juice
Orthodontist Judgment
overjet (type of maloclusion)
OL open label
OLMC online medical control
OLSNA Orthopaedic Laser Society of North America
OLT orthotopic liver transplantations
OM obtuse marginal artery
occupational medicine
omental (adipose tissue)
osteopathic manipulation
otitis media
OMCTS octamethylcyclotetrasiloxane
OME acute otitis media with effusion
OMS organic mental syndrome
osteomyelosclerosis
ON optic neuritis
ONC oncology
ONDCP Office of National Drug Control Policy
ONFH osteonecrosis of the femoral head
ONIHL occupational noise-induced hearing loss
OO osteoid osteoma
OOB out of bed
OOH out of hospital
OOP out of plaster
O'p-DDD mitotane
Op. operation
OP occiput posterior
opening pressure
operation
opponens pollicis
oropharynx
out patient
O/P out patient
O+P ova and parasite
OPA orthogonal projection approach
OPC oculopalatocerebral (syndrome)
outpatient clinic
OPCA olivopontocerebellar atrophy
OPCD olivopontocerebellar degeneration
OPCOS oligomenorrheic polycystic ovary syndrome
OPD obstetric prediabetic
optical path difference
otopalatodigital (syndrome)
outpatient department
outpatient dispensary
p-phetiylenediamine
OpDent operative dentistry
OPDG ocular plethysmodynamography
opg opening
OPG ocular pneumoplethysmography
orthopantomograin
osteoprotegerin
oxypolygelatin
OPH obliterative pulmonary hypertension
ophthalmia
Oph ophthalmology
ophthalmoscopy
ophthalmoscope
OPHC Office of Prepaid Health Care
OphD Doctor of Ophthalmology
Ophth ophthalmology
OPI obliteration prediction index
oculoparalytic illusion
Omnibus Personality Inventory
opiates
osteoblastic proliferation index
overproduction inhibition
OPIDN organophosphorus-induced delayed neuropathy
OPK optokinetic
OPL other party liability
outer plexiform layer
ovine placental lactogen

OPLL ossification of posterior longitudinal ligament
OPM occult primary malignancy
Office of Personnel Management
ophthalmoplegic migraine
OPN ophthalmic nurse
osteopontin
OPO Organ Procurement Organization
opp opposite
OPP opposite
osmotic pressure of plasma
oxygen partial pressure
OPPA vincristine, procarbazine, prednisone, adriamycin
OPPG oculopneumoplethysmography
OPRD opiate receptor delta
OPRK opiate receptor kappa
OPRR Office of Protection from Research Risks
OPRT orotate.. phosphoribosyltransferase
OPRTase orotate phosphoribosyltransferase
OPS operations
optical position sensor
osteoporosis-pseudolipoma syndrome
outpatient service
outpatient surgery
OPSA ovarian papillary serous adenocarcinoma
OpScan optical scanning
OPSI overwhelming postsplenectomy infection
OPSR Office of Professional Standards Review
opt best *(Lat: optimus)*
optics
optician
OPT outpatient
outpatient treatment
OPTHD optimal hemodialysis
OPU organophosphate utilization
OPV oral polio vaccine
OPV (cont.) oral poliovirus vaccine
OPWL opiate withdrawal
Or orbitale
OR (o)estrogen receptor
odds ratio
oil retention (enema)
open reduction
operating room
optic radiation
oral rehydration
orosomucoid
orthopedic
orthopedic research
open reduction
operating room
oriented
oxidoreductase
rate of outflow
O-R oxidation-reduction
ORA opiate receptor agonist
Orthopaedic Rehabilitation Association (AAOS Specialty Societies)
ORALABX oral antibiotics
ORANS Oak Ridge Analytical System
ORBC ox red blood cell
ORBD-NRC Osteoporosis and Related Bone Diseases - National Resource Center
ORC oculo-reno-cerebellar [syndrome]
Orcb orchitis
ORD optical rotatory dispersion
oral radiation death
ORDS Office of Research, Demonstration, and Statistics
ORE oil retention enema
OREF open reduction, external fixation
Orthopaedic Research and Education Foundation
ORF open reading frame
OR+F open reading frame
open reduction and fixation

org, Org organic
orif orifice
ORIF open reduction, internal fixation (sample operative report)
OrJ orange juice
ORJF open reduction jaw fracture
ORL otorhinolaryngology
ORM orosomucoid
other regulated material
oxygen ratio monitor
ORMC oxygen ratio monitor controller
Orn ornithine
ORN operating room nurse
orthopedic nurse
ORNL Oak Ridge National Laboratoiy
ORO oil red O
OROS oral osmotic
ORP operating room personnel
oxidation-reduction potential
ORPM orthorhythmic pacemaker
ORS olfactory reference syndrome
oral rehydration solution
oral surgeon
oral surgery
Orthopaedic Research Society (also: AAOS Specialty Societies)
orthopedic surgeon
orthopedic surgery
oxygen radical scavengers
ORSA osteoclast resorption stimulating activity
ORS-ROC Orthopedic Research Society, Republic of China
ORT object relations technique
operating room technician
oral rehydration therapy
operating room technician
orth, ortho orthopedics
orthopedic
Ortho orthopedics
Ortho. orthopaedic surgery
ORTHO orthopedics
ORV Orthopaedic Research of Virginia
ORW Osler-Rendu-Weber (syndrome)
ORY occludin-related gene
os opening
mouth
bone
Os occipitosacral
occupational safety
office surgery
Omenn syndrome
opening snap
operating system
oral surgery
organ specific
orthopedic surgeon
orthopedic surgery
Osgood-Schlatter [disease]
osmium
osteogenic sarcoma
osteosarcoma
osteosclerosis
oubain sensitivity
overall survival
oxygen saturation
OS bone
by mouth *(Lat: os)*
left eye *(Lat: oculus sinister)*
mouth or other opening *(Lat: os)*
oculus sinister
opening snap (heart sound)
oral surgery
osteogenic sarcoma
overall survival
ozone safe
OSA obstructive sleep apnea
Office of Services to the Aging
Optical Society of America
ovarian sectional area
OSAE Orthopaedic Special Assessment Examination (for AAOS members: Medical Education Section)
OSAS obstructive sleep apnea syndrome

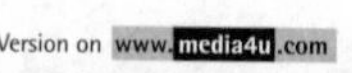

osc oscillation
OSC original sampling connections
outer subcutaneous (adipose tissue)
OSCAR on-line survey, certification and reporting system
OSCC oral squamous cell carcinoma
OSCE objective structured clinical examination
OSEM ordered subset expectation maximization
OSF organ system failure
osteoclast-stimulating factor
outer spiral fiber
overgrowth stimulating factor
OSH Act Occupational Safety and Health Act of 1970
OSHA Occupational Safety and Health Adminstration
OSI open systems interconnection [reference model]
osm osmole
osmosis
osmotic
OSM ovine submaxillary mucin
oxygen saturation meter
OSMED otospondylometaphyseal dysplasia
Osm/kg osmoles per kilogram
Osm/l osmoles per liter
osmo osmolality
osmol osmole
OSR oilseed rape
OSRD Office of Scientific Research and Development
oss osseous
OSS over-the-shoulder strap
OST object sorting test
Office of Science and Technology
osteo osteoarthritis
osteomyelitis
osteopathy
OSTOP Osteoporosis Society of British Columbia
OSUK Ophthalmological Society of the United Kingdom
OSV Orbis Sigma Valves Type I
ot. ear
Ot otolaryngology
OT objective test
oblique talus
occlusion time
occupational therapist
occupational therapy
ocular tension
office therapy
old term (in anatomy)
old tuberculin (Koch's old tuberculin) or Koch's original tuberculin
olfactory threshold
optic tract
orientation test
original tuberculin
ornithine transcarbamylase
orotracheal
orthopedic treatment
otolaryngology
otology
oxytocin
oxytryptamine
O+T operations and training
OTA occupational therapy assistant
Office of Technology Assessment
ornithine transaminase
Orthopaedic Trauma Association (Newsletter) (also: AAOS Specialty Societies)
orthotoluidine arsenite
OTC over the counter (a drug that can be obtained without a prescription)
OTM orthodontic tooth movement
os tibiale mediale
Oto otolaryngology
otology

OTRPC osm TRPC
OU both eyes, each eye *(Lat: oculus uterque)*
OV office visit
OWL Orthopaedic Web Links
OXT oxytocin
oz ounce(s)

P

p parent
pathological
$\bar{p}$ after, post
p24 viral protein specific to HIV virus
p53 a tumor suppressor gene
P after (post)
parent
periarteriolar lymphocyte sheath (about spleen)
phosphorus
plan
pressure
pulse
para
product
proline
P: plan
P2 second pulmonic heart sound
PA patient
pernicious anemia
phagocytic activity
physician assistant
polyactive
posteroanterior (x-ray)
pulmonary artery
P+A percussion and auscultation
P-A posteroanterior
PAB PBS/bovine serum albumin/azide buffer
PAC porous apatite ceramics
premature atrial contraction
PACAP Pituitary adenylate-cyclase-activating polypeptide
PaCO2 carbon dioxyde partial pressure in arterial blood
partial pressure of carbon dioxide in arterial blood
PACU post anesthesia care unit
PAD palmar adductors
peripheral arterial disease
peripheral arteriosclerotic disease
preliminary anatomic diagnosis
PADP pulmonary artery diastolic pressure
PAEDP pulmonary artery end-diastolic pressure (normal range 4-13 mmHg)
P(a-ET)CO2 arterial-end tidal PCO2 difference (should be less than 7 mmHg)
PAF paroxysmal atrial fibrillation
platelet-activating factor
PAGE polyacrylamide gel electrophoresis
PAH polycyclic aromatic hydrocarbon
PAHO Pan American Health Organization
PAI physical activity index
PAL posterior axillary line
palp. palpable
palpate
palpated
PALS pediatric advanced life support (training course)
periarteriolar lymphocyte sheath
PAM Potential Acuity Meter
PAN polyarteritis nodosa
p-ANCA perinuclear antineutrophil cytoplasmic antibodies
PAO periarticular ossification
PaO2, PAO2 alveolar oxygen
partial pressure of oxygen in arterial blood
peripheral arterial oxygen content
PAOD peripheral arterial occlusive disease
PAOP pulmonary artery occluded pressure

PAOP (cont.) pulmonary artery occlusive pressure (a.k.a.PCWP)
Pap Papanicolaou smear
PAP peroxidase antiperoxidase
prostatic acid phosphatase
pulmonary artery pressure (normal mean 9-19 mmHg)
para number of pregnancies
Para prior births
paraplegic
pares. paresthesias
PARP poly (ADP-ribose) polymerase
PARQ Parent-Adolescent Relationship Questionnaire
Parental Acceptance/Rejection Questionnaire
Physical Activity Readiness Questionnaire
physical activity recall questionnaire
PARU post anesthesia recovery unit
PAS primosome assembly site
pulmonary artery systolic pressure
PASG pneumatic anti-shock garment
PASI psoriasis area and severity index induration (scoring of erythema, scaling and involved area)
PA(S)P pulmonary artery (systolic) pressure
PAT paroxysmal atrial tachycardia
Path pathology
PAWP pulmonary artery wedge pressure
Pb lead
PB phenobarbital
peripheral blood
PBB polybrominated biphenyls (intoxication cause disorders of immune function)
PBC primary biliary cirrhosis
PBD Pick body dementia
PBI protein bound iodine
PBL primary brain lymphoma
problem-based learning
PBMC peripheral blood mononuclear cells
PBN phenyl-N-tert-butyl nitrone
pBNP porcine brain natriuretic peptide
PBO placebo
PBOSRF Palm Beach Orthopaedic and Spinal Research Foundation
PBP Penicillin-binding Protein
PBPC peripheral blood progenitor cells
PBS phosphate buffered saline
postprandial blood sugar
PBSC peripheral blood stem cell
PBT persistent bioaccumulative and toxic
pc post cenam, after meals
p/c., p.c. after meals
PC after meals
personal computer
pheochromocytoma
phone call
plasma cells
posterior cervical
present complaint
PCA patient controlled analgesia
pCai -log10 intracellular Ca2+ concentration
PCAI passive cutaneous anaphylaxis inhibition
penetrating coronary artery injury
per capita annual income
plasma cell apoptotic index
posterior cerebral artery infarction
primary chronic adrenal insufficiency
PCB polychlorinated biphenyls, toxic used in manufacture of electrical transformers
postcoital bleeding
production cell bank
PCBA printed circuit board assembled
PCC primary cell culture
PCCE pseudostratified ciliated columnar epithelium

PCD	percutaneous catheter drainage
	programmed cell death
PCF	posterior cervical fusion
PCG	pancreatico-cholangiography
	paracervical ganglion
	phonocardiogram
	preventive care group
	primate chorionic gonadotropin
	pubococcygeus
PCH	paroxysmal cold hemoglobinuria
PCI	parturition to conception interval
	percutaneous coronary intervention
PCIOL	posterior chamber intraocular lens
PCKD	all parameters rechecked
	polycystic kidney disease
PCL	posterior cruciate ligament
	primary cerebral lymphoma
	primary cutaneous lymphoma
PCLI	bone marrow plasma cell labeling index
PCN	penicillin
PCNA	proliferating cell nuclear antigen
PCNSL	primary central nervous system lymphoma
PCO	polycystic ovaries
PCO2	partial pressure of carbon dioxide
PCOD	polycystic ovarian disease
PCP	phencyclidine
	Pneumocystis carinii pneumonia
	primary care physician
PCR	polymerase chain reaction
PCT	procalcitonin
	proximal convoluted tubule
PCU	Policy Coordination Unit
PCV	packed cell volume (hematocrit)
PCW	pulmonary capillary wedge
PCWP	pulmonary capillary wedge pressure (normal range: 5 to 12 mmHg)
PD	Paget's disease
	Parkinson's disease
PD (cont.)	partial denture
	per diem
	perinatal death
	peritoneal dialysis
	Police Department
	presenile dementia (Alzheimer)
	progressive disease
	psoriatic diatheses
	pulmonary disease
	pupillary distance
2PD	two point discrimination
PD50	protective dose 50 %
PDA	patent ductus arteriosus
	posterior descending artery
PDAg	Pennsylvania Department of Agriculture
PDAT	pre-senile dementia of Alzheimer type
PDD	pervasive developmental delay
PDE	phosphodiesterase
PDGF	platelet derived growth factor
PDH	pigment-dispersing hormone
PDL	periodontal ligament
PDLLA	poly D,L-lactic acid
PDLL-D	diffuse poorly-differentiated lymphocytic lymphomas
PDLL-N	nodular poorly-differentiated lymphocytic lymphomas
PDMM	poorly differentiated malignant mesothelioma
PDMS	polydimethylsiloxane
PDN	private duty nurse
PDOH	Pennsylvania Department of Health
PDPC	poorly differentiated papillary carcinomas of papillary thyroid carcinomas
PDQ	Parkinson's disease questionnaire
	Physician's Data Query (CancerNet)
pdr.	powder
PDR	Physician's Desk Reference
	polydioxanone

PDR (cont.) poly-p-dioxanone or polydioxanone suture (commercial synthetic absorbable suture)

PDS Progressive Deterioration Scale

PDT photodynamic therapy

PDTC pyrrolidine dithiocarbamate

Pe pressure on expiration

PE Edinburgh Pharmacopoeia
Norway's electrical inspection agency
pancreatic extract
paper electrophoresis
partial epilepsy
pelvic examination
penile erection
pericardial effusion
peritoneal exudate
personal edition
pharyngoesophageal
phase encoded
phenylephrine
phenylethylamine
phenytoin equivalent
phosphatidylethanolamine
photographic effect
phycoerythrin (fluorescent dye used in flow cytometry)
physical education
physical engineering
physical examination
physical exercise
physician extender
physiological ecology
pigmented epithelium
pilocarpine epinephrine
placental extract
plant engineering
plasma exchange
plating efficiencies
platinum etoposide
pleural effusion

PE (cont.) point of entry
polyethylene
post-exponential growth
potential energy
powdered extract
preeclampsia
preexcitation
present evaluation
pressure equalization
presumptive eligibility
prior to exposure
probable error
professional engineer
program evaluation
proportional error
pseudoexfoliation
Pseudomonas exotoxin
pulmonary edema
pulmonary embolism
pulmonary embolus
pyrogenic exotoxin

PEA pelvic examination under anesthesia
phenylethyl alcohol
phenylethylamine
polysaccharide egg antigen
pulseless electrical activity (cardiac)

PEAC Pharmaceutical Education Advisory Committee

PEAP positive end airway pressure

PEAR phase encoded artifact reduction

PEARL Personnel Expertise and Resource Listing
pupils equal and reactive to light

PEB cisplatin, etoposide and bleomycin

PEC peritoneal exudate cells
Petri Enteropathogen Count (plate)

PECAM-1 platelet endothelial cell adhesion molecule (CD-31)

peds pediatrics

Ped., Peds Pediatrics

PEEK polyetheretherketone

PEEP positive end-expiratory pressure
PEF peak expiratory flow
PEFR peak expiratory flow rate
PEG percutaneous endoscopic gastrostomy
pneumoencephalogram
PEG-PE poly(ethylene glycol)-modified phosphatidylethanolamine
PEI percutaneous ethanol injection
PEL permissible exposure limit
primary effusion lymphoma
PEM protein-energy malnutrition
PEN parenteral nutrition
penicillin
PEP phosphoenol-pyruvate
postexposure prophylaxis
primer-extension preamplification
PEP A peptidase A isozyme
PEP B peptidase B isozyme
PEP C peptidase C isozyme
PEP D peptidase D isozyme
PEPEC pig enteropathogenic E.coli
PEP/ET preejection to ejection time
pep M24 pepsin extract of type-24 M protein
PEPP Payment Error Prevention Program
PEP S peptidase S isozyme
per by
PerCP peridinin chlorophyll A protein (fluorescent dye used in flow cytometry)
Peri around or about (e.g. perirenal = around the kidney)
perineal
PERLA pupils equal, reactive to light + accommodation
per/os by mouth
PER OS by mouth
PERRL pupils equally round and reactive to light
PERRLA pupils equally round and reactive to light and accommodation
PES prenatal environmental stress
PET positron emission tomography
psychosocially enhanced treatment program
PETE polytetrafluoroethylene
pev peak electron volts
PEV peak expiratory velocity
potentiel évoqué visuel (french)
PE tube pressure equalization tube
PF Purkinje fibers
push fluids
PF4 platelet factor 4
PFC persistent fetal circulation
PFCx prefrontal cortex
PFFD proximal femoral focal deficiency (virtual support group)
PFJ patellofemoral joint
PFO patent foramen ovale
PFOLA Prescription Foot Orthotic Laboratory Association
PFPS patellofemoral pain syndrom
PFS progression free survival
PFT pulmonary function tests
pg picogram - 0.000000000001 gram
PG phosphate yeast glucose (a broth used in microbiology)
prostaglandin
proteoglycan
pseudogout (chondrocalcinosis)
PGA polyglycolic acid
PGC pregastricin
primordial germ cell
PGD2 endoperoxide-D-isomerase
6-PGD 6-phosphogluconate dehydrogenase
PGD,6- 6-phosphogluconate dehydrogenase
PGE prostaglandin E
PGE1 Prostaglandin E1
PGE2 endoperoxide-E-isomerase
PG(E) Prostaglandin (E)
PGF paternal grandfather
PGF2 endoperoxide-F-isomerase

PGH	pituitary growth hormone
PGI2	prostacyclin
PGL	persistent generalized lymphadenopathy
PGM	paternal grandmother
Pgp	P-glycoprotein
PGP	progressive general paralysis
PGR	progesterone receptor
pH	hydrogen-ion concentration - acid / alkaline
Ph1	Philadelphia chromosome
PH	past history
	plasmactytic hyperplasia
	pulmonary HTN (pulmonary hypertension)
PHA	phytohemagglutinin
pharm	pharmacy
PhD	Doctor in Philosophy
Phe	phenylalanine
PHI	peptide histidine isoleucine
PHM	peptide histidine methionine
pHn	nutrient pH
	pH values measured by NMR
	phenacetin
	photoreceptors
Phn	phenazinium
PhN	pharyngeal branch of the vagus nerve
	phenylnitrene
	phrenic nerve
PHn	pleckstrin homology
PHN	(phenyl)hydroxy-naftopidil
	headphone
	papillary Hurthle cell neoplasms
	paraventricular hypothalamic nucleus
	passive Heymann nephritis
	pelvic hematoma necessitans
	perihypoglossal nucleus
	periventricularis hypothalami
	phenanthrene
	phentolamine
PHN (cont.)	phenylephrine
	phenylisothiocyanate
	p-hydroxynefazodone
	p-hydroxynorephedrine
	poly-3-hydroxynonanoate
	portal hypertension
	post-herpetic neuralgia
	preferred Health Network
	Public Health Nursing
	Public Health Nutrition
	pulmonary hypertension
PHNs	public health nurses
Photo DSC	photo differential scanning calorimeter
PHPT	primary hyperparathyroidism
PHPV	poly-3-hydroxy-5-phenylvalerate
PHS	periarthropatia homero scapularis (periarthritis humeroscapularis)
	phenytoin hypersensitivity syndrome
PHSC	pluripotential hematopoietic stem cell
PHTLS	prehospital trauma life support
PHX	past history
phy	phytane isoprenoid
PHYS.	physical
	physiology
PHYSO	physostigmine
Pi	inorganic orthophosphate
PI	permanently implantable
	personal injury
	positive indices
	present illness
	protease inhibitor
	pulmonic insufficiency (disease)
PIA	performance incentive award
	posterior interosseous artery
PIB	para-iodobenzoate
PIBIDS	Syndrome: photosensitivity, ichthyosis, brittle hair, impaired intelligence, decreased fertility
PIC	peripherally inserted catheter

PIC (cont.) products of incomplete combustion
PICA postero-inferior cerebellar artery
PICC peripherally inserted central catheter
PICU pediatric intensive care unit
pulmonary intensive care unit
PiD Pick's disease
PID pelvic inflammatory disease (CDC documentation)
prolapsed intervertebral disc
PIE Practical Incidence Estimators
Problem-Intervention-Evaluation (system)
pulmonary infiltration with eosinophilia
PIG-A phosphatidylinositol glycan-class A (gene)
phosphatidylinositolglycan A
PIH pregnancy-induced hypertension
pyridoxal isonicotinoyl hydrazone
PIL peripheral intravenous line
PIM pre-installation maintenance
PIN posterior interosseous nerve
PIP proximal interpalangeal
proximal interphalangeal joint
PIP2 phosphatidylinositol-4,5-biphosphate
PIPC piperacillin
PIPJ proximal interphalangeal joint
Pit. Pitocin
PIV peripheral intravenous (line)
PJC premature junctional contraction
PK pain killer
PKD polycystic kidney disease
PKU phenylketonuria
PL posterolateral
PLA phospholipases
polylactic acid
Plac. placenta
PLAP placental alkaline phosphatase
PLC Pariboy Pari LC+ jet nebulizers
PLF posterior lumbar fusion
PLGA polylactic/glycolic acid
PLIF posterolateral interbody fusion
PLL prolymphocytic leukemia
Plm plasmepsin
PLm plantar muscles
PLM peplomycin
periodic leg/limb movements
permeation liquid membrane
phospholemman or phospholipomannan
polarized light microscopy
Population, Labour Force and Migration (Pakistan)
PLND pelvic lymph node dissection
PLNs peripheral lymph nodes
PLO-SL polycystic lipomembranous osteodysplasia with sclerosing leukoencephalopathy (Nasu-Hakola syndrome)
PLR pupillary light reflex
plt paucity of lymph node T cell mutation
PLT platelet(s)
post-liver transplantation
primary lymphoplasmacytic lymphoma
primed lymphocyte tests
psittacosis-lymphogranuloma-trachoma group viruses
plts. platelets
pm afternoon
PM paramedic (for Paramedic licensure level)
petit mal
polymyositis
postmenopausal
post meridian (afternoon)
postmitotic cells
postmortem
post-nasal
P.M. afternoon
post-mortem

PMA Pharmaceutical Manufacturers Association
positive mental attitude
progressive muscular atrophy
PMB postmenopausal bleeding
PMBL primary mediastinal B-cell lymphoma
PMD private medical doctor
PMDD premenstrual dysphoric disorder
PMH past medical history
pMI mitotic index of proliferating cell population
previous myocardial infarction
PMI maxillary primary incisors
pacemaker implantation
pain management index
Pain Management Inventory
painless myocardial infarction
panoramic mandibular index
past medical illness
paternal meiosis I
perioperative myocardial infarction
phosphomannose isomerase
placental membrane inflammation
plasma membrane integrity
point of maximum impact
pollen mitosis one
posterior myocardial infarctions
postmortem interval
power motion imaging
Pressure Management Indicator
Prevention Marketing Initiative
prolonged mechanical inspiration
prostate malignancy index
psoas minor muscle
PMII paternal meiosis II
PMK primary monkey kidney
PML promyelocytic leukemia and its gene on chromosome 15 (previously named myl)
promyelocytic leukemia protein
PMMA polymethylmethacrylate
PMN polymorphonuclear leukocyte
PMP previous menstrual period
PMP22 Peripheral myelin protein 22
PM+R Physical Medicine and Rehabilitation
PMR physical medicine and rehabilitation
polymyalgia rheumatica
protonic magnetic resonance (analysis)
psychomotor retardation
PMS premenstrual syndrome
premenstrual tension syndrome (late luteal phase dysphoric disorder)
Profile of Mood States
Pn Pneumonia
PN pain
pneumonia
poorly nourished
practical nurse
P+N psychiatry and neurology
PNA protein equivalent of total nitrogen appearance
PNC postnecrotic liver cirrhosis
prenatal care
PND paroxysmal nocturnal dyspnea
post nasal drip
postnatal day
PNES psychogenic nonepileptic seizures
PNET primitive neuroectodermal tumor
pneu. pneumo
pneumonia
PNF proprioceptive neuromuscular facilitation
PNH paroxysmal nocturnal hemoglobinuria
PNI peripheral nerve injury
PNMT phenylethanolamine-N-methyl-transferase
PNP pooled normal plasma
PNS peripheral nervous system

PNS (cont.) Porta-Neb Sidestream jet nebulizers
Pnv neck vein pressure
PNV neomycin sulfate and vancomycin hydrochloride
phenoxymethylpenicillin
phoneutria nigriventer spider venom
polymyxin B sulfate
Porta-Neb Ventstream jet nebulizers
postchemotherapy nausea and vomiting
postinfusion nausea and vomiting
postoperative nausea and vomiting
practical normal value
predictive negative value
prenatal vitamins
protein nutritional value
PNX pneumothorax
p.o., po by mouth
PO by mouth *(Lat: per os)*
orally
per os
postoperative
postovulatory
P/O patient in office
PO2 pressure of oxygen
partial pressure of oxygen
Poa p IX Poa pratensis group IX allergen
POC point-of-care
postoperative care
product of conception
p.o.d. postoperative day
POD postoperative day
postovulatory day
POEMS Syndrome: polyneuropathy, organomegaly, endocrinopathy, monoclonal gammopathy, and skin lesions
POG Pediatric Oncology Group (USA)
poly prefix for multiple
poly(P) polyphosphate
polys polymorphonuclear cells
polymorphonuclear leukocytes
POME persistent otitis media effusion
POMR problem oriented medical record
PONF Paediatric Oncology Nurses Forum (UK)
Pop popliteus tendon
POP pain on palpation
plaster of Paris
poplit. popliteal
pos positive
POS Piedmont Orthopaedic Society
POSI Paediatric Orthopaedic Society of India
POSNA Pediatric Orthopaedic Society of North America (AAOS Specialty Societies)
poss. possible
post, post. posterior
postop postoperative
post op postoperative
post-op post-operative(ly)
POSTOP postoperative
PO sus rel PO (by mouth) sustained release
POTS postural orthostatic tachycardia syndrome
POV privately owned vehicle
POX point of exit
pulse oximetry
pp postpartum
postprandial
PP per protocol
Peyer's patches
phosphoprotein phosphatase
positive pressure
presenting problem
private physician
pulsus paradoxus
PP+A palpation, percussion and auscultation
PPA primary progressive aphasia

PPAR-alpha peroxisome proliferator activated receptor-alpha
PPAR-gamma peroxisome proliferator activated receptor-gamma
PPBS post prandial blood sugar
PPD packs per day
permanent partial disability
purified protein derivative (of tuberculin)
P+PD percussion and postural drainage
PPE personal protective equipment
PPF protein plasma fractional
PPG peristomal pyoderma gangrenosum
portosystemic pressure gradient
PPH past pertinent history
post-partum hemorrhage
primary pulmonary hypertension
PPHN persistent pulmonary hypertension of the newborn
PPK polyphosphate kinase
PPLO pleuropneumonia-like organisms
ppm parts per million
PPMC physician practice management companies
PPMS primary progressive multiple sclerosis
PPN peripheral parenteral nutrition
PPND pallido-ponto-nigral degeneration
PPP peripheral pulses present
pregnancy-prevention program
PPPE persistent pigmented purpuric eruption
PPPG post prandial plasma glucose
PPRI periparturient relaxation of immunity
pps phosphoenolpyruvate synthase gene
PPs peroxisome proliferators
Peyer's patches
phosphoprotein phosphatases
PPS pachyman polysaccharides
pelvic pain syndrome
PPS (cont.) pentosan polysulfate
peripheral pulmonary stenosis
Personal Preference Scale
physician, patient and society
plasminogen-plasmin system
polyvalent pneumococcal polysaccharide
poor progesterone surge (cycles)
popliteal pterygium syndrome
postpartum psychiatric syndromes
postpartum sterilization
postperfusion syndrome
postpericardiotomy syndrome
post-polio syndrome
postpump syndrome
potentiating paired stimulation
prenatal psychological stress
preputial separation
primary acquired preleukemic syndrome
professional practice standards
prospective payment system
prospective pricing system
protein plasma substitute
pulse per second
PPSH pseudovaginal perineoscrotal hypopospadias
PPS/PCO pelvic pain syndrome/polycystic ovaries
P-PST-1 phenol-sulfating form of sulfotransferases
ppt part per trillion
PPT Physical Performance Test
plasma pregnancy test
postpartum thyroiditis
PPT-B Preprotachykinin B
PPTL postpartum tubal ligation
PPV positive predicitive value
positive pressure ventilation device
p.r. per rectum
PR partial response / partial remission
perirenal (adipose tissue)

PR (cont.)	per rectum *(Lat)*
	proctology
	progress record
	pulse rate
PR3	proteinase 3
PRA	plasma/peripheral renin activity
PRAMS	Pregnancy Risk Assessment Monitoring System
PRAS	prereduced anaerobically sterilized (media)
pRb	product of Rb (retinblastoma) gene
PRBC	packed red blood cells
PR(B)C	packed red (blood) cells
PRb-P	phosphorylated (inactivated) product of Rb (retinblastoma) gene
PRC	packed red blood cells
	pregnancy risk category
	proximal row carpectomy
PRCA	pure red cell aplasia
PRE	progressive resistance exercises
preop	preoperative
pre op	preoperative
pre-op	pre-operative(ly)
prep	preparation
	prepare as
prep.	prepare for
pri	pristane isoprenoid
Pri	isopropanol
	primary
PRI	PACAP receptor I
	pain rating index
	pain rating intensity score
	patient review instrument
	Pediatric Risk Index
	performance rating instrument
	perinatal respiratory insufficiency
	Pharyngeal Retention Index
	phenol red impurity
	phosphate reabsorption index
	phosphoribose isomerase
	phosrestin I
PRI (cont.)	photochemical reflectance index
	placental ribonuclease inhibitor
	placental RNase inhibitor
	platelet reactivity index
	point respiratory inversion
	post recurrence induction
	postpartum resumption interval
	post-radiosurgical imaging
	post-remission intensification
	power ratio index
	preinoculation
	premarital residential independence
	pre-response interval
	preservation-reperfusion injury
	pressure relief index
	primates
	primidone
	prinedil
	Pristinamycin
	ProFile Ni-Ti rotary instruments
	progressive renal insufficiency
	proliferation rate index
	protease inhibitors
	protein intake
	proximal promoter region I
	Psychopathy Resemblance Index
	root-inducing plasmids
PRI-100	Personal Reaction Inventory
PRIAS	Packard Radioimmunoassay System
PRICE	protection, relative rest, ice, compression, elevation
PRICEMM	protection, relative rest, ice, compression, elevation, modalities, medication
PRICES	physician modalities, rehabilitation, injections, cross training, evaluation, salicylates
	protection, rest, ice, compression, elevation, support
PRIDE	Parents Resource Institute for Drug Education

OP

PRIH prolactin release inhibiting hormone
PRII proximal promoter region II
PRIM+R Public Responsibility in Medicine & Research
PRIM primase
PRIME plankton reactivity in the marine environment
PRIME-MD Primary Care Evaluation of Mental Disorders
PRIMEX primary care extender
primip. primipara
first pregnancy
Primip primipara
primiparity
PRIMOS prime operating system
PRINCE projects in controlled environments (UK)
PRIND prolonged reversible ischemic neurologic deficit
PRION proteinaceous infectious particle
PRIS pain rating intensity score
PRISM The Paediatric Risk of Mortality (score)
PRIST paper radioimmunosorbent test
Prl prolactin
p.r.m. according to circumstances
p.r.n. pro re nata - as required, as needed
prn, PRN pro re nata - as required, as needed
Pro proline
PRO prophylaxis
prod. productive
Prog. prognosis
PROM passive range of motion
premature rupture of membranes
ProMACE-CytaBOM prednisone, methotrexate, doxorubicin, cetoposidey-clophosphamide, cytarabine, bleomycin, vincristine, methotrexate
pron. pronator
pronation
pros. prostate
prostatic
prosth. prosthesis
prot protocol
prot. protein
protestant
pro. time prothrombin time
Pro time prothrombin time
PrP prion protein
PRP penicillase-resistant penicillin
pityriasis rubra pilaris
PRRE pupils round, regular and equal
Prss14 protease, serine, 14, a gene
PRT patient refused test
PRUJ proximal radioulnar joint
PRUL proximal radioulnar ligament
PS parasegment
paraspinous
pathologic stage
physical status
plastic surgery
present symptoms
psychotic
pulmonary stenosis
P+S permanent and stationary
PSA polysubstance abuse
prostate-specific antigen
PSC primary sclerosing cholangitis
PSCR peripheral stem cell rescue
PSCT peripheral stem cell transplant
PSD passive sampling devices
PSEF Plastic Surgery Educational Foundation
P-selectin (GMP140) adhesion molecule on endothelial cells and platelets
PSF peak scatter factor
posterior spinal fusion
post-sophomore fellow
PSG polysomnography
progressive subcortical gliosis
PSGN post streptococcal glomerulonephritis

PSH past surgical history
psi pounds per square inch
PSIS posterior superior iliac spine
PSMA progressive spinal muscular atrophy
PSP phenylsulfonphthalein test
posterior spinous process
PSS Perceived Stress Scale
progressive systemic sclerosis
PSSV pre-study site visit
pST porcine somatotropin
Pst phosphate-specific transporter
PST palmar skin temperature
paroxysmal supraventricular tachycardia
problem-solving therapy
proximal straight tubule
proximal straight tubules
pulse separation time
PSTH poststimulus time histograms
PSTT placental site trophoblastic tumor
PSUR periodic safety update report
PSV peak systolic velocity
PSVT paroxysmal supraventricular tachycardia
Psych. psychiatry
PsyD Doctor in Psychiatry
pt. patient, pint
PT paroxysmal tachycardia
patient
permanent and total
physical therapy
pneumothorax
prothrombin time
P.T. physical therapy
posterior tibial artery pulse
PTA percutaneous transluminal angioplasty
prior to admission (medication)
phosphotungstic acid
prior to admission/arrival
PTAH phosphotungstic acid hematoxylin
PTB patellar tendon bearing
PTC percutaneous transhepatic cholangiography
PTCA percutaneous transluminal coronary angioplasty
PTD permanent total disability
PTE pulmonary thromboembolism
PTEN phosphate and tensin homolog (gene on 10q23)
PTFE polytetrafluoroethylene
PTGC progressively transformed germinal centers
PTH, Pth parathyroid hormone
phenylthiohydantoin
PTHc C-terminal parathyroid hormone
PTHC percutaneous transhepatic cholangiography
posttransfusion hepatitis C
PTHrP parathyroid hormone-related peptide
PTK protein tyrosine kinases
PTL preterm labor
PTLD post-transplant lymphoproliferative disorder
PTM pretibial myxedema
PTMC percutaneous transvenous mitral commissurotomy
PTMR percutaneous transmyocardial revascularization
PTO portal triad occlusion
PTOA post-traumatic osteoarthritis
PTP Professional Team Physicians
PTR patellar tendon reflex
PTS phosphotransferase system
PTSD Post-Traumatic Stress Disorder (National Center for PTSD)
PTT partial thromboplastin time
PTU propylthiourcil (antithyroid drug)
PTW play-the-winner
PTX pneumothorax
PTZ pentylenetetrazol
PU passed urine
peptic ulcer

O P

PU (cont.)	polyurethane
	pregnancy urine
PUCP	maximum urethral closure pressure
PUD	peptic ulcer disease
	peri-urethral diathermy (associated with superficial bladder cancer)
	pulmonary disease
PUFA	polyunsaturated fatty acids
pulv	powder
Pulv	pulvinar
PuLv	ventral part of the lateral pulvinar
Pulv-LP	pulvinar-posterior-lateral complex
PuM	medial pulvinar
PUO	pyrexia of unknown origin
PUPPP	pruritic urticarial papules and plaques of pregnancy
PV	examination per vaginam
	paravertebral
	peripheral vascular
	pemphigus vulgaris
	plasma volume
	polycythemia vera
	portal vein
PVA	polyvinyl alcohol fixative
PVASI	pelvic vascular injury
PVB	paravertebral block
	premature ventricular beat
PVB19	parvovirus B19
PV bleed	per vagina bleed
PVC	premature ventricular contraction
	pulmonary venous congestion
PVD	peripheral vascular disease
	pre-senile vascular dementia
PVN	paraventricular nuclei
PVNS	pigmented villonodular synovitis
PvO2	mixed venous oxygen tension
PVR	peripheral vascular resistance
	post-void residual
	pulmonary vascular resistance
	pulse volume recorder
PVST	paraventriculospinal tract
PVST (cont.)	paroxysmal supraventricular tachycardia
pvt-1	plasmacytoma variant translocation-1 gene (on chromosome 15)
PVT	paroxysmal ventricular tachycardia
	periprostatic vein thrombosis
	polymorphic ventricular tachycardia
	popliteal vein transplant
	portal vein thrombosis
PWB	partial weight bearing
P,W+D	pink, warm and dry
PWP	pulmonary wedge pressure
PWS	Prader-Willi syndrome
Px	physical examination
PX	papular xanthoma
	physical examination
	pinealectomy
	prescription
	prognosis
PXE	pseudoxanthoma elasticum
py	pack years (of cigarettes)
PZI	protamine zinc insulin - a long acting insulin

Q

q	*(Lat: quaque)* - every, each
Q	glutamine
QA	quality assurance
QALY	quality-adjusted life year
qam	every morning
QAM	every morning
QA/QC	quality assurance/quality control
QAR	quantitative autoradiography
QC	quality control
QCA	quantitative coronary angiography
QCT	quantitative computed tomography

qd once a day, every day *(Lat: quaque in die)*
q.d. once a day, every day *(Lat: quaque in die)*
qh every hour
q.h. every hour
QD every day
q2h, q2H every two hours
Q2H every two hours
q4h, q4H every four hours
Q6H every six hours
QH every hour
qhs every night at bedtime
qid four times a day
q.i.d. four times a day
QID four times a day
q.i.w. four times a week
ql, q.l. as much as pleased *(Lat: quantum libet)*
qm every morning
QM every morning
QMI Q-wave myocardial infarction
QMT quantitative muscle testing
qn, q.n. every night *(Lat: quaque nox)*
QN every night *(Lat: quaque nox)*
qns, q.n.s. quantity not sufficient
QNS quantity not sufficient
qod every other day
q.o.d. every other day
QOD every other day
QOH every other hour
QoL quality of life
q.o.n. every other night
QON every other night
QP as much as desired
at will
qpm every afternoon
QPM every afternoon
q.q., QQ each
every
qqh, q.q.h. every four hours *(Lat: quaque quarta hora)*
q.s., qs quantity sufficient
QS as much as will suffice *(Lat: quantum sufficit)*
quantity sufficient *(Lat: quantum satis)*
sufficient quantity
QS21 saponin purified from Quillaja saponaria used as immunoadjuvant
Qs/Qt shunt fraction
qt. quart
QT quantity
quart
quiet
total cardiac output
quad. quadriplegic
quant. quantitative
quantity
qv, q.v. as much as desired
as much as you like *(Lat: quantum vis)*
QV as much as desired
as much as you like *(Lat: quantum vis)*
q.w. every week

R

r. rectal
right
roentgen
x-ray
R arginine
rectal
residual tumor after treatment
resistance
respiration (also resp)
right
roentgen
x-ray
R. rub

R. (cont.)	rectal temperature
Ra	radium
RA	refractory anemia rheumatoid arthritis right atrium room air
RAAP	right atrial appendage pacing
RACS	Royal Australasian College of Surgeons
rad	radiation absorbed dose radiotherapy
rad.	radial
RAD	reactive airway disease right axis deviation
RAE	right atrial enlargement
RAEB	refractory anemia with excess blasts
RAF	rapid atrial fibrillation Royal Air Force
RAG-1/2	recombinase-activating gene 1/2
RAI	radioactive iodine uptake
RAIU	radioactive iodine uptake
r.a.m.	rapid alternating movements
RAO	recurrent aortic occlusions right anterior oblique
RAO2 sat	room-air oxygen saturation
RAP	resident assessment protocol right atrial pressure
RAPD	relative afferent pupillary defect
RAR-α	retinoic acid receptor-alpha (gene on chromosome 17)
RAS	renin-angiotensin system
R.A.S.	right arm sitting
RAST	serum radioallergosorbent test (test for milk sensitivity)
RATx	radiation therapy
Rb	retinoblastoma gene (located on chromosome 13q14)
RBBB	right bundle branch block
rbc	red blood cell red blood count
RBC	red blood cells/count
RBD	REM behavioral disorders
RBE	relative biological effects
RBF	renal blood flow
RBILD	respiratory bronchiolitis interstitial lung disease
RBP	retinol-binding protein
RBS	red blood cell
RBWC	randomly bred White Carneau pigeons
RCA	right coronary artery
RCA1	Ricinus communis agglutinin
rCBF	regional cerebral blood flow
RCI	respiratory control index
RCJ	radiocarpal joint
RCM	right costal margin
RCMD	refractory cytopenia with multilineage dysplasia
RCMI	red blood cell morphologic index
RCP	Royal College of Physicians
RCPSC	Royal College of Physicians and Surgeons of Canada
RCR	respiratory control ratio
RCS	reticulum cell sarcoma
RCSED	Royal College of Surgeons of Edinburgh
RCSENG	Royal College of Surgeons of England
RCSI	Royal College of Surgeons in Ireland
RCT	randomized controlled trial
RCU	respiratory care unit
RCX	right circumflex
R.D.	registered dietician
RD	respiratory disease respiratory distress reaction to degeneration
RDA	recommended dietary allowance
RDI	recommended daily intake respiratory disturbance index # of apneas/hypopneas per hour of sleep (aka, AHI, apnea/hypopnea index)

RDP3 respiratory-dependent pacemakers
RDS respiratory distress syndrome
RDW red cell distribution width
re: regarding
RE reconditioning exercise
right eye
REAL Revised European American Classification
REB squats with rebound
rect. rectum
rectal(ly)
rectus muscle
REEs rare earth elements
reg, reg. regular
Reg regular(ly)
Reg. registrar
rehab. rehabilitation
REL release
REM rapid eye movement
REP repair
repeat
REPS repetitions
REQ required
RER replication error (phenotype)
RES reticuloendothelial system
RESNA Rehabilitation Engineering and Assistive Technology Society of North American
resp respiration
Resp respiration, respiratory
REV Reticuloendotheliosis virus
RF renal failure
rheumatic fever
rheumatic factor
rheumatoid factor
risk factor
RFA radiofrequency ablation
RFA ratio of fat area
right frontoanterior
RFFIT rapid fluorescent focus inhibition test
RFI renal failure index: UNa/(UCr/PCr)
RFLP restriction-fragment length polymorphism
RFP right frontoposterior
RFS relapse free survival
RFT right frontotransverse
RGD arginine-glycine-asparagine (aminoacid sequence responsible for cell-binding properties of fibronectin, vitronectin, fibrinogen, laminin, collagen)
r/g/m rubs, gallops, murmurs
RGO reciprocating gait orthosis
RH, Rh, Rh. Rhesus (monkey) factor
RH relative humidity
Reproductive Health
RHA right hepatic artery
rhBMP-2 recombinant human bone morphogenetic protein
RHD renal hypertensive disease
rheumatic heart disease
RHF right heart failure
RHIA registered health information administrator
RHIT registered health information technician
Rh neg. Rhesus factor negative
Rh- Rhesus factor negative
Rh pos. Rhesus factor positive
Rh+ Rhesus factor positive
RHT right hypertrophia
RI relative fluorescence index
resistive index
reticulocyte index = (%reticulocyte x pt Hct)/45 x (1/shift correction factor); (shift correction factor = 1.5 for Hct 35%; 2 for Hct 25%; 2.5 for Hct 15%); if RI <2% = hypoproliferative anemia, if RI 2% = excessive destruction or loss
RIA radioimmunoassay
Rib riboflavin
ribose

RICE rest, ice, compression, and elevation
RIF lymphocyte E-rosette inhibitory factors
RIH right inguinal hernia
RII radioimmunoimaging
RIND reversible ischemic neurologic deficit
RIP radioimmunoprecipitation
rapid information processing
rat insulin promoter
receptor-interacting protein
reflex inhibiting pattern
regulated intramembrane proteolysis
repeat-induced point mutation
replication initiation point
respiratory inductance plethysmography
rest in peace
ribosome-inactivating protein
RNA III-inhibiting peptide
RIP-mOVA membrane ovalbumin under the control of the rat insulin promoter
RIS Risperidone
RJOS Ruth Jackson Orthopaedic Society (also: AAOS Specialty Societies)
RK rabbit kidney
RL right lateral
right leg
right lung
Ringer's lactate
RIa laryngeal resistance
RLA Rancho Los Amigo Scale
Resident Legal Advisor
RLD reference lumen diameter
RLE rabbit limbal epithelial
rabbit liver esterase
rat liver epithelial cells
rat lung epithelial cells
right lower extremity
RLF retrolental fibroplasia
RLFP remaining lifetime fracture probability
RLL right lower lobe (lung)
RLQ right lower quadrant (abdomen)
RLS restless legs syndrome
RLS-PLM restless legs-periodic leg movements during sleep
RM routine maintenance
RMA refuse/s medical assistance
right mentoanterior
RML right middle lobe (lung)
right mediolateral
RMP right mentoposterior
RMR resting metabolic rate
RMS root mean square
RMSF Rocky Mountain spotted fever
RMT right mentotransverse
RN registered nurse
RNA ribonucleic acid
RNVG radionuclide ventriculography
RO rule out
R/O rule out
ROA right occiput anterior
ROC receiver operating curve analysis
ROD removal of drain
ROI region of interest
ROM range of motion (of joint)
right otitis media
rupture of membranes
ROMI Rating of Medication Influences scale (psychiatry)
rule-out myocardial infarction
ROP retinopathy of prematurity
right occiput posterior
ROS reactive oxygen species
removal of sutures
review of symptoms
review of systems
ROT right occiput transverse
rule of thumb
RP red pulp
retrograde pyelogram

rPA reteplase
RPA recursive partitioning analysis
RPD ERP dispersion
RPE retinal pigment epithelium
RPF renal plasma flow
RPG retrograde pyelogram
RPGN rapidly progressive glomerulonephritis
RPH retroperitoneal hematoma
RPI reticulocyte production index
RPP rate pressure product
rpr rapid plasma reagin
RPR rapid plasma reagin
R.P.R. rapid plasma reagin
RPT register physical therapy
RQ respiratory quotient
RR relative risk
respiratory rate
risk ratio
R.R. recovery room
R2R Reach to Recovery ACS program
RRE, RR+E round, regular, and equal
RRF residual renal function
RRMS relapsing remitting multiple sclerosis
RROM resistive range of motion
RROSR RoundupReady* oilseed rape
rrp genes encoding response regulators
rRP recombinant ribosomal P
Rrp receptor related protein
RRp ribosome receptor protein
RRP radiation-related pericardial effusion
radical retropubic prostatectomy
rapid repeat pregnancy
rate responsive pacing/pacemakers
raw rock phosphat
readily releasable pool (of vesicles)
recurrent rectal prolapse
recurrent respiratory papillomatosis
reduced renal perfusion pressure
Refugee Resettlement Program

RRP (cont.) regA-regulated protein
relative refractory period
relative rest period
relatively resistant to penicillin (Neisseria meningitidis strains)
relaxed resting posture
re-replacements
respiratory-related power (spectrum)
resting rectal pressure
restraint reduction program
retrograde refractory period
reverse redistribution pattern
reversible radical pair model
rhomboid-related protein
rivalry-related potential
RRPs reaction related potentials
RNA-dependent RNA polymerases
RRR regular rate and rhythm
Rrs respiratory resistance
RRs response regulators
RRT random response technique
Registered Respiratory Therapist
relative retention time
RRU respiratory resistance unit
RRV-TV rhesus rotavirus vaccine-tetravalent
Rs Rauwolfia serpentina
systemic resistance
R/s roentgens per second
RS radioscaphoid
random sample
rating schedule
Raynaud syndrome
recipient's serum
reclassification sensitivity
rectal sinus
rectal suppository
rectosigmoid
reducing substance
Reed-Sternberg cells characteristic for Hodgkin's disease

RS (cont.) reinforcing stimulus
Reiter syndrome
relative stimulus
renal specialist
respiratory syncytial (virus)
response to stimulus
resting subject
reticulated siderocyte
retinoschisis
Rett syndrome
review of symptoms
Reye syndrome
Richter's syndrome (transformation of CLL in DLCL)
right sacrum
right septum
right side
right stellate (ganglion)
Ringer solution
Roberts syndrome
Rous sarcoma

Rsa systemic arterial resistance

RSA rabbit serum albumin
regular spiking activity
relative specific activity
relative standard accuracy
reticulum cell sarcoma
right sacroanterior (fetal position)
right subclavian artery
roentgenographic stereogrammetric analysis

RSB Rapid Shallow Breathing Index
rectal suction biopsy
recurrent sinus barotrauma
reticulocyte standard buffer
retinal Schiff base
right sternal border
roasted soybeans

RSC rat spleen cell
rested state contraction
reversible sickle-cell
right subclavian

RScA right scapuloanterior (fetal position)

RSCN Registered Sick Children's Nurse

RScP right scapuloposterior (fetal position)

RSD reflex sympathetic dystrophy
relative standard deviation (Srel)

RSDS reflex sympathetic dystrophy syndrome

RSE rapid spin-echo

RSEP right somatosensory evoked potential

RSES Rosenberg Self-Esteem Scale

RSH Royal Society of Health

RSI rapid sequence induction
rapid sequence intubation
repetition strain injury

RSIC Radiation Shielding Information Center

R-SIRS Revised Seriousness of Illness Rating Scale

RSJVP rapid-sequence intravenous pyelography

RSL radioscapholunate ligament
right sacrolateral (fetal position)

RSLD repair of sublethal damage

RSM restriction site mutation
risk screening model
Royal Society of Medicine

RSMR relative standard mortality rate

RSN restin
right substantia nigra

RSNA Radiological Society of North America

rSO2 regional oxygen saturation

RSO radiation safety officer
Resident Surgical Officer
right salpingo-oophorectomy
right superior oblique (muscle)

RSP removable silicone plug
ribose-5-phosphatase
right sacroposterior (fetal position)

RSPCA Royal Society for the Prevention of Cruelty to Animals
RS3PE remitting seronegative symmetrical synovitis with pitting edema
RSPH Royal Society for the Promotion of Health
RSPK recurrent spontaneous psychokinesis
rSr an electrocardiographic complex
RSR regular sinus rhythm
relative survival rate
right superior rectus (muscle)
RSS rat stomach strip
rectosigmoidoscopy
Russell-Silver syndrome
RSSE Russian spring-sununer encephalitis
RSSR relative slow sinus rate
RST radiosensitivity test
reagin screen test
right sacrotransverse (fetal position)
rubrospinal tract
RSTI Radiological Service Training Institute
RSTL relaxed skin tension lines
RSTMH Royal Society of Tropical Medicine and Hygiene
RSTS retropharyngeal soft tissue space
RSU radiological sciences unit
RSV respiratory syncytial virus
right subclavian vein
Rous sarcoma virus
RSVC right superior vena cava
RSVP retired senior volunteer program
rt right
right lateral *(Lat)*
rt. right
r/t related to
rT ribothymidine
Rt right
total resistance
Rt. right
RT radiologic technologist
radiotelemetry
radiotherapy
radium therapy
rapid tranquilization
reaction time
reading test
reciprocating tachycardia
recreational therapy
rectal temperature
reduction time
Registered Technician
renal transplantation
resistance transfer
respiratory therapist/therapy
response time
rest tremor
retransformation
reverse transcriptase
reverse transcription
right thigh
room temperature
Rubinstein-Taybi (syndrome)
R/T related to
RT3 rT3 reverse triiodothyronine
RTA ray tracing algorithm
renal tubular acidosis
reverse transcriptase assay
road traffic accident
RTAD renal tubular acidification defect
RT(ARRT) Radiologic Technologist certified by the American Registry of Radiologic Technologists
rtc return to clinic
RTC random control trial
rape treatment center
regional trauma center
renal tubular cell
residential treatment center
return to clinic
round the clock

RT-CT radiotherapy dedicated computed tomography
Rtd retarded
RTD renal tubular defect
routine test dilution
RTECS Registry of Toxic Effects of Chemical Substances
RTF resistance transfer factor
respiratory tract fluid
RTG-2 rainbow trout gonadal tissue cells
rTHF recombinant tumor necrosis factor
RTI respiratory tract infection
reverse transcriptase inhibition
RTK receptor-tyrosine kinase: rhabdoid tumor of the kidney
rtl rectal
RTM registered trademark
rTMS repetitive transcranial magnetic stimulation
RTN renal tubular necrosis
RT(N)(ARRT) Radiologic Technologist (Nuclear Medicine) certified by the American Registry of Radiologic Technologists
RTO return to office
right toe off
RTOG Radiation Therapy Oncology Group
radiation therapy oncology group
R to L+A react to light and accommodation
RTP radiation treatment planning
renal transplantation patient
reverse transcriptase-producing (agent)
rtPA recombinant tissue plasminogen activator
rt-PA recombinant tissue plasminogen activator
rTPA recombinant tissue plasminogen activator
RTPCR reverse transcriptase polymerase chain reaction
RT-PCR reverse transcriptase polymerase chain reaction
RTR Recreational Therapist, Registered
red blood cell turnover rate
retention time ratio
RT(R)(ARRT) Registered Technologist, Radiography certified by the American Registry of Radiologic Technologists)
RTs reaction times
relaxation times
residence times
respiratory therapists
reverse transcriptases
RTS real time scan
respiratory tract secretions
Rett syndrome
revised trauma score
revised trauma scores
right toestrike
Rothmund-Thomson syndrome
Rubinstein-Taybi syndrome
RT(T)(ARRT) Radiologic Technologist (Radiation Therapy) certified by the American Registry of Radiologic Technologists
RT3U resin T3 uptake
RU resin uptake
routine urinalysis
RU 486 antiprogesterone used for abortion in early gestation
RUC regular uterine contraction
RUE right upper extremity
RUG retrograde urethogram
RUGS resource utilization groups
RUL right upper lobe (lung)
RUP regulated ubiquitin/proteasome-dependent processing
RUQ right upper quadrant (abdomen)
RUT rapid urease test
RV residual volume of lung
right ventricle

RVAS right ventricular assist system
RVD regulatory volume decrease
RVDC right ventricle diastolic collapse
RVF right ventricular failure
RVG radionuclide ventriculography
RVH right ventricular hypertrophy
RVLM rostral ventrolateral medulla
RVMI right ventricle myocardial infarction
RVP reduced vascular response
resting venous pressure
right ventricular pressure
RVO relaxed vaginal outlet
RVR respiratory rate: tidal volume ratio
RVT renal vein thrombosis
RWM regional wall motion
Rx drug
prescription (*Lat: recipe*)
recipe
treatment
Rxn reaction
RXR retinoid receptors
RYCH-J Roux-Y choledocho-jejunostomy

S

$\underline{s}$ without (*Lat: sine*)
s without
S DNA synthesis phase of a cell cycle
serine
sensation
sensitive
serum
sleep attacks
specialist (physician)
susceptibility
$S_1 \dots S_4$ heart sounds, 1st to 4th
SA salicylic acid
sinoatrial node
sleep attacks
suicide attempt
SA (cont.) surface area (see BSA)
Sa. saline
S-A sinoatrial
SAA synthetic amino acid
SAB spontaneous abortion
SAD seasonal (schizo-) affective DO
SAE serious adverse event
SAFHS sonic accelerated fracture healing system
SAH subarachnoid hemorrhage
systemic arterial hypertension
SAL saline
SAM sulfur-adenosylmethionine
SaO2 systemic arterial oxygen saturation (%)
SAPO systemic arterial pressure oscillation
SAR specific absorption rate (MRI)
suspected adverse reaction
structure-activity relationship
SARSS suspected adverse reaction surveillance scheme
SAS signs and symptoms (also S/S)
statistical analysis system
SASOC the Social Acceptability Scale of Occlusal Conditions
SAT South African territories
SATO Sociedad Andaluza de Traumatologia y Ortopedia (Andalusian Society of Traumatology + Orthopaedics)
Sau3A restriction enzyme from Staphylococcus aureus 3A
S. aureus staphilococcus aureus
SB stillborn
sudan black
SBB sudan black B
SBC screening-detected breast cancer
SBCP Sociedade Brasileira de Cirurgia Plastica (Brazilian Society of Plastic Surgery)
SBE shortness of breath on exertion

SBE (cont.)	subacute bacterial endocarditis
SBFT	small bowel follow through series
SBM	soybean meal
SBO	side branch occlusion (in coronary artery stenting)
	skull base osteomyelitis
	small bowel obstruction
	soybean oil
SBOT	Sociedade Brasileira de Ortopedia e Traumatologia (Brazilian Association of Orthopaedics and Traumatology)
SBP	systemic blood pressure
	systolic blood pressure
SBR	styrene butadiene rubber
SC	scaphocapitate
	sickle cell
	stratum corneum
	subclavian
	subcutaneous
	synaptonemal complexes
s.c.	subcutaneous
SCAI	The Society for Cardiac Angiography and Interventions
SCAN	suspected child abuse or neglect
SCC	sickle cell crisis
	squamous cell carcinoma
	standard clinical criteria
SCCA	squamous cell carcinoma antigen
SCCOT	Colombian Society for Orthopaedics and Traumatology
SCD	sequential compression device
	sickle cell disease
	spinocerebellar degenerations
	sudden cardiac death
SCDs	scalp current densities
	sickle cell diseases
	steroid contraceptive drugs
SCDS	Seychelles Child Development Study
	Sheffield child development study
	sudden cardiac death syndrome
SCE	sister-chromatid exchange
	stem cell factor
SCFE	slipped capital femoral epiphysis (case report)
SCGX	superior cervical ganglionectomy
SCHIP	State Children's Health Insurance Program
schiz	schizophrenia
SCI	spinal cord injury
SCICU	spinal cord intensive care unit
SCID	severe combined immunodeficiency disease
SCIWORA	spinal cord injury without radiologic abnormality (Wheeless Textbook: Fractures)
SCJ	squamocolumnar junction
SCLC	Small cell lung cancer
SCOI	Southern California Orthopaedic Institute
SCORS	Social Cognition and Object Relations Scale
SCr	serum creatinine
SCR	sister-chromatid recombination
SCS	spinal chord stimulation
	Spinal Cord Society
SCTN	Scottish Cancer Therapy Network
SCU	special care unit
SD	shoulder disarticulation
	signal detection
	sleep deprivation
	spatial disorientation
	stable disease
	standard deviation
SDAT	senile dementia of Alzheimer's type
S-DD	dose-dependent susceptibility
SDH	sorbitol deshydrogenase
	subdural hematoma
SDL	step-down latency
SDS	Shwachman-Diamond syndrome
	Shy-Drager syndrome
S-DSA	stepping digital subtraction angiography

SDS-PAGE sodium dodecyl sulfate-polyacrylamide gel electrophoresis
SDTI systolic delay time index
SDU source delivery unit
standard deviation units
SDV Source Data Verification
SE spin echo (MRI)
staphylococcal enterotoxins
SEB staphylococcal enterotoxin B
sec second
SEC spontaneous echo contrast
SECOT Sociedad Espanola de Chirurgia Ortopedica y Traumatologia (only Spanish)
sed rate sedimentation rate
segs polymorphonuclear neutrophil
SEHCS silicones environmental health and safety concil
SELDI surface enhanced laser desorption/ ionization mass spectroscopy
SEM scanning electron microscopy
standard error of the mean
systolic ejection murmur
SEMI subendocardial MI
sem. ves seminal vesicles
Sens. sensory
sensation
sep. separated
Sept. AB septic abortion
Ser serine
Serol. serology
serological test
Serpins serin protease inhibitors
SES sick euthyroid syndrome
socioeconomic status
SETTLE spindle epithelial tumor with thymus-like differentiation
SeV Sendai viruses
SF swine fever
Sf9 Spodoptera frugiperda cells
SFA French Society of Arthroscopy score
SFA (cont.) saturated fatty acids
screen-film angiography
spike frequency adaptation
spindle frequency activity
standing foot angle
superficial femoral artery
SFB saphenofemoral bypass
SFG spotted fever group
SFOP French Paediatric Oncology Society
SG specific gravity
Swan-Ganz
SGA small-for-gestational age
SGC salivary gland carcinoma
SGDM Study Group on Data Management
SGGT serum gamma-glutamyl transpeptidase
SGI somatogravic illusion
s.gl. without correction (without glasses)
sGMM synthetic glucose monomycolate
SGO Society of Gynecologic Oncologists
SGOT serum glutamic-oxalacetic transaminase (see AST)
SG-P silica glass powder
SGPT Serum glutamic-pyruvic transaminase (see ALT)
SH social history, serum hepatitis
Society for Hematopathology
SHAFT Sad, Hostile, Anxious, Frustrating, Tenacious Syndrome
SHBG sex hormone binding globulin
SHG sonohysterography
SHO Senior House Officer
SHR spontaneously hypertensive rats
SHx social history
SI sacroiliac joint
International System of Units
serum iron
shock index
Steel (mouse)
stroke index

SI (cont.)	syncytium-inducing viral phenotype
SIADH	syndrome of inappropriate antidiuretic hormone secretion
sib, sib.	sibling
SICOT	International Society of Orthopaedic Surgery and Traumatology (AAOS Specialty Societies: SICOT US Chapter)
SICU	surgical intensive care unit
SIDS	Sudden Infant Death Syndrome (SIDS Network)
SIER	sonication-induced epitope retrieval
SIF	serum inhibition factors
sig	instructions or directions
SIg	surface immunoglobulins
SIL	squamous intraepithelial lesions
SIM	Society of the Internet in Medicine
SIMA	small intestinal mucinous antigen
SIMV	synchronous intermittent mandatory ventilation
SIOP	International Society of Paediatric Oncology
SIOT	Societa Italiana di Ortopedia e Traumatologia (Italian Society of Orthopaedics and Traumatology)
SIR	standardized incidence ratio
SIROT	Societee Internationale de Recherche Orthopeique et Traumatologie
SIRP	signal-regulatory proteins
SIRS	systemic inflammatory response syndrome
sis	simian sarcoma proto-oncogene
SIS	small intestinal submucosa (hernia repair)
SITOP	Societa Italiana di Ortopedia e Traumatologia Pediatrica (Italian Society of Paediatric Orthopaedics and Traumatology)
SIVD	subcortical ischemic vascular disease
SJM	St. Jude Medical (heart valves)
SJR	standing vertical jump and reach
sk	trx skeletal traction
SK	streptokinase
S-K	Sauve Kapandji (procedure)
skel.	skeletal
SKSD	SK-SD streptokinase-streptodomase
sl	in a broad sense *(Lat: sensu lato)*
	stemline
	sublingual
SL	sarcolemma
	scapholunate
	sclerosing leukoencephalopathy
	secondary leukemia
	segment length
	sensation level
	sensory latency
	septal leaflet
	short-leg (brace)
	Sibley-Lehninger (unit)
	signal level
	Sinding Larsen (syndrome)
	Sjogren-Larsson (syndrome)
	slit lamp
	small lymphocyte
	sodium lactate
	solidified liquid
	sound level
	stabilized liposomes
	Stein-Leventhal (syndrome)
	streptolysin
	sublingual
	systolic wave, latent
S/L	sublingual
SL1	segment length, inferior
SL5	segment length, septal
SLA	left sacroanterior (fetal position) *(Lat: sacrolaeva anterior)*
	segment length, anterior

SLA (cont.) single-cell liquid cytotoxic assay
slide latex agglutination
soluble liver antigen
superficial linear array
surfactant-like activity

SLAC scapholunate advanced collapse (wrist)

SLAM scanning laser acoustic microscope
systemic lupus erythematosus activity measure

SLAP serum leucine aniinopeptidase
superior labrum anterior posterior (lesion)

SLAT simultaneous laryngoscopy and abdominal thrusts

SLB short-leg brace

SLC secondary lymphoid organ chemokine
short leg cast

SLCC short-leg cylinder cast

SLD SLDH serum lactate dehydrogenase
sublethal damage

SLDR sublethal damage repair

SLE slit lamp examination
St.Louis encephalitis
systemic lupus erythematosus

SLEA sheep erythrocyte antibody

SLEDAI systemic lupus erythematosus disease activity index

SLEP short latent evoked potential

SLEV St.Louis encephalitis virus

SLG synthetic latex gloves

SLHR sex-linked hypophospbatemic rickets

SLI selective lymphoid irradiation
somatostatin-like immunoreactivity
splenic localization index

SLIC scanning liquid ionization chamber

SLIDRC Student Loan Interest Deduction Restoration Coalition

SLIL scapholunate interosseous ligament

SLIM synovial-like interface membrane

SLIP serial line interface protocol

SLIR somatostatin-like immunoreactivity

SLK superior limbic keratoconjunctivitis

SLKC superior limbic keratoconjunctivitis

SLL segment length, lateral
small lymphocytic lymphoma

SLM sound level meter

SLMC spontaneous lymphocyte-mediated cytotoxicity

SLN sentinel lymph node
sublentiform nucleus
superior laryngeal nerve

SLNB sentinel lymph node biopsy

SLNWBC short-leg non-weight bearing cast

SLNWC short-leg nonwalking cast

SLO Smith-Lemli-Opitz syndrome
streptolysin O

SLOS Smith-Lenili-Opitz syndrome

SLP left sacroposterior (fetal position) *(Lat: sacrolaeva posterior)*
segmental limb systolic pressure
sex-limited protein
short luteal phase
subluxation of the patella

SLPI secretory leukocyte protease inhibitor

SLPP serum lipophosphoprotein

SLR Shwartzman local reaction
single lens reflex
straight leg raising (Lasègue)

SLRT straight leg raising test

SLS segment long-spacing
short-leg splint
single limb support
Sjogren-Larsson syndrome
stagnant loop syndrome
Stein-Leventhal syndrome

S

SLT left sacrotransverse (fetal position) *(Lat: sacrolaeva transversa)*
single lung transplantation
smokeless tobacco
solid logic technology

SLUD salivation, lacrimation, urination, defecation

SLUDGE salivation, lacrimation, urination, defecation, gastrointestinal upset, emesis

SLWC short-leg walking cast

sm an small animal
smear

sm, sm. small

sM suckling mouse

Sm samarium
Serratia marcescens
Smith (antigen)

SM Master of Science
sadomasochism
self-monitoring
silicon microphysiometer
simple mastectomy
skim milk
smooth muscle
somatomedin (insulin-like growth factors)
space medicine
sphingomyelin
splenic macrophage
sports medicine
streptomycin
Strumpell-Marie (syndrome)
submandibular
submaxillary
submucous
suckling mouse
sucrose medium
suction method
superior mesenteric
surgical microscope
surrogate mother

SM (cont.) sustained medication
symptoms
synaptic membrane
synovial membrane
systemic mastocytosis
systolic motion
systolic murmur

S/M sadomasochism

SMA sequential multiple analysis or analyzer
sequential multichannel autoanalyzer
simultaneous multichannel autoanalyzer
smooth muscle antibody
Society for Medical Anthropology
somatomedin A
spinal muscular atrophy
spontaneous motor activity
Sport Medicine Australia
standard method agar
superior mesenteric artery
supplementary motor area

SM-A somatomedin A

SMA-6 Sequential Multiple Analysis in-six different serum tests

SMA-14 routine admission chemistry

SMABF superior mesenteric artery blood flow

SMaC Surrogate Marker Cost-Efficacy

SMAC Sequential Multiple Analyzer Computer
soluble membrane attack complex
sorbitol MacConkey agar
superior mesenteric arterial conductance

SMAE superior mesenteric artery embolism

SMAF smooth muscle activating factor
specific macrophage arming factor

SMAG Special Medical Advisory Group

SM-AHNMD systemic mastocytosis with associated clonal hematopoietic non-mast cell lineage disorder
SMAL serum methyl alcohol level
SMAO superior mesenteric artery occlusion
S/MARs scaffold/matrix attachment regions
SMART simultaneous multiple angle reconstruction technique
SMAS submuscular aponeurotic system
superficial musculo-aponeurotic system
superior mesenteric artery syndrome
SMAST Short Michigan Alcoholism Screening Test
sMb suckling mouse brain
SMB selected mucosal biopsy
standard mineral base
SMBFT small bowel follow-through
SMBG self-monitored blood glucose
SMC Scientific Manpower Commission
smooth muscle cell
somatomedin C
succinylmonocholine
SM-C Sm-C somatomedin C
somatomedin C
SMCA smooth muscle contracting agent
suckling mouse cataract agent
SMCD senile macular choroidal degeneration
systemic mast cell disease
systemic meningococcal disease
SM-C/IGF somatomedin C/insulin-like growth factor
SMCR Smith-Magenis chromosome region
SMD senile macular degeneration
spondylometaphyseal dysplasia
submanubrial dullness
SMDA Safe Medical Devices Act (of 1990)
starch methylenedianiline
SMDC sodium-N-methyl dithiocarbamate
standards for medical device communication
SMDM Society for Medical Decision Making
SMDS secondary myelodysplastic syndrome
SME severe myoclonic epilepsy
SMED spondylometaphyseal dysplasia
SMF secondary myelofibrosis
S-Mgb serum myoglobin
SMO slips made out
Sociedad Mexicana de Ortopedia (only Spanish)
SMP sympathetic maintained pain
SMR sexual maturity ratings
submucous resection
SMS solitary myofibroma(tosis) of the skin
SMTP Stachybotrys microspora triprenyl phenol
SMX sulfamethoxazole
SMY Syh-Mo-Yin (prescription of Traditional Chinese Medicine for liver disease)
SN séroneutralization
SNA sambucus nigra agglutinin
sympathetic nerve activity
SNARF-1 carboxy-seminaphthorhodafluor
SND striatonigral degeneration
SNF skilled nursing facility
SNLG Scottish and Newcastle Lymphoma Group
SNP single nucleotide polymorphism
sodium nitroprusside
SNS Syh-Nih-San (prescription of Traditional Chinese Medicine for liver disease)
sympathetic nervous system
SNV sin nombre virus (hantavirus)
SO standing order OR significant other
superior oblique

SO4	sulfate
SOA	Southern Orthopaedic Association
SOAP	symptoms, objective, assessment, and plan
S.O.A.P.	subjective, objective assessment plan
SOB	shortness of breath
SOBCOT	Societee Belge de Chirurgie Orthopédique et de Traumatologie (Belgian Society of Orthopaedics and Traumatology)
SOCITRAS	Societa Italiana di Traumatologia della Strada (Italian Society of Road Traumatology)
sod.	sodium
SOFCOT	French Society of Orthopaedics and Trauma Surgery
SOFIGO	The International Association of Supporters of FIGO
sol, Sol.	solution
SOL	soleus muscle
SOMOS	Society of Military Orthopaedic Surgeons (AAOS)
sono.	sonogram
SOP	standard operating protocol
sos	if necessary
S.O.S.	repeat once if urgent
SOTOCAV	Sociedad de Ortopedia y Traumatologia de la Comunidad Autonoma Valenciana (only Spanish)
SOTRS	Sociedade de Ortopedia e Traumatologia do Rio Grande do Sul (only Portuguese)
sp.	spine
	spinal
SP	substance P
	suprapubic
	systolic pressure
S/P	no change
	status post
SP-1	pregnancy-specific beta-1-glycoprotein
SP-A	surfactant protein A
SPC	septal perforator compression
	soybean phosphatidylcholine
	sphingosylphosphorylcholine
	spleen cells
	spontaneous phasic contractions
	Summary of Product Characteristics
	systemic to pulmonary collaterals
sp.cd.	spinal cord
SPD	phase difference method
spec, spec.	specimen
SPECT	single photon emission computed tomography
SpEP	sphenoidal evoked potential
	spinal somatosensory evoked potentials
SPEP	serum protein electrophoresis
S-PEP	peplomycin emulsion in saline
	self-administered positive expiratory pressure
SPET	single photon emission tomography
SPEU	segmented polyurethane
SPF	specific-pathogen-free
	S-phase fraction
	sun protection factor
sp.fl.	spinal fluid
spg.	sponge
sp. gr.	specific gravity
sp+H	speech and hearing
S-phase	proliferative index % of tumor cells actively dividing at a given time
spin.	spine
	spinal
SPIO	superparamagnetic iron oxide MRI enhancement
SPM	synchronous pacemaker

SPME-MS-MVA	solid-phase microextraction, mass spectrometry, and multivariate analysis
S-PMI	subendocardial perioperative myocardial injury
SPN	stiatopallidonigral
SpO2	oxygen saturation by pulse oximeter
SPOHNC	Support for People with Oral and Head and Neck Cancer
spont.	spontaneous
SPT	skin prick test
sq	squamous
	subcutaneous
SQ	subcutaneous
SQW	Shieh-Qing-Wan (prescription of Traditional Chinese Medicine for liver disease)
SR	sedimentation rate
	Show Racer pigeons
	stimulus response
	superior rectus muscle
	sustained release
	systems review
SRA	(14C)-serotonin-release assay (for diagnosis of HIT)
SRBD	sleep-related breathing disorders
SRFD	South Rockwood Fire Department
SRH	sleep-related hallucinations
SRIF	somatotropin release-inhibiting factor (somatostatin)
SROM	spontaneous rupture of membrane
SRP	signal recognition particle
SRS	Scoliosis Research Society (also: AAOS Specialty Societies)
ss	one half
SS	Salmonella-Shigella agar
	social service
	systemic sclerosis
S/S	signs and symptoms (also SAS)
S+S	signs and symptoms
SSA	sewage sludge ashes
	Social Security Administration (US)
SSC	side scatter (flow cytometry term)
SsCEP	somatosensory cerebral evoked potentials
SSCP	substernal chest pain
SSD	sexual size dimorphism
	shaded-surface display
	side-to-side duodenoplasty
	single saturating dose
	single-strand damage (DNA)
	Social Security disability
	source-skin distance
	source-surface distance
	speech-sound discrimination
	succinate semialdehyde dehydrogenase
	sum of square deviations
	syndrome of sudden death
SSE	soap suds enema
	Spine Society Of Europe
SSEP	somatosensory evoked potentials
SSER	somatosensory evoked response
ss. gl.	without glasses (or corrective lenses)
SSKI	saturated solution of potassium iodine
SSM	Southern Sports Medicine (+ Orthopaedic Center)
	Superficial Spreading Melanoma
SSMAL	Shuffling Similarities with Multiple Alignments
SSNT	single supernumerary teeth
Sso	sulfolobus solfataricus
SSPE	subacute sclerosing panencephalitis
SSR	signal sequence receptor
	sympathetic skin response
SSRI	selective serotonin reuptake inhibitor
SSS	scalded skin syndrome
	sick sinus syndrome

SSS (cont.)	superior sagittal sinus
SSSS	staphylococcal scalded-skin syndrome
SstII	restriction enzyme from Streptomyces stanford
S + sx	signs and symptoms
st.	stage of disease stomach
st	stage of disease
ST	esotropia scaphotrapezial sinus tachycardia sulfotransferases syncytiotrophoblast
Staph	Staphylococcus
Staph.	Staphylococcus
StAR	steroidogenic acute regulatory
stat, stat.	immediately *(Lat: statim)*
STAT	immediately *(Lat: statim)* signal transducers and activators of transcription
STC	secondary thyroid carcinoma
Std	sexually transmitted disease
STD	sexually transmitted disease skin test dose standard
STH	somatotropin
STI	severe torso injury systolic time intervals
STIs	soft tissue infections
STLN	soft tissue lateral neck
STM	soft tissue mobilization
stom.	stomach
STR	single twitch response (EMG) slow-twitch red (skeletal muscle)
Strep, strep.	Streptococcus
STRPC	short TRPC
STS	serological test for syphilis single twitch stimulation (EMG) Society of Thoracic Surgeons
S.T.S.	serological test for syphilis
STSG	split thickness skin graft
STT	scapho-trapezo-trapezoidal
STZ	streptozotocin
subcu.	subcutaneous
subling.	sublingual
subq	subcutaneous (sub cutis)
Subq	subcutaneous (sub cutis)
SUDAAN	software for statistical analysis of correlated data
SUDS	single-use diagnostic system
SUFE	slip of the upper femoral epiphysis (radiograph)
sulf.	sulfate
sup.	superior
supin.	supination
supp	suppository
suppos	suppository
surg, surg.	surgical
SUs	substance users
susp	suspension
SUVs	unilamellar vesicles
Sv	sievert
SV	overall survival simian virus stroke volume supraventricular
SV40	simian vacuolating virus no. 40
SVA	sequential ventriculo-atrial pacing shell vial assay sinus of Valsalva aneurysms supraventricular arrhythmia
SVA-IFA	shell vial assay-indirect immunofluorescent assay
SVC	superior vena cava
SVCS	superior vena cava syndrome
SVD	spontaneous vaginal delivery Swine Vesicular Disease
SVe	stroke volume echocardiography
SVE	of soil vapor extraction saline volume expansion seminal vesicle epithelium Sendai virus envelopes serum vitamin E

SVE (cont.) significant villous edema
small volume expansion
sports vision evaluations
sterile vaginal examination
Stressful Vital Events
subcortical vascular encephalopathy
supraventricular ectopy
supraventricular extrasystole
surveillance examinations
sustained volume expansion

SVG saphenous vein graft

SVI stroke volume index

SvO2 mixed venous hemoglobin saturation

SVR systemic vascular resistance

SVT supraventricular tachycardia

SW social worker
software

SWA slow-wave activity

SWD short wave diathermy

SWI surgical wound infection

SWOG Southwest Oncology Group

SWPS Social Welfare Policy + Services

SWT systolic wall thickening

Sx signs and symptoms
symptom(s)

SX sulfisoxazole

SXR steroid and xenobiotic receptor

Sxr locus a part of the Y chromosome

sys. system

syst. systolic

SYSTERS SYSTEmatic Re-Searching (protein sequence cluster set)

Sz, SZ schizophrenia
seizure

T

T extent of primary tumor
temperature
thoracic, to be followed by number designating specific thoracic vertebra
threonine
thymine

T0, T1-3 size of tumor in staging cancers

T1 – T12 thoracic nerves 1 through 12
thoracic vertebrae 1 - 12 (spine e.g. T1 = 1st thoracic vertebra)

T3 triiodothyronine

T4 thyroxine

TA technical assistance
tendon Achilles
tibialis anterior
tolfenamic acid

T+A tonsillectomy and adenoidectomy
tonsils and adenoids

TAANOS The American Academy of Neurological and Orthopaedic Surgeons

tab. tablet

tab(s), Tabs tablet(s)

TAC transient amplifying cells (cells that have the potential to complete a limited number of divisions before differentiating)
Trauma Association of Canada

TACE transcatheter arterial chemo-embolization

TACHY tachycardia

TAE transarterial embolization

TAH total abdominal hysterectomy

TAM total active motion
tamoxifen

TAO thyroid associated ophthalmopathy

TAPVC total anomalous pulmonary venous connection

T

TaqI	heat stable polymerase isolated from Thermus aquaticus
TAs	triggered activations
TAT	tetanus antitoxin
	thematic apperception test
T.A.T.	tetanus antitoxin
Taw	airway wall temperature
TAw	water titration alkalinity
TAW	temporal acoustic window
	thoracoabdominal wounds
	traction-absorbing wiring
	twice a week
TAW-925	a human B lymphoblastoid cell line
TB	tuberculosis
tbc.	TB, tuberculosis
TBD	to be determined
TBF	tail blood flow
	tentacle ball formation
	terbinafine
	thyroid blood flow
	tick-borne fever
	tissue blood flow
	total body fat
	tumor blood flow
TBG	thyroid binding globulin
Tbi	initial body temperature
	intermediate tectobulbar pathway
TBI	total body irradiation
	T- and B-cell epitopes containing immunogen
	tetrapolar bioelectrical impedance
	thiazolobenzimidazole [1-(2,6-difluorophenyl)-1H,3H-thiazolo[3,4-a] benzimidazole]
	Thromboplastin Bilbao
	thrombotic brain infarction
	thyrotropin binding inhibition
	thyroid binding index
	thyroxine binding index
	time-based injection
	Tissue Banks International
	toe brachial index
TBI (cont.)	tooth brushing instruction
	total bilirubin
	total binding index
	total body impedance
	total body iron
	total body irradiation
	total bone index
	trabecular bone index
	transbronchial injection
	transbullar injections
	translid binocular interactor
	traumatic brain injury
	triamcinolone acetonide benzoyl-beta-amino-isobutyrate
	2,4,5-tribromoimidazole
TBLC	term birth living child
TBMM	total body muscle mass
TBS	The Bethesda System
	to be scheduled
TBSA	total body surface area
tbsp, tbsp.	tablespoon
TBVF	trabecular bone volume fraction
TBW	total body water
T+C	type and crossmatch
TCA	thymus-derived chemotactic agent
	tricyclic antidepressant
TCD	transcranial doppler
TCDB	turn, cough, deep breath
TCF	tissue cage fluid
TCI	to come in (hospital)
TCID50	Tissue Culture Infectious Dose 50%
TCM	traditional Chinese medicine
TCP	transcutaneous pacing
TCPC	tricalcium phosphate ceramic
TCR	T-cell receptor
TCRBCL	T-cell-rich B-cell lymphoma
TCRBJ	TCR J beta
TCRGR	T-cell receptor gene rearrangement (study)
TCs	technical components
TCT	thrombin clotting time
TCU	transitional care unit

TCV tall-cell variant of papillary thyroid carcinomas
turnip crinkle virus
Td adult tetanus toxoid and reduced-dose diphtheria toxoid
TD tardive dyskinesis
texture-defined
tolerance dose
transdermal
TDA toluenediamines
Trade and Development Agency
TDI toluene diisocyanate (a highly volatile chemical known to cause occupational asthma in exposed workers)
TDLU terminal-duct-lobular-units
TdT terminal deoxynucleotide transferase
TDT tooth decay test
transmission disequilibrium test
TDTH cells a functional subset of T helper cells that are involved in delayed-type hypersensitivity reactions
TDY Temporary Duty
TE echo time (MRI)
TEC thromboembolic complications
transient erythroblastopenia of childhood
transluminal extraction atherectomy
TECA-LBO total ear canal ablation-lateral bulla osteotomy
TEDs Thromboembolic Deterrent Stockings
TEDS timed exposure diffusive sampler
transoesophageal echo-Doppler system
Treatment Episode Data Set
TEE transesophageal echocardiogram
TEF tracheoesophageal fistula
TEIL tobacco EIN3-like
Tele telemetry
TEM Technical Error Measurement
transmission electron microscopy
temp, temp. temperature
Temp. T, temperature
TEN-IBC Trans-European Network-Integrated Broadband Communications
TENS transcutaneous electrical nerve stimulation
transient electric nerve stimulation
TES Toxocara canis excretory/secretory antigen(s)
transcranial electrical stimulation
TESD total end systolic diameter
TF tail-flick
thoracic fluid content
T.F. tuning fork
TFA trifluoroacetic acid
TFCC triangular fibrocartilage complex
TFF tangential flow filtration
TFPI tissue factor pathway inhibitor
Tfree free testosterone
TFT thin-film transistor
thrombus formation time
thyroid function test
tight filum terminale
trifluorothymidine
TG triglycerides
TG(6-) 6-Thioguanine (anti cancer drug)
TGA transient global amnesia
transposition great vessels
TGE transmissible gastroenteritis
TGF transforming growth factors
TGF-α tumor growth factor alpha
TGF-β tumor growth factor beta
TGV thoracic gas volume
transposition of great vessels
THAM T cell-activating molecule
TH1 T helper type 1 cell
TH2 T helper type 2 cell
T+H type and hold
THA tacrine hydrochloride

T

THA (cont.) total hip arthroplasty (sample operative report)
THBR thyroid hormone binding ratio
THBSO total hysterectomy with bilateral salpingo-oophorectomy
THC delta-9-tetrahydrocannabinol the psychoactive substance in Cannabis sativa
transhepatic cholangiogram
THERAP. therapy
therapeutic
thor. thorax
thoracic
THP thoracic impedance
total hip prosthesis
Thr threonine
THR total hip replacement
total hip revision (sample operative report)
THV terminal hepatic venule (central vein)
Thy-1 a highly abundant glycoprotein on the surface of thymocytes and neurons
TI tricuspid insufficiency
TIA thanks in advance
transient ischemic attacks
TIBC, TIBS total iron-binding capacity
t.i.d. tid, three times a day
tid three times a day *(Lat: ter in die)*
TIFA Trade and Investment Framework Agreement
TIG tetanus immune globulin
TIGR The Institute for Genomic Research
TIL tumor-infiltrating lymphocytes
TIMI Thrombolysis in Myocardial Infarction
TIMP tissue inhibitor of metalloproteinase
TiO2 titanium dioxide
TIP terminal interphalangeal (joint)
TIPS transjugular intrahepatic portosystemic shunt
TIPSS transjugular intrahepatic portosystemic stent shunts
TIS titanium interbody spacers
TIUP term intrauterine pregnancy
tiw three times a week
t.i.w. three times per week
TJ tetrajoule
triceps jerk
triceps reflex
TJ-10 Saiko-keishi-to, herbal medicine
TJ-41 Hochu-ekki-to (a Japanese herbal medicine)
TJ-43 Liu-Jun-Zi-Tang, a herbal medicine exerting gastroprotective action
TJ-48 Juzen-taiho-to, a kampo medicine
TJ-9 Sho-saiko-to, a herbal medicine
TJ-96 saiboku-to (a herbal preparation)
TJ-960 sho-saiko-to-go-keishi-ka-shakuyakuto (Japanese herbal medicine), a compound known to have free radical scavenging activity
TJA total joint arthroplasty
TJD transient job disability
traumatic joint disease
TJs tight junctions
TK tyrosine kinase
TKA total knee arthroplasty
TKE total knee extension
TKN total Kjeldahl nitrogen (waste waters treatment)
TKO to keep open
TKR total knee replacement/revision
TLA three letter abbreviation/acronym (ha)
TLC tender loving care
thin-layer chromatography
total lung capacity
TLCK N-tosyl-L-lysine chloromethyl ketone

TLD thermoluminescent dosimeters
TLI thymidine labeling index
total lymphoid irradiation
TLR target lesion revascularization
TLSO thoracolumbosacral orthosis
TLV threshold limit values
TM transmembrane
tympanic membrane
T.M. tympanum membrani (ear drum)
TMA thrombotic microangiopathy
tissue microarray infostructure
transmetatarsal amputation
TMA-Gly:CPH poly[trimellitylimidoglycine-co-1,6-bis(carboxyphenoxy)hexane] - a novel class of polymers
TMAO trimethylamine N-oxide
TMD transient myeloproliferative disorder
TMDC transverse magnetization decay curve
TMEP telangiectasia macularis eruptiva perstans
TMG toxic multinodular goiter
TMGA tetramethylene glutaric acid
TMJ (temporalist mandibulae junctio)
temporomandibular joint
TMP trimethoprim
TMP-SMX trimethoprim-sulfamethoxazole
TMR transmyocardial revascularization
TMS transcranial magnetic stimulation
TMV tobacco mosaic virus
TNF tumor necrosis factor
TNI total needed irradiation
total nodal irradiation
TNM tumor, nodes, metastases
TNT trinitrotoluene
TNTC too numerous to count
t.o. telephone order
TO telephone order
TOA Texas Orthopaedic Association
tubo-ovarian abscess
to AA to affected areas
TOC total organic carbon
TOD target organ damage
third-order dispersion
TOF train-of-four (EMG)
T of F tetralogy of Fallot
top topical(ly)
TOP termination of pregnancy
TOPV oral attenuated poliovirus with types 1, 2, and 3
trivalent oral polio vaccine
TOR total outflow resistance
TORCH congenital infections with T = toxoplasmosis, O = other, R = rubella, C = cytomegalic inclusion disease, H = hepatitis B and herpes
TOS thoracic outlet syndrom
Tox toxic
toxicology
toxicologic
TP term pregnancy
thyropharyngeus muscle
total pancreatectomy
total platinum
TP-5 thymopentin
TPA thrombo proteolytic activity
tissue plasminogen activator
TPI Treponema pallidum immobilization test
T-PMI transmural perioperative myocardial infarction
TPN thalamic projection neuron
total parenteral nutrition
transition protein
triphosphopyridine nucleotide
TPNAC total parenteral nutrition-associated cholestasis
Tpo thrombopoietin
TPP thiamin pyrophosphate
TPPA Treponema pallidum
TPR temperature, pulse, respirations
total peripheral resistance
TPUR transperineal urethral resection

tr	trace
tr.	tinct., tincture
TR	Texas red
trach	tracheal
	tracheostomy
TRAM-flap	one type of breast reconstruction
TRAP	tartrate resistant acid phosphatase
	telomeric repeat amplification protocol
TRH	thyrotropin-releasing hormone
TRIS	tris(hydroxymethyl)aminomethane
TRK	transketolase
Trp	tryptophan
TRP	transient receptor potential
TRPA	tryptophan-rich prealbumin
TRPC	transient receptor potential channel proteins
TrPl	treatment plan
TRP II	tricho-rhino-phalangeal syndrome type II
TRPM	testosterone-repressed prostate message
TRPO	tryptophan oxygenase
TRPS	trichorhinophalangeal syndrome
TRPT	theoretical renal phosphorus threshold
TRR	total respiratory resistance
TrS	trauma surgery
TRS	testicular regression syndrome
	total reducing sugars
	tubuloreticular structure
TRSV	tobacco ringspot virus
TRT	testosterone replacement therapy
	thoracic radiotherapy
	transfer ribonucleic acid threonine
TR/TE	repetition time/echo time
TRU	task-related unit
	turbidity-reducing unit
	transrectal ultrasonography
T3RU	triiodothyronine resin uptake
TRV	tobacco rattle virus
TRVV	total right ventricular volume
trx	mammalian homologue of the Drosophila trithorax gene
TRX	thioredoxin trx traction
Tryp	tryptophan
Ts	skin temperature
	tosylate
	tsp, teaspoon
TS	T suppressor (cell)
	Takayasu syndrome
	Tay-Sachs (disease)
	temperature, skin
	temporal stem
	tensile strength
	test solution
	thermal stability
	thoracic surgery
	thymidylate synthetase
	time required to complete the S phase of the cell cycle
	tissue space
	total solids (in urine)
	Tourette syndrome
	toxic substance
	toxic syndrome
	tracheal sound
	transferrin saturation
	transitional sleep
	transsexual
	transverse section
	transverse sinus
	trauma score
	treadmill score
	triceps surae
	tricuspid stenosis
	triple strength
	tropical sprue
	trypticase soy (plate)
	tuberous sclerosis
	tumor-specific
	Turner syndrome
	type-specific
T/S	transverse section

T+S type and screen
T4SA thyroxine-specific activity
TSA technical surgical assistance
toluene sulfonic acid
total shoulder arthroplasty
total solute absorption
toxic shock antigen
transcortical sensory aphasia
trypticase-soy agar
tumor surface antigen
tumor-specific antigen
type-specific antibody
thyroid-stimulating antibody
TSAP toxic-shock-associated protein
TSAS total severity assessment score
TSAT tube slide agglutination test
TSB total serum bilirubin
trypticase soy broth
tryptone soy broth
TSBA total serum bile acids
TSBB transtracheal selective bronchial brushing
TSC technetium sulfur colloid
thiosemicarbazide
transverse spinal sclerosis
tuberous sclerosis
TSCA Toxic Substances Control Act
TSCS Tennessee Self-Concept Scale
TSD target-skin distance
Tay-Sachs disease
theory of signal detectability
TSE testicular self-examination
tissue-specific extinguisher
total skin examination
trisodium edetate
TSEB total skin electron beam
T sect transverse section
TSEM transmission scanning electron microscopy
TSES Target Symptom Evaluation Scale
T-set tracheotomy set
TSF testicular feminization syndrome
TSF (cont.) thrombopoiesis-stimulating factor
total systemic flow
triceps skinfold
TSG tumor-specific glycoprotein
TSGP tumor-specific glycoprotein
TSH thyroid stimulating hormone
transient synovitis of the hip
TSHA thyroid-stimulating hormone, alpha chain
TSHB thyroid-stimulating hormone, beta chain
TSHR thyroid-stimulating hormone receptor
TSH-RF thyroid-stimulating hormone-releasing factor
TSH-RH thyroid-stimulating hormone-releasing hormone
TSI thyroid stimulating immunoglobulin
triple sugar iron
TSIA total small intestine allotransplantation
triple sugar iron agar
tSIDS totally unexplained sudden infant death syndrome
TSL terminal sensory latency
TSM type-specific M protein
tsp, tsp. teaspoon
Tsp teaspoon
TSP testis-specific protein
thrombin-sensitive protein
thrombospondin
total serum protein
total suspended particulate
trisodium phosphate
tropical spastic paraparesis
TSPA thiotepa
TSPAP total serum prostatic acid phosphatase
TSPL transplant
TSPP tetrasodium pyrophosphate
TSR target site restenosis

TSR (cont.)	theophylline sustained release
	thyroid to serum ratio
	total systemic resistance
TSS	total suspended solids
	toxic shock syndrome
	tropical splenomegaly syndrome
TSSA	tumor-specific cell surface antigen
TSSE	toxic shock syndrome exotoxin
TSST	toxic shock syndrome toxin
TSST-1	toxic shock syndrome toxin-1
TST	thiosulfate sulfur-transferase
	thromboplastin screening test
	total sleep time
	transforming sequence, thyroid
	treadmill stress test
	tricipital skinfold thickness
	tumor skin test
TSTA	toxoplasmin skin test antigen
	tumor-specific tissue antigen
	tumor-specific transplantation antigen
TSU	triple sugar urea (agar)
TSV	total stomach volume
TSVR	total systemic vascular resistance
TSY	trypticase soy yeast
TT	tablet triturate
	tactile threshold
	tendon transfer
	tetrathionate
	therapeutic touch
	tolerance test
	total time
	tube thoracostomy
	tuberculoid (in Ridley-Jopling Hansen disease classification)
	tactile tension
	test tube
	testicular torsion
	tetanus toxin
	tetanus toxoid
	tetrazol
	thrombin time
TT (cont.)	thrombolytic therapy
	thymol turbidity
	tibial tubercle
	tilt table
	total thyroxine
	transferred to
	transient tachypnea
	transit time
	transthoracic
	transtracheal
	tuberculin test
	tumor thrombus
	turnover time
T+T	time and temperature
	touch and tone
TT2	total diiodothyronine
TT3	total triiodothyronine
TT4	total thyroxine
TTA	tetanus toxoid antibody
	timed therapeutic absence
	total toe arthroplasty
	transtracheal aspiration
TTAP	threaded titanium acetabular prosthesis
TTB	third trimester bleeding
TTC	triphenyltetrazolium chloride (stain for lactic dehydrogenase)
	triphenyltetrazolium chloride
	T-tube cholangiogram
TTD	tissue tolerance dose
	temporary total disability
	transient tic disorder
	transverse thoracic diameter
	trichothio-dystrophy
TTE	transthoracic echocardiography
TTF-1	thyroid transcription factor 1
TTFD	tetrahydrofurfuryldisulfide
TTG	T-cell translocation gene
	telethermography
	tellurite, taurocholate, and gelatin
TTGA	tellurite, taurocholate, and gelatin agar

TTH thyrotropic hormone
tritiated thymidine

TTI tension-time index
timepto-intubation
time-tension index
torque-time interval
total thromboplastin index
transtracheal insufflation

TTN transient tachypnea

ttot total time (of pungency)

Ttot total testosterone

TTP thrombotic thrombocytopenic purpura

TTR transthyretin

T-Tube cholangiogram

TTV therapeutic trial visit

TTWB toe touch weight bearing

TTX tetrodotoxin

TU tuberculin units (in Mantoux test)

TUIP transurethral incision of the prostate

TULIP transurethral ultrasound-guided laser induced prostatectomy

TUMT transurethral microwave thermotherapy

TUNA transurethral needle ablation (prostatic)

TUNEL TdT-mediated-dUTP nick end labeling, enzymatic labeling of DNA fragments in apoptotic cells

TUR transurethral resection

TUR (P/BT) transurethral resection (of prostate/bladder tumor)

TURB transurethral resection of bladder

TURBT transurethral resection of bladder tumor

TURP transurethral resection of the prostate
tubular undulating row photobioreactors
transurethral prostatectomy

TV tidal volume

TV (cont.) total volume

TVA temporal (beat-to-beat) variability of repolarization in amplitude

TvC treatment versus control

TVC timed vital capacity
total viable cells
total viable count (a measurement of the number of organisms in a sample that are viable in the chosen nutrient medium, in a microbiological test. measured in cfu/ml or cfu/g etc. cfu = colony forming units)
total volume capacity
transvaginal cone
triple voiding cystogram
true vocal cord

TVF target vessel failure

TVH total vaginal hysterectomy
turkey virus hepatitis

TVR target vessel restenosis
target vessel revascularization
tricuspid valve replacement

TvT treatment versus treatment

TVT target value tailored apheresis
temporal (beat-to-beat) variability of repolarization in time
tension-free vaginal tape
thermal vascular test
total ventilation time
Transmissible venereal tumour
Trivittatus
tunica vaginalis testis

TVUS transvaginal ultrasound

tw twice a week

TW tap water

TWb wet bulb temperature

TWB terminal warm blood cardioplegia
total worm burden
tower building
translator's work bench
treponemal Western blot

TWB (cont.)	trough whole blood
	turing-wave bifurcation
TWG	total weight gain
Tx	therapy
	traction
	transplant
	treatment
TXA2	thromboxane A2
TXB2	thromboxane B2
Tyr	tyrosine

U

u	unified atomic mass unit
	velocity
U	congenital limb absence
	in electrocardiography, an undulating deflection that follows the T wave
	internal energy
	International Unit of enzyme activity
	Mann-Whitney rank sum statistic
	potential difference (in volts)
	ulcer
	ulna
	ultralente (insulin)
	umbilicus
	uncertain
	unerupted
	unit(s)
	universal application (residency)
	unknown
	unsharpness
	upper
	uracil
	uranium
	urea
	urethra
	uridine
	uridylic acid
U (cont.)	urinary concentration
	urine
	urology
	uterus
	uvula
	volume velocity
U.	unit
U/2	upper half
U/3	upper third
ua	urinalysis
UA	absorption unsharpness
	ultra-audible
	ultrasonic arteriography
	umbilical artery
	unauthorized absence
	unit of analysis
	unstable angina
	upper airways
	upper arm
	uric acid
	uridylic acid
	urinalysis
	urine analysis
	urinary aldosterone
	uronic acid
	uterine aspiration
U/A	uric acid
	urinalysis
UAC	umbilical artery catheter
	uracil-adenine-cytosine codon for tyrosine
	uric acid
UA/C	uric acid creatinine (ratio)
UAE	unilateral absence of excretion
	urine albumin excretion
UAEM	University Association for Emergency Medicine
UAI	uterine activity interval
U-AMY	urinary amylase
UAN	uric acid nitrogen
UAO	upper airway obstruction
UAP	unlicensed assistive personnel

UAP (cont.)	unstable angina pectoris
	urinary acid phosphatase
	urinary alkaline phosphatase
UAPA	unilateral absence of pulmonary
UAR	upper airway resistance
	uric acid riboside
UAS	upper abdomen surgery
	upstream activation site
UASA	United Amputee Services Association
UAU	uracil-adenine-uracil codon for tyrosine
	uterine activity unit
UB	ultimobranchial body
	Unna boot
	upper back
	urinary bladder
UBA	undenaturated bacterial antigen
UBB	ubiquitin B
UBBC	unsaturated vitamin B12 binding capacity
UBC	ubiquitin C
	University of British Columbia (brace)
UBE	ubiquitin-activating enzyme
UBG	Ubg urobilinogen
UBI	ultraviolet blood irradiation
UBJ	uretero-bladder junction
UBL	undifferentiated B-cell lymphoma
UBN	urobilin
UBO	unidentified bright object
	upper body obesity
UBP	ureteral back pressure
UBS	unidentified bright signal
UBW	usual body weight
UC	ulcerative colitis
	ultracentrifugal
	umbilical cord
	unchanged
	unclassifiable
	unconscious
	undifferentiated cells
UC (cont.)	unit clerk
	unsatisfactory condition
	untreated cells
	urea clearance
	urethral catheterization
	urinary catheter
	urine concentrate
	urine culture
	uterine contractions
U+C	urethral and cervical
	usual and customary
UCA	uracil-cytosine-adenine codon for serine
UCB	unconjugated bilirubin
UCBC	umbilical cord blood culture
UCC	uracil-cytosine-cytosine codon for serine
UCD	urine collection device
	usual childhood diseases
UCDS	uniform clinical data set
UCE	urea cycle enzymopathy
UCG	ultrasonic cardiography
	urinary chorionic gonadotropin
UCHD	usual childhood diseases
UCI	unusual childhood illness
	urethral catheter in
	urinary catheter in
UCK	uridine-cytidine kinases
UCL	ulnar collateral ligament
	upper collateral ligament
	upper confidence limit
	upper control limit
	urea clearance
UCLP	unilateral cleft of lip and palate
UCO	ultrasonic cardiac output
UCOD	underlying cause of death
UCP	uncoupling protein
	urinary coproporphyrin
	urinary C-peptide
UCPT	urinary coproporphyrin test
UCR	unconditioned response

UCR (cont.)	usual, customary, and reasonable (fees)
ucs	unconscious
UCS	unconditioned stimulus
	unconscious
	uterine compression syndrome
UCT	urological care table
uCTD	undifferentiated connective tissue disease
UCTD	undifferentiated (unclassifiable) connective tissue disease
UCU	uracil-cytosine-uracil codon for serine
UCV	uncontrolled variable
ud	as directed
UD	ulcerative dermatosis
	ulnar deviation
	underdeveloped
	undetermined
	unit dose
	urethral dilatation
	urethral discharge
	uridine diphosphate
	uroporphyrinogen decarboxylase
	uterine delivery
UDC	usual diseases of childhood
UDCA	ursodeoxycholic acid
UDH	usual ductal hyperplasia
Udil	urethral dilatation
UDKase	uridine diphosphate kinase
UDN	ulcerative dermal necrosis
UDO	undetermined origin
UDP	uridine diphosphate
UDPG	uridine diphosphate glucose
	urine diphosphoglucose
UDPGA	uridine diphosphate glucuronic acid
UDPGT	uridine diphosphate glucuronosyl transferase
UDR-BMD	ultradistal radius bone mineral density
UDRP	urine diribose phosphate
UDS	ultrasound Doppler sonography
	uniform data system
	unscheduled deoxynucleic acid synthesis
UDUN	under developed under nourished
UE	uncertain etiology
	under elbow
	uninvolved epidermis
	upper esophagus
	upper extremity
uE~	unconjugated estriol
UEG	ultrasonic encephalography
	unifocal eosinophilic granuloma
UEHB	uniform effective health benefits
UEL	upper explosive limit
UEM	universal electron microscope
UEMC	unidentified endosteal marrow cell
UES	upper esophageal sphincter
U+Es	urea and electrolytes
u/ext	upper extremity
UF	film unshapness
	ultrafiltration
	ultrafine
	ultrafiltrate
	ultrasonic frequency
	universal feeder
	unknown factor
	urinary formaldehyd
UFA	unesterified fatty acid
	unifactorial analysis
UFB	urinary fat bodies
UFC	urinary free cortisol
UFD	ultrasonic flow detector
	unilateral facet dislocation
UFFI	urea formaldehyde foam insulation
UFL	upper flammable limit
UFP	ultrafiltration pressure
UFR	ultrafiltration rate
	urine filtration rate
uFSH	urinary follicle-stimulating hormone
UG	geometric unsharpness

UG (cont.) upward gaze
urogastrone
urogenital
UGC uracil-guanine-cytosine codon for cysteine
UGD uniglandular disease
urogenital diaphragm
UGDP University Group Diabetes Project
UGF unidentified growth factor
UGG uracil-guanine-guanine codon for tryptophan
UGH uveitis-glaucoma-hyphema (syndrome)
UGH+ uveitis-glaucoma-hyphema plus vitreous hemorrhage (syndrome)
UGI upper gastrointestinal
upper gastrointestinal series
upper gastrointestinal tract
UGIB upper gastrointestinal biopsy
upper gastrointestinal bleeding
UGIH upper gastrointestinal hemorrhage
UGIS upper gastrointestinal series
UGT uridine diphosphate-glucuronosyltransferase
UGU uracil-guanine-uracil codon for cysteine
UH unfractionated heparin
UH 82 universal billing document (1982)
UHDPE ultra-high-density-polyethylene
UHF ultra high frequency
uterine blood flow
UHMWPE ultra-high molecular weight polyethylene
UICC Union Internationale Contre le Cancer - International Union Against Cancer
UIP usual interstitial pneumonia
UL upper lid
uln ulnar
ULN upper limits of normal
ULQ upper left quadrant
ultra ultrasound
umb. umbilicus (navel)
UMCD uremic medullary cystic disease
UMLS Unified Medical Language System
UMN upper motor neuron (signs)
UNDP United Nations Development Program
UN-E ulnar neuropathy at the elbow
UNFPA United Nations Family Planning Association
ung, ung. ointment
unilat. unilateral
unk unknown
UNK unknown
u/o under observation for
urine output
UO urethral catheter out
urinary catheter out
urinary output
UP ultrafilterable platinum
unipolar
u-PA urokinase-like plasminogen activator
u-PAR, uPA-R urokinase-like plasminogen activator receptor
UPDRS Unified Parkinson's Disease Rating Scale
UPEP urine protein electrophoresis
UPJ ureteropelvic junction
UPOJ University of Pennsylvania Orthopaedic Journal
UPPP uvulopalatopharyngoplasty
UPR unfolded protein response
unipolar recurrent depression
UPr/C urine protein-to-creatinine ratios
UPSI unprotected sexual intercourse
UPT urinary pregnancy test
ur., Ur. urine
Urd uridine
URD ultrarapid opioid detoxification
unrelated donors
upper respiratory disease

U V

URD-BMT unrelated donor bone marrow transplantation
URI upper respiratory tract infection
Urol. urology
URQ upper right quadrant
URTI upper respiratory tract infection
U/S, u/s ultrasound
US ultrasound
USA unstable angina
USAN United States Adopted Names
USDA US Department of Agriculture
USH usual state of health
USI urinary stress incontinence
USN ultrasonic nebulizer
USP US pharmacopeea
USP. United States Pharmacy
USPHA United States Public Health Administration
USPHS United States Public Health Service
USSTC unstimulated short-time cultures
UST ultrasound therapy
UTD up to date
UTI urinary tract infection
UTL unable to locate
UTMDACC University of Texas M. D. Anderson Cancer Center
UTZ ultrasound ultrasonography
UUA uracil-uracil-adenine codon for leucine
urokinase urine activity
UUC uracil-uracil-cytosine codon for phenylalanine
UUG uracil-uracil-guanine codon for leucine
UUN urinary urea nitrogen
UUU uracil-uracil-uracil codon for phenylalanine
UV ultraviolet
UVI ultra violet index
ultraviolet irradiation
ultraviolet laser therapy
ultraviolet light illumination
UVI (cont.) unaided visual inspection
unequal ventilation index
UVJ ureterovesical junction
UVL ultraviolet light
UVR ultra violet radiation
UWUN underweight undernourished

V

V valine
vein
venous invasion
V2 second compartment volume
V3 third compartment volume
VA alveolar volume
valproic acid
ventriculoatrial
Veterans Administration (US)
visual acuity
VAC ventriculoatrial conduction
VACTERL Syndrome: abnormalities of vertebrae, anus, cardiovascular tree, trachea, esophagus, renal system, and limb buds associated with administration of sex steroids during early pregnancy
VaD vascular dementia
VAD ventricular assist device
vincristine, doxorubicin and dexamethasone
VAERS Vaccine Adverse Events Reporting System (FDA)
VAFS vaccine-associated feline sarcoma
vag vaginal(ly)
VAHS virus-associated hemophagocytic syndrome
VAIN vaginal intraepithelial neoplasia
Val valine
VAS vibroacoustic stimulation
visual analogue scale

VATER vertebral defects, anal atresia, tracheoesophageal fistula with esophageal atresia, and radial and renal anomalies
VATS video-assisted thoracic surgery
VB B chain variable (gene segments of T-cell receptor)
vaginal bleeding
VBAC vaginal birth after cesarean
VBD vertebral bone density
VBG venous blood gas
VBH Vogele-Bale-Hohner head holder
VBI vertebrobasilar insufficiency
VC colored vision
vital capacity
VCA viral capsid antigen (in EBV-IM)
VCAM vascular cell adhesion molecule (endothelial cell adhesion molecule)
VCAM-1 vascular cell adhesion molecule 1
VCD vocal cord dysfunction
VCE vaginal administration of conjugated equine estrogens
VCE smear a cytologic smear of material obtained from the vagina, ectocervix, and endocervix
VCFS velocardiofacial syndrome
VCS vasoconstrictor substance
VCU voiding cystourethrogram
VCUG voiding cystourethrogram
Vd void
VD venereal disease
vessel diameter
VD-GC vacuum distillation gas chromatography
VDRL Venereal Disease Research Laboratory (test for syphilis)
VE vaginal examination
VEF ventricular ejection fraction
VEGF vascular endothelial cell growth factor
vent, vent. ventilator
VEP visually evoked potentials
VER visual evoked response
v-erb viral avian erythroblastosis oncogene
vert. vertical
VF ventricular fibrillation
ventricular flutter
visual field
field of vision
VFC Vaccines for Children program
v-fes viral feline sarcoma oncogene
Vfib Ventricular fibrillation
V-fib Ventricular fibrillation
VG vein graft
VH vaginal hysterectomy
variable region of the Ig heavy chain genes
VHA Veterans Health Administration (US)
VHD valvular heart disease
ventricular heart disease
VHL von Hippel-Lindau disease gene (located on chromosome 3p25)
VI volume index
V.I. vaginal irrigation
Via by way of
Vibrio ABE-1 psychrophilic marine bacterium Vibrio sp. strain ABE-1
VIE vincristine, ifosfamide and epirubicin
VIP etoposide, ifosfamide and cisplatin (chemotherapy)
vasoactive intestinal peptide
vasoinhibitory peptide
venous impedance plethysmography
ventricular inotropic parameter
visual impact performance
voluntary interruption of pregnancy

VIPS	voluntary interruption of pregnancy and sterilization service
VISI	volar intercalary wrist instability
vit.	vitamin
VJ	vertical jump
VKH	Vogt-Koyanagi-Harada's disease
VLA-4	very late antigen 4 (adhesion molecule)
VLACS	very long-chain acyl-CoA synthetase
VLDL	very low density lipoprotein
VLH	ventrolateral hypothalamus
VLO	ventrolateral outflow
VM	ventricular muscle
	vestibular membrane
VM-26	Teniposide (anti cancer drug)
VMA	vanillylmandelic acid (urine levels concordant to serum catecholamine levels)
VMCH	Vinyl acetate - maleic acid - vinyl chloride copolymer
VMO	vastus medialis obliquus (a muscle)
	visiting medical officer
VN	visiting nurse
VNS	visiting nurse service
vo	verbal order
VO	verbal order
	voice order
VOD	vision right eye
vol	volume
v-onc	viral oncogene
VOS	vision left eye
VP	venous pressure
VP-16	Etoposide (anti cancer drug)
VPA	valproate
VPC	ventricular premature contractions
VPF	vascular permeability factor
VPL	ventral posterolateral
VPM	ventral posteromedial
VPN	vocational practice nurse
VPPIM	Vinyl polysiloxane putty impression material
VPRC	volume packed red cells
VQ	ventilation/perfusion scan
V/Q	ventilation-perfusion ratio
VRE	vancomycin-resistant enterococcus
vri	vrille (a transcription factor essential for embryonic development)
VRI	variable region I
	vascular resistance index
	venous reflux index
	ventricular response interval
	Veterinary Research Institute
	violence-related injuries
	viral respiratory infection
	vocational rehabilitation index
	volume regulatory increase
VRI-33	fowl adenovirus serotype 8
VRI 86-1	a monoclonal antibody raised against third stage Trichostrongylus colubriformis
VRO	vertical ramus osteotomy
vs	visit
VS	vertical shear
	vs, vital signs
V.S.	vital signs
VSA	vital signs absent
VSD	ventricular septal defect
v-sis	viral simian sarcoma oncogene
VSO	vertical sagittal split osteotomy
VSP	variable screw placement
VSS	vital signs stable
VT	tidal volume
	ventricular tachycardia
V+T	volume and tension (pulse)
V-tach	ventricular tachycardia
VTE	venous thromboembolism
VTEC	verotoxin producing enteropathogenic Escherichia coli
VTNR	vessel-to-tissue noise ratio
VTP	velocity/time profile

VTX vertex
VV varicose veins
VVI fixed-rate ventricular single-chamber systems
VVIR ventricular single-chamber synchronous pacemakers
VWD von Willebrand Disease
VWF von Willebrand factor
Vx. vertex presentation
VZIG varicella-zoster immune globulin
VZV varicella-zoster virus

W

W tryptophan
widowed
white
w/ with
w/a when awake
W/A while awake
WAGR (syndrome) Wilms' tumor, aniridia, genotourinary anomalies, and mental retardation syndrome
WAIS Wechsler Adult Intelligence Scale
Wass. Wassermann
WB Western blot
whole blood
WBAA whole blood acetaldehyde assay
WBAT weight bearing as tolerated
WBBMC whole body bone mineral content
wbc white blood cells
white blood count
w.b.c. white blood cell
white blood count
WBC white blood cell
white blood count
WBGT wet bulb globe temperature
WBS skin wound breaking strength
WBT weight bearing to tolerance
w/c, W/C wheelchair
WC white cells
white collar
whole cell
WC-2 White Carneau pigeons
WCB welders and caulker/burners
wet corn bran
whole canine blood
whole cord blood cells
worker's compensation benefits
workers' compensation board
working cell bank
WCC white cell count
WCGF wet corn gluten feed
WCI Washington Cancer Institute
WC/rCTB whole cell/recombinant B subunit cholera vaccine
WD ward
well-developed
wound
W+D warm and dry
WDE wound dressing emulsion
WDHA watery diarrhea, hypokalemia, and achlorhydria
WDWN well-developed well-nourished
WE, W-E wide excision
WF white female
word fluency
W/F white female
WFL Wistaria floribunda
within functional limits
WG Wegener's granulomatosis
wh, wh. wheelchair
WHO World Health Organization
Whp whirlpool
WIC Special Supplemental Food Program for Women, Infants, and Children
WISC Wechsler Intelligence Scale for Children
wk week(s)
WLD Wulong Dan
WLE wide local excision

WLT Warthin-like papillary carcinoma of the thyroid
W-MPP water MPP (multipurpose phantoms)
WMSH white matter signal hyperintensities
WM white male
Waldenström's macroglobulinemia
W/M white male
WN well-nourished
West Nile virus
w/n within
WNL within normal limits
w/o without
WOA Western Orthopaedic Association
WOC World Orthopaedic Concern
Wow Weakener of white (a locus is described in Drosophila melanogaster that modifies the expression of the white eye color gene)
WOW-1 a novel monovalent ligand-mimetic antibody
WPD warm, pink, dry (skin signs)
WPOA Western Pacific Orthopaedic Association (Australian Chapter)
WPW weighted Play-the-Winner
Wolff-Parkinson-White
WRT with relation to
WSCA Washington State Chiropractic Association
wt, wt. weight
WT-1 Wilms tumor gene (located on chromosome 11p13)
WTO World Trade Organization
w/u workup
w/v weight by volume
WW white woman

X

x times
X cross
except
for (duration)
multiplied by times
times
x/12 x number of months
x/24 x number of hours
x/40 x number of gestation weeks
x/52 x number of weeks
x/7 x number of days
XIP x-ray in plaster
XLD xylose lysine deoxycholate agar
XLPRA X-linked progressive retinal atrophy
XML extensible markup language
XP xeroderma pigmentosa
XR x-ray
XRD x-ray diffraction
XRN X-linked recessive nephrolithiasis
XRT external radiation therapy
radiation therapy
radiotherapy
XT exotropia
XX female sex chromosome
XY male sex chromosome

Y

y	classification after initial multimodal treatment
	year(s)
Y	tyrosine
	Y chromosome
	yttrium, tyrosine, pyrimidine nucleoside
	Yttrium
Y-90	Yttrium 90
YAC	yeast artificial chromosome
YAG	yttrium-aluminum-garnet (laser)
Yb	ytterbium
Yd.	yard
YES	Youth Exchange Scheme
YFEC	Youth Forum of the European Communities
y/o, y.o.	years old
Y/O	years old
yoa	years of age
YOB	year of birth
YPLL	years of potential life lost
yr.	year
Yr	year
yrs.	years
YRBS	Youth Risk Behaviour Survey
YST	Yolk sac tumor
YVS	Yorkshire Veterinary Society (UK)

Z

ZAI	Zero Administrative Initiative
ZAP	zoster associated pain
ZAP-70	tyrosine kinase involved in signal transduction
ZBB	Zero Base Budgeting
ZDF	Zucker diabetic fatty (rat)
ZDV	Zidovudine
ZE	Zollinger-Ellison
ZEEP	zero end-expiratory pressure
ZES	Zollinger-Ellison syndrome
ZFW	Health insurance sickness scheme for employees (Netherlands)
ZIF	Zero Insertion Force
ZIFT	Zygote Intrafallopian Transfer
ZIG	zoster immune globulin
ZIP	Zigzag In-line Package
	Zoster Immune Plasma
ZL	Central Laboratory of Pharmacists (Germany)
Zn	zinc
ZNS	zonisamide
Zr	zirconium
ZSE	Zoological Spongiform Encephalopathy
ZSL	Zoological Society of London
ZSR	zeta sedimentation rate
ZZ	ZZ genotype (deficiency of a 1-antitrypsin)

Symbols

Arrows, Angles

↑	above
	alive
	elevated
	elevation
	enlarged
	gas
	greater than
	high
	improved
	increase
	increased
	more than
	rising
	raised
	superior
	up
	upper
↑g	increasing
	rising
∧	above
	and
	diastolic blood pressure
	elevated
	greater than
	increased
	superior
	upper
↗	deviated
	displaced
	increasing
↓	below
	dead
	decrease
	deficiency
	deficit
	depressed
	depression
	deteriorated
	diminished
	down
	falling
	inferior
	less than
	lower
	lowered
	normal plantar reflex
	precipitate
	restricted
↓g	decreasing
	diminishing
	falling
	lowering
∨	below
	deficiency
	depressed
	inferior
	less than
	systolic blood pressure
↘	decreasing
→	causes
	demonstrates
	direction of flow
	distal
	due to
	followed by
	indicates
	greater than
	leads to
	no change
	produces
	progressing
	radiating to
	results in
	shows
	to
	to the right
	toward
	transfer to
	vector
	yields
←	caused by
	derived from
	direction of flow
	due to
	less than
	produced by
	proximal
	resulting from
	secondary to
	to the left
↔	normal
	same as
	stable
	steady
	unchanging
	widened
	width
↓↓	down bilaterally
	flexor
	plantar response (Babinski sign)
	testes descended
↑↑	extensor
	extensor response (Babinski sign)
	testes undescended
⇌	reversible chemical reaction
	reversible reaction
∠	angle
	flexion
	flexor
Γ	right upper quadrant
L	right lower quadrant
┐	left upper quadrant
┘	left lower quadrant

Marks, Numbers

@	at
‖	parallel
	parallel bars
*	birth
	not verified
	presumed
	supposed
†	dead
	death
	deceased
	died
#	fracture
	gauge
	number
	pound
	weight
/	divided by
	extension
	fraction
	of
	per
	to
:	divided by
	is to
	ratio
√	check
	flexion
	observe for
	urine
	voided
√d	checked
	observed
+	acid reaction
	add
	added to
	and
	convex lens
	excess
	increased
	plus
	positive
	present
(+)	significant
(+)ive	positive
-	absent
	alkaline reaction
	concave lens
	decreased
	deficiency
	minus
	negative
	none
	subtract
	without
(-)	insignificant
-ve	negative
±	doubtful
	equivocal
	indefinite
	more or less
	plus or minus
	positive or negative
	possibly significant
	questionable
	suggestive
	variable
	with or without
(±)	possibly significant
=	equal
	equal to
≠	not equal to
≡	identical
	identical with
~	about
	approximate
	difference
	proportionate to
	similar
≃	approximately equal to
	similar or equal
≈	approximately equal to
	nearly equal
>	causes
	greater than
	left ear-bone conduction threshold
	more severe than
	worse than
≥	greater than or equal to
≯	not greater than
<	caused by
	less severe than
	less than
	right ear-bone conduction threshold
≤	less than or equal to
≮	not less than
∴	therefore
∵	because
	since
∷	as
	proportionate to
°	degree
	hour
	severity of burns
	severity of wounds
	temperature
′	foot
	minute
	univalent
″	bivalent
	ditto
	inch
	second
Ø	no
	none
	without
♥	heart
?	doubtful
	not tested
	possible
	questionable
	question of

	suggested
	unknown
0	completely absent (pulse)
	no contraction (musc.)
	no response (reflexes)
1°	first degree
	one hour
	primary
1+	low normal reflexes
	markedly impaired pulse
1x	once
1:1	one-to-one
2°	because of
	due to
	secondary
	second degree
	two hours
2+	average reflexes
	moderately impaired pulse
2x	twice
3°	tertiary
	third degree
	three hours
3+	brisk reflexes
	slightly impaired pulse
3x	three times
4+	normal pulse
	very brisk reflexes

Greek Symbols

α	alpha particle
	angular acceleration
	proportional to
	optical rotation
	prefix (first in a series)
α-CD	alpha-chain disease
α-GLUC	alpha-glucosidase
α-LP	alpha-lipoprotein
β	beta particle
	prefix (second in a series)
	photon
β-2m	beta2 microglobulin
γ	done
	globulin
	plasma protein
	prefix (third in a series)
γ-G	immunglobulin G
γ-HCDT	gamma heavy chain disease
Δ	anion gap
	change
	delta gap
	diagnosis
	heat
	increment
	sulfur
	temperature
Δ A	change in absorbance
Δ dB	change in decibels
Δ p	change in pressure
Δ pH	change in pH
Δ t	time interval
δ	prefix (fourth in a series)
ε	dielectric constant
η	absolute viscosity
	dynamic velocity
θ	negative (theta)
	temperature interval
κ	magnetic susceptibility
λ	homosexuality
	junction of lambdoid and sagittal sutures
	wavelength
μ	micro (10^{-6})
	mutation rate
	statistical mean
μA	microampere
μb	microbar
μg	microgram
μL	microliter
μm	micrometer
μs	microsecond
μV	microvolt
μW	microwatt
ν	frequency (nu)
π	3.1416
	osmotic pressure
ρ	correlation coefficient
	electric charge density
	mass density
Σ	foaminess
	sigmoid
	sum of
	summary
	syphilis
σ	conductivity
	difference
	standard deviation
	stress
	surface tension
	wave number
σ^2	variance (normal distribution)
τ	life (drug, radioactive isotope)
	mean life
	relaxation time
	transmisison coefficient
τ1/2	half-life (drug, radioactive isotope)
ϕ	phenyl (phi)
	thyroid
χ^2	chi-square (statistical test)
Ψ	psychiatric (psi)
ψ	pseudo
ω	angular frequency/velocity

Circles, Rectangles

- ○ female; living female; respiration; right ear-masked air conduction threshold
- ● affected female; deceased female; pulse rate
- □ brother; father; left ear-masked air conduction threshold; living male; male; son
- ■ affected male; deceased male
- ◇ sex unknown

- Ⓐ axilla (temperature)
- (IM) intramuscular
- (IV) intravenous
- Ⓛ left
- Ⓜ by mouth; murmur; oral
- Ⓞ by mouth; oral
- Ⓡ rectal; rectum; right

- ⊙ annual; gold; start of operation; sun
- ⊗ end of anesthesia; end of operation
- ⊖ normal
- ♀ copper; female; female sex
- ♂ male; male sex

Positions

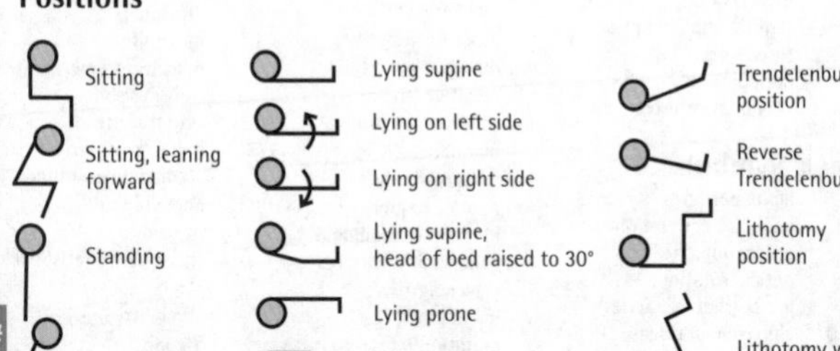

Roman Numbers

I	i	1	**XVII**	17	**C**	100
II	ii	2	**XVIII**	18	**CI**	101
III	iii	3	**XIX**	19	**CL**	150
IIII	iiii	4	**XX**	20	**CC**	200
IV	iv	4	**XXIII**	23	**CD**	400
V	v	5	**XXIV**	24	**D**	500
VI	vi	6	**XXVII**	27	**DC**	600
VII	vii	7	**XXVIII**	28	**M**	1000
VIII	viii	8	**XXXIX**	29	**MDLVIII**	1558
IX	ix	9	**XXX**	30	**MDCXXV**	1625
X	x	10	**XL**	40	**MDCCCIV**	1804
XI	xi	11	**L**	50	**MCM**	1900
XII	xii	12	**LIX**	59	**MCMLXII**	1962
XIII	xiii	13	**LX**	60	**MIM**	1999
XIV	xiv	14	**LXX**	70	**MM**	2000
XV	xv	15	**LXXX**	80		
XVI	xvi	16	**XC**	90		

Greek Letters

Α	α	alpha	Ι	ι	iota	Ρ	ρ	rho
Β	β	beta	Κ	κ	kappa	Σ	σ	sigma
Γ	γ	gamma	Λ	λ	lambda	Τ	τ	tau
Δ	δ	delta	Μ	μ	mu	Υ	υ	upsilon
Ε	ε	epsilon	Ν	ν	nu	Φ	ϕ	phi
Ζ	ζ	zeta	Ξ	ξ	xi	Χ	χ	chi
Η	η	eta	Ο	ο	omicron	Ψ	ψ	psi
Θ	θ	theta	Π	π	pi	Ω	ω	omega

Phonetic Alphabet

	NATO	Old US
A	Alfa	Abel
B	Bravo	Baker
C	Charlie	Charlie
D	Delta	Dog
E	Echo	Easy
F	Foxtrot	Fox
G	Golf	George
H	Hotel	How
I	India	Item
J	Juliet	Jig
K	Kilo	King
L	Lima	Love
M	Mike	Mike
N	November	Nan
O	Oscar	Oboe
P	Papa	Peter
Q	Quebec	Queen
R	Romeo	Roger
S	Sierra	Sugar
T	Tango	Tare
U	Uniform	Uncle
V	Victor	Victor
W	Whisky	William
X	X-ray	X-ray
Y	Yankee	Yoke
Z	Zulu	Zebra

Sign Language

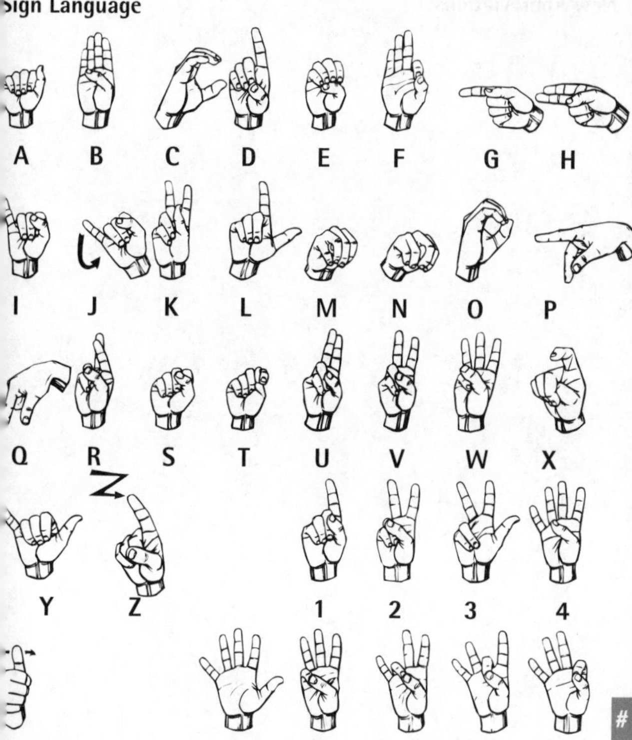

#

New Abbreviations

New Abbreviations

New Abbreviations

New Abbreviations

#

Index

A

Aarskog-Scott syndrome 7
abbreviated 8
abbreviation 8
- three letter 162
abdere abdomen 9
abdomen 9
- adhere 9
- left upper quadrant 102
- right lower quadrant 144
- surgery upper 169
abdominal 8, 9, 20
- aortic aneurysm 5
- circumference 10
- hysterectomy 15
- hysterectomy, total 159
- sonography emergent 67
- trauma blunt 29
- X-ray 28
abdominal series
- acute 7
abducens nucleus 9
abduction 9
abductor
- pollicis 14
- pollicis brevis 10, 21
- pollicis longus 10, 22
- vocal cord paralysis, bilateral 29
abductors
- dorsal 56
Abelson virus transformed 25
aberrant
- ventricular conduction 26
aberration
- chromosomal 37
ablation
- nephropathy 9
- radiofrequency 143
able to work 27
abnormal 8, 9
- cannabidiol 10
- glucose tolerance test 15
- uterine bleeding 25
- vasopressin 27
abnormalities
- asymptomatic urinary 25
- intraretinal microvascular 94
- myelo-vertebral 114
- no apparent 114
- no significant 120
abnormality 9
- chromosome, of a 9
- electrophysiological 66
abnormally
- contracting region 12
abortion 8
- elective 66
- incomplete 92
- inevitable 92
- living, full term premature 75
- septic 151
- spontaneous 149
about 180
above 179
- elbow (cast), long 98
- knee 17, 18
- knee amputation 18
- the elbow 14
- the knee (amputation) 18
- waist 27
abrupt withdrawal 27
Abrus precatorius agglutinin 21
abscess
- tubo-ovarian 163
abscissic acid 8
absence
- genetic, epilepsy rat 77
- of excretion, unilateral 168
- of pulmonary, unilateral 169
- of skin, congenital localized 46
absent 10, 180
- completely 181
- vital signs 174
absolute
- basophil count 8
- bone conduction 8
- catabolic rate 12
- error, median 103
- neutrophil count 19
- retention time 23
- viscosity 181
absorbance
- change 181
absorbed radiation dose 56
absorbent cover dressing 10
absorptiometry
- dual energy X-ray 65
absorption
- rate (MRI), specific 149
- test, conglutinating complement 40
- test, fluorescent treponemal antibody 76
- total solute 165
- unsharpness 168
abstinence syndrome 7
abuse
- intravenous drug 95
- polysubstance 138
abvolt 26
academic
- aptitude test 7
- health care 15
- health center 15
acalculous biliary colic 8
acantholysis
- focal suprabasal 76
accelerated
- fracture healing system, sonic 149
- ventricular rhythm 27
acceleration
- angular 181
- mean orthostatic 110
- time 13
acceleromyography 19
acceptable daily intake 14
acceptance quality level 22
access
- fixed scheduled 76
- multiple module 109
- permit 21
accessory
- conduction pathway 12
- pathway 21
accident 10
- automobile 7
- cerebrovascular 55
- date 55
- motor vehicle 114

- road traffic 147
accidental
- hypothermia 15
- incurred 17
- injury 17
accidentally
- incurred 88
accommodation 10
according to circumstances 138
according to custom 25
account
- flexible spending 76
- medical materials 109
accountable health plan 16
accounts payable 21
accuracy
- relative standard 146
Ace bandage 8
acetabular
- prosthesis, threaded titanium 166
acetaldehyde
- assay, whole blood 175
acetaminophen 11, 21
acetazolamide 13
acetone
- butanol-ethanol 9
acetyl
- aminofluorene 5
- choline 11
- choline, receptor 11
- ethyleneimine 14
- L-tyrosine ethyl ester 19
- salicylic acid 23
Achard-Thiers syndrome 25
achievement
- check list 11
- counseling, treatment 13
achilles tendon 24
- reflex 24
- reflex test 23
acid
- agropinic 15
- aspiration syndrome 7
- balance control 8
- base equilibrium 9
- base ratio 8
- citrate-dextrose 10
- deficient, linoleic 98
- detergent fiber 14
- dodecanedioic 58
- equivalent ceftiofur free 43
- fast bacilli 14
- homocysteic 84
- mesoxalic 110
- mevalonic 114
- mevinolinic 114
- N-acetylneuraminic 115
- N-acetylneuraminic, storage disorders 120
- output maximal 104
- phosphatase 12, 21
- phosphatase, prostate-specific 12
- phosphate 11
- reaction 180
- test solution 25
- uric 168
acid-fast 14
acidic
- cytokeratin 45
- fibroblast growth factor 15
- protein, glial fibrillary 78
acidification
- defect, tubular renal 147
acidosis
- chronic metabolic 48
- renal tubular 147
acids
- crystalline amino 38
aciduria
- mevalonic 114
acinar parenchyma 21
aconite-belladonna-chloroform 8
acoustic 12
- canal, internal 88
- microscope, scanning laser 153
- window, occipital 121
- window, temporal 160
acoustics 12
acquired
- hepatocellular degeneration 15
- hepatocerebral degeneration 15
- hypertrichosis lanuginosa 16
- immune deficiency syndrome 85
- immune deficiency syndrome with Kaposi's sarcoma 18
- immune deficiency syndrome with opportunistic infection 18
- immune deficiency syndrome, beliefs and behavior questionnaire 8
- immunodeficiency disease 17
- immunodeficiency syndrome 18
- valvular disease 26
- valvular heart disease 26
- valvular heart syndrome 26
acquisition
- multigated 113
acral
- pseudolymphomatous angiokeratoma of childhood 21
acriflavine 12
acrocallosal syndrome 13
acrocephalopolysyndactyly 12
acrocephalosyndactyly 13
acromioclavicular joint 10, 11
acronym
- three letter 162
acrylic 12
actin 13
- depolymerizing factor 14
- filamentous 72
actinomycin 13
- vincristine-Platinol 27
action
- democracy 13
- potential 21
- potential, compound muscle (or motor) 48
- potentials, motor unit 113
activated
- clotting time 13
- protein C 21
activating
- factor, smooth muscle 154
activation
- maximal voluntary 113
- protein(s), fatty acid 72

- site, upstream 169
active 13, 14
- antiretroviral therapy, highly 83
- assertive range of motion 7
- assisted range of motion 7
- avoidance reaction 7
- bilaterally 8
- bulimia nervosa (BN) 9
- hepatitis, chronic 38
- hostility index 16
- ingredient 17
- motion 13
- motion, total 159
- pepsin 21
- range of motion 23
- resistance 22
- resistance, exercise 22
- substance, compact colony-forming 41
- vasodilator 26
activities 84
activities, daily living 14
activity 13
- antibacterial 8
- before exercise 9
- colony-stimulating 53
- electrical 66
- electrical control 67
- electrical response 70
- focal epileptic 74
- growth-promoting 81
- index, physical 127
- interval, uterine 168
- of antiactivator in plasma 5
- osteoclast resorption stimulating 125
- phagocytic 127
- pulseless electrical 130
- regular spiking 146
- relative specific 146
- surfactant-like 153
- sympathetic nerve 155
- thyroxine-specific 165
- unit uterine 169
- vector analysis 26
- water 27
actual
- base excess 9
- body weight 10
acuity
- mesopic visual 114
- visual 172
acute 10
- anterior uveitis 7
- articular rheumatism 7
- bacterial endocarditis 9
- bacterial exacerbations of chronic bronchitis 9
- bacterial nephritis 9
- brachial neuritis 9
- brachial neuropathy 9
- cardiovascular disease 13
- cerebrospinal meningitis 11
- cervical sprain 13
- cervical strain 13
- cervical trauma syndrome 13
- chest syndrome 13
- conditioned neurosis ventilation 11
- confusional state 13
- coronary insufficiency 11
- coronary occlusion 12
- disseminated encephalomyelitis 14
- disseminated encephalopathy 14
- fatty liver of pregnancy 15
- flaccid paralysis 15
- glomerulonephritis 15
- granulocytic leukemia 15
- hazardous events (database) 15
- heart disease 15
- heart failure 15
- hemolytic uremic (syndrome) 17
- hemorrhagic conjunctivitis 15
- hemorrhagic cystitis 15
- hemorrhagic encephalomyelitis 15
- hemorrhagic leukoencephalitis 16
- hemorrhagic pancreatitis 16
- hepatitis 15
- herpetic gingival stomatitis 16
- hypoxemic respiratory failure 16
- infectous disease 17
- intensive treatment 18
- interstitial pneumonia 18
- ionization detector 17
- laryngotracheobronchitis 19
- left ventricular failure 19
- leukemia, hypocellular 83
- life-threatening event 19
- lumbar strain 19
- lumbar trauma syndrome 19
- lymphoblastic leukemia 18
- lymphoblastic leukemia antigen, common 38
- lymphoblastic leukemia, B-cell 28
- lymphocytic leukemia 18
- motor axonal neuropathy 19
- motor sensory axonal neuropathy 19
- myeloblastic leukemia 19
- myelogenous leukemia 19
- myocardial infarction 19
- necrotizing hemorrhagic encephalopathy 19
- nerve irritation 20
- non-lymphocytic leukemia 20
- otitis media 20
- otitis media with effusion 123
- pancreatitis 21
- peritoneal dialysis 21
- phase 20
- pneumonia 21
- proliferative 21
- renal failure 22
- respiratory disease 22
- respiratory distress syndrome 22
- respiratory failure 22
- retinal necrosis bilateral 29
- rheumatic fever 22
- tubular necrosis 24
- ulcerative gingivitis 25
- undifferentiated leukemia 25

- upper gastrointestinal hemorrhage 25
- vasomotor nephropathy 27
- viral hepatitis 26
- viral respiratory infection 27

acyl carrier protein 12
ad usum 25
adaptation
- spike frequency 151

add 180
added to 180
addiction 14
adduct 14
adduction 14
adductors
- palmar 127

adenine 5
adeno-associated virus 7
adenocarcinoma 14, 18
- infiltrating pancreatic ductal 93
- ovarian papillary serous 124

adenomas
- hepatic cell 84

adenomatosis
- colon, rectum 12
- multiple endocrine 105

adenomatous polyposis 21
- coli 21
- familial 73

adenosine diphosphate 14
adenosyl homocysteine 15
adenylate
- cyclase-stimulating activity 13
- cyclase-stimulating protein 13

adhesion molecule
- E-selectin (on endothelial cell) 69
- intercellular 89
- L-selectin 98
- on endothelial cells and platelets 138
- platelet endothelial cell 130

adhesion regulator
- cell matrix 48

adipose
- tissue, brown 29
- tissue, middle subcutaneous 112

adiposity index 17
adjacent 14
adjoining 14
adjunct 14
adjust 14
adjusted
- annual per capita cost 6
- average per capita cost 6
- community rate 12

adjustment
- facility, enhanced structural 70

adjuvant chemotherapy 14
administration department
- corporate services 53

administrative
- initiative, zero 177

admission 14
- date 56
- discharge 13
- discharge-transfer 14
- hospital 83

admitting
- diagnosis 13
- room 22

adolescent
- idiopathic scoliosis 18
- psychiatry 21

adrenal
- androgen stimulating hormone 7
- cortex 10
- hyperplasia, congenital lipoid 46
- insufficiency, primary chronic 128

adrenarche
- idiopathic premature 93

adrenocortical polypeptide 12
adrenocorticotropic
- hormone 13
- hormone receptor 13

adrenocorticotropin
- like immunoreactivity 13

adriamycin 14
- and vincristine 26
- cyclophosphamide, methotrexate 11

adult
- basic education programs 9
- caucasian 37
- children 10
- children of alcoholics 12
- congregate living facility 11
- disease 13
- female 14
- female, caucasian 38
- granulosa cell tumor 15
- Intelligence Scale, Wechsler 175
- male 19
- male, Caucasian 38
- medically indigent 107
- onset diabetes mellitus 14, 20
- respiratory distress syndrome 22
- T-cell leukemia 24
- T-cell lymphoma 24
- tetanus toxoid 161
- thymectomy 25

advanced
- breast cancer 8
- cardiac life support 11
- collapse (wrist), scapholunate 153
- coronary treatment 13
- life support 19
- life support, pediatric 127
- nurse practitioners 20
- pediatric life support 22
- registered nurse practitioner 22
- trauma life support 24

adverse
- clinical event, major 103
- drug reaction 14
- effect 14
- effect level, no observable 118
- event 14
- event, serious 149
- reaction, suspected 149

advice
- against medical 19

advised 14

advisor
- medical 103
aerosol pentamidine 21
aerospace medicine 19
afferent pupillary defect
- relative 142
affinity
- electric 66
aflatoxicol 15
- M1 15
aflatoxin 14
African
- American 5
- horse sickness 16
- swine fever 23
after 127
- hyperpolarization 16
- meals 128
- parturition 21
afterdepolarization
- early 67
aftereffect
- motion 103
afternoon 133
against
- all risks 7
- medical advice 19
agar
- bacteroides bile esculin 30
- cefotoxin-cycloserine fructose 41
- cystine-lactose-electrolyte-deficient 46
- eosin methylene blue 69
- Hektoen enteric 84
- Kliger iron 97
- medium, Mueller-Hinton 107
- salmonella-shigella 157
- sorbitol MacConkey 154
- standard method 154
- tellurite, taurocholate, and gelatin 166
- triple sugar iron 165
- triple sugar urea 166
- trypticase-soy 165
- xylose lysine deoxycholate 176
age
- bone 28
- chronological 37
- educational 66
- mental 103
- standardized rate 24
agent
- chimpanzee coryza 40
- echocontrast 67
- mycoplasma removal 111
agglutination
- assay, granulocyte 77
- chick cell 40
- slide latex 153
- test, antilactoferrin latex bead 100
- test, chick cell 40
- test, tube slide 165
agglutinin
- abrus precatorius 21
- isolated 114
- Marasmius oreades 110
- ricinus communis 142
- sambucus nigra 155
aggravation 15
aggregated
- human gammaglobulin 16
- human globulin 16
- human IgG 17
aggregates
- multivesicular 114
aggregation
- half time 17
- index 17
aggressive
- systemic mastocytosis 23
agnogenic
- myeloid metaplasia 19
- myeloid metaplasia with myelofibrosis 19
agonist
- carbachol, cholinergic 41
agropinic acid 15
aid
- first 72
aid to the blind 8
AIDS
- dementia complex 14
- related complex 22
air
- adsorption, high-efficiency particulate 84
- and bone conduction 8
- at atmospheric pressure 6
- at high pressure 16
- conduction 10
- dose 65
- evacuation, medical 103
- expired 66
- greater than bone (conduction) 8
- velocity 26
- velocity index 26
airflow
- obstruction, chronic 38
- resistance, nasal 119
airway 27
- breathing, circulation 8
- disease, chronic obstructive 49
- disease, reactive 142
- obstruction, upper 168
- pressure, biphasic intermittent positive 32
- pressure, continuous positive 50
- pressure, distal 56
- pressure, positive end 130
- resistance, upper 169
- wall temperature 160
airways
- upper 168
alanine 5, 18
- aminotransferase 7, 18, 19
- codon 78
- transaminase 18
albendazole 18
Albright
- Butler-Bloomberg syndrome 8
- hereditary osteodystrophy 16
albumin 18
- calcium-magnesium 11
- egg 66
- estradiol bound to 9
- excretion, urine 168
- formaldehyde-treated 76
- globulin ratio 15

- guinea pig 81
- human serum 87
alcian blue 8
alcohol 18, 20
- and drug abuse data system 13
- blood 28
- concentration, blood 28
- consumption, early detection 68
- ethylene-vinyl 71
- fixative, polyvinyl 140
- level, blood 28
- on breath 20
- phenylethyl 130
- use disorders identification test 25
- useilnventory 25
- users 25
- withdrawal 27
alcoholic
- abstinence syndrome 7
- ketoacidosis 18
- liver disease 18
alcoholics
- anonymous 5
- screening test, children 38
Alcon closure system 13
aldolase
- fructose-six phosphate 76
aldosterone
- urinary 168
alert 6, 12, 20
- and orientated 20
- verbal, painful, unresponsive 27
alert and oriented 20
alertness behavior 8
alfalfa mosaic virus 19
algoneurodystrophy 19
algorithm
- ray tracing 147
alimentary papilloma virus
- bovine 29
alimentation
- enteral 66
alive 19, 179
- and well 27
alkaline
- phosphatase 18, 21
- phosphatase, bacterial 28
- phosphatase, leukocyte 98
- protease inhibitor, barley 28
- reaction 180
alkalinity
- water titration 160
alkali-treated bound niacin 9
alkylating agent therapy 7
all
- parameters rechecked 129
- subjects treated 24
Allan-Herndon-Dudley syndrome 15
Allen vision test 27
allergen
- group IX, Poa pratensis 135
allergenic
- unit 25
allergic
- alveolitis, extrinsic 66
- autoimmune neuritis, experimental 67
- bronchopulmonary aspergillosis 8, 10
- contact dermatitis 10
- contact dermatitis, eczematous 67
- encephalomyelitis, experimental 67
- vasculitis 26
allergies 19
allergy 18
- and immunology 17
- cow's milk 48
- relief medicine 22
allogeneic
- stem-cell transplantation 18
allophycocyanin 21
allotransplantation
- total small intestine 165
all-trans-retinoic acid 24
allylisopropylacetamide 17
allyloxycarbonyl 18
alpha
- 1-antitrypsin 7
- 2,6 sialyltransferase 19
- 2HS-glycoprotein 16
- 2-macroglobulin 19
- 2u-globulin 25
- amylase 2 19
- amylase subtilisin inhibitor 29
- chain, disease 181
- D-glucose pentaacetate 15
- fetoprotein 15
- glucosidase 181
- hydrazine analog, histidine 16
- hydroxybutyric acid 15
- keto acid dehydrogenase, branched-chain 31
- L-arabinofuranosidases 9
- lipoprotein 181
- methyl-p-tyrosine 18
- particle 181
- particles, kinetic energy 66
- synuclein 23
- thalassemia-mental retardation 24
- Z polypeptide. guanosine nucleotide-binding 80
also known as 18
alternate 19
- hours 19
- site-testing 24
alternating
- current 10
- days 13
alternative
- birth center 8
- level of care 18
altitude 19
alum
- blood and charcoal 8
- blood and clay 8
- precipitated 21
aluminum tartrate 19
alumni
- porous 18
alveolar
- capillary membrane 11
- capillary membrane permeability 11
- concentration, minimum 103
- hypoventilation syndrome 16
- macrophage, human 83
- macrophages 19
- oxygen 127

- volume 172
- wall 27
- wall basement membrane 27
alveolectomy and odontectomy 121
alveolitis
- extrinsic allergic 66
alveolo-arterial
- carbon dioxide tension difference 6
- oxygen tension 6
- oxygen tension difference 7
Alzheimer
- amyloid precursor protein 22
- disease 13
- disease, assessment scale 14
ambient
- temperature and pressure saturated 24
ambulate 19
ambulating 19
ambulation 19
ambulatory 19
- acute care unit 13
- Holter monitor 16
- peritoneal dialysis, continuous 38
- surgery unit 24
- venous pressure 27
- visit group 26
American
- standard test method 24
amine
- precursor uptake and decarboxylation 22
amino
- acid, branched chain 30
- acid, carrier, excitatory 66
- acid, decarboxylase 5
- acid, essential 66
- acid, excitatory 66
- acid, pool, free 72
- acid, sequence 7
- acids, crystalline 38
- adipic acid 5
- antipyrine 6
- benzamide 8
- benzoate 9
- cyclopentane carboxylic acid 12
- ethyl carbazol 14
- ethylisothiouronium bromide hydrobromide 14
- imidazole, carboxamide 17
- imidazole, carboxamide ribonucleotide 17
- isobutyrate 17
- isobutyric acid 17
- peptidase 21
- phenylphosphorylcholine 22
- purine 20
- terminal fragment 24
- transferase, alanine 18, 19
amiodarone neuropathy 20
Ammon's horn 38
amnesia
- transient global 161
amniocentesis 19
amnion
- deficit, spectrum 67
- deficit, syndrome 67
amniotic
- fluid 14
- fluid cortisol 14
- fluid index 15
amount 19
ampere 19
ampere/volt 26
amphetamine 19
- induced locomotion 18
Amplatzer
- septal occluder 23
amplification
- protocol, telomeric repeat 164
amplifier
- endocardio graphic 66
amplitude
- clipping, infinite 88
ampoule 19
amputation 19
- above elbow 14
- above knee 18
- below knee 33
- knee bearing 97
- transmetatarsal 163
amygdala
- medical 103
amygdalohippocampal complexes 15
amylase
- alpha 19
- inhibitor activity 17
- urinary 168
amylogenesis imperfecta 17
amyloid
- angiopathy, cerebral 38
- beta 9
- beta-peptides 24
- of unknown origin 25
- p-component 21
- precursor protein 22
- precursor protein, cytoplasmic tail 22
amyloidosis
- idiopathic 18
- reactive 5
amyotrophic lateral sclerosis 19
ana 5
anaerobic
- digestion test, high solids 87
- system, membrane 104
anaesthetic/anesthesia
- general 77
anal
- sphincter 23
analgesia
- electroacupuncture 66
- patient controlled 128
analgesic 19
analicular
- system, open 122
analogue
- scale, visual 172
analyser
- defibrillation systems 63
analysis
- automated image 17
- error grid 69
- frozen section 76
- full-spectrum data 76
- gastric 77
- medical management 109
- multiple correspondence 104
- multivariate 114

- of variance 20
- program, F-actin image 72
- protonic magnetic resonance 134
- recursive partitioning 145
- roentgenographic stereogrammetric 146
- sequential multiple 154
- solid-phase microextraction, mass spectrometry, and multivariate 157
- unifactorial 170
- urine 168

analytic
- hierarchy process 16

analytical
- system, oak ridge 124

analyzer
- blood color 30
- sequential multiple 154

anaphase
- first meiotic 17

anaphylatoxin inactivator 17

anaphylaxis inhibition
- passive cutaneous 128

anaplastic
- astrocytomas / oligodendrogliomas 5
- large cell 18
- lymphoma kinase 18

anastomosis
- arteriovenous 26
- diamond-shaped, duodenoplasty 57
- entero 66
- microvascular 114
- ring, biofragmentable 29

anatomic
- diagnosis, preliminary 127

and 71, 179, 180

androgen
- binding protein 10
- stimulating hormone 7

anemia 5
- chronic disease 10
- congenital dyserythropoietic 43
- congenital hypoplastic 44
- Fanconi's 72
- hemolytic 83
- iron deficiency 90
- microangiopathic hemolytic 103, 107
- pernicious 127
- refractory 142
- with excess blasts, refractory 142

anesthesia 19
- continuous lumbar epidural 46
- intravenous regional 96
- local 98
- post, recovery unit 128

aneuploidy
- mosaic variegated 114

aneurysm
- abdominal aortic 5
- of atrial septum 7

aneurysmal
- bone bone cyst, aneurysmal 8

angina
- microvascular 114
- pectoris 20, 21
- pectoris, unstable 169
- unstable 168, 172

angiocardiography 11

angiogenesis inhibitor 17

angiography
- digital substraction 63
- magnetic resonance 111
- quantitative coronary 140
- screen-film 151
- stepping digital subtraction 150
- three-dimensional magnetic resonance 61

angioimmunoblastic lymphadenopathy 18

angiokeratoma
- of childhood, acral pseudolymphomatous 21

angiopathy
- cerebral amyloid 38

angioplasty
- balloon catheter 30
- multiple vessel 114
- percutaneous transluminal 139
- percutaneous transluminal coronary 139

angiotensin 17
- converting enzyme 10
- converting enzyme inhibitors 10
- I, converting enzyme 17

angle 19, 179
- center-edge 43
- costovertebral 55
- greatest flexion 15
- min of visual 113
- minimum audible 103
- minimum visible 114
- of aorta 20
- radiograph 43

Angstrom
- unit 25

angular
- acceleration 181
- frequency 181
- velocity 181

anion
- binding exosite 9
- gap 15, 181

anisotropy
- chemical shift 53

ankle
- foot orthoses 15
- jerk 18
- platform system, biomechanical 28
- to brachial index 9

ankylosing spondylitis 23

annulus fibrosis 20

anodal
- closure contraction 10
- closure odor 12
- closure sound 13
- closure tetanus 13

anode
- break excitation 9

anomalies
- extra-cardiac structural or karyotypic 67

anomalous pulmonary venous connection
- total 159

anomaly
- branchial cleft 30
anonymous
- alcoholics 5
anosmia 16
antacid of choice 6
ante
- cenam 10
- partum 20, 21
anteflexed 26
anterior 20
- and posterior 21
- aortic wall 8
- auditory field 5
- axillary line 5
- BNST lesions 9
- capsulolabral reconstruction 11
- cervical discectomy 10
- cervical discectomy and fusion 10
- cervical fusion 10
- chamber 10
- cingulate cortex 10
- clavicular line 11
- communicating artery 12
- cruciate ligament 11
- descending (coronary artery), left 98
- descending artery 13
- dynamized system 14
- fascicular block, left 98
- hypothalamic preoptic area 16
- inferior cerebellar artery 17
- inferior communicating artery 17
- inferior iliac spine 18
- interosseous nerve 18
- ischemic optic neuropathy 18
- lateral myocardial infarction 18
- medullary velum 19
- nasal discharge 19
- pituitary 21
- pituitary hormone 22
- polar cataract 21
- spinal fusion 23
- spinal/scoliosis system, Kaneda 97
- superior spine 24
- tibial 24
- urethral valve 25
- uveitis 25
- wall 27
- wall of aortic root 27
antero
- colic transposition 13
- lateral, rotatory instability 19
- lateral, sclerosis 19
- medial 19
- posterior 21
- posterior and lateral 22
- posterior compression 21
- posterior diameter 21
- ventral 26
- ventral, cochlear nucleus 26
- ventral, third ventricle 27
anteroposterior 20
anteversion 26
anteverted 26
anthrax
- anti serum 7
anthrylvinyl-labeled phosphatidylcholine 22
antiactivator
- in plasma, activity 5
anti-alkaline phosphatase 21
anti-arteriosclerosis polysaccharide factor 6
antibacterial
- activity 8
anti-basement membrane antibody disease 9
antibiotic 8, 10
- associated pseudo-membranous colitis 6
- associated pseudomembranous colitis 6
- oral 124
antibodies
- antineutrophil cytoplasmic 19
- cytoplasmic antineutrophil cytoplasmic 38
- hepatitis associated 83
- maternal derived 103, 105
- monoclonal 110
- perinuclear antineutrophil cytoplasmic 127
antibody 8
- absorption test, fluorescent treponemal 76
- against Ki-67 107
- anticardiolipin 11
- anti-Forssman glycolipid 75
- anti-immunoglobulin 17
- anti-insulin 17
- anti-microphthalmia transcription factor 55
- antimitochondrial 19
- antinuclear 19
- antiviral 26
- dependent cell-mediated cytotoxicity 14
- disease, anti-basement membrane 9
- embryonic 66
- erythrocyte 66
- fluorescent 72
- human bladder carcinoma 32
- nitrogen 9
- novel monovalent ligand-mimetic 176
- sheep erythrocyte 153
- smooth muscle 154
- test, direct fluorescent 59
- test, fluorescent antinuclear 73
- testing, direct 56
- tetanus toxoid 166
- thyroid-stimulating 165
- titer, heterophil 83
- type-specific 165
anticardiac myosin 11
anticardiolipin 11
antichymotrypsin 13
anticipatory vomiting 26
anticoagulant therapy 13
anticonstipation regimen 12
antidepressant
- tricyclic 160
antidiuretic
- hormone 14
- hormone, inappropriate secretion 88

- hormone, syndrome, inappropriate secretion 88
antidromic potential 21
anti-Forssman glycolipid antibody 75
antigen 15
- 1 100
- 1-lymphocyte function-associated 100
- antiglobulin reaction 7
- Australia 25
- australia 25
- australia hepatitis-associated 25
- basal-cell 30
- binding 8
- binding, capacity 8
- breast cancer 30
- carcinoembryonic 43
- cell surface 53
- cephalin cholesterol 40
- circulating cathodic 40
- common acute lymphoblastic leukemia 38
- enterobacterial common 67
- Epstein-Barr nuclear 67
- fibroblast specific 76
- Goodpasture 81
- hepatitis B surface 83
- human leukocyte 86
- human leukocyte associated 86
- lymphocyte function-associated 100
- polysaccharide egg 130
- presenting cells 21
- proliferating cell nuclear 129
- prostate-specific 138
- protein, invasion plasmid 93
- small intestinal mucinous 152
- soluble liver 153
- squamous cell carcinoma 150
- toxic shock 165
- toxoplasmin skin test 166
- tumor specific transplantation 166
- tumor surface 165
- tumor-specific 165
- tumor-specific cell surface 166
- tumor-specific tissue 166
- undenaturated bacterial 169
- viral capsid 173
antiheart muscle autoantibody 16
antihemophilic
- factor 16
- factor C 15
- globulin 16
- globulin factor 16
antihuman
- gammaglobulin 16
- globulin 16
- lymphocyte globulin 16
- lymphocyte serum 16
- thymocyte globulin 17
- thymocyte plasma 17
- thymus serum 17
antihyaluronidase 15
- reaction 16
- titer 17
antihypertensive drug 15
anti-immunoglobulin antibody 17
anti-inflammatory
- drugs, non-steroidal 120
anti-insect agent 117
antiinsulin
- antibody 17
- serum, guinea pig 81
anti-isoleucyl-tRNA synthetase 20
antilactoferrin
- latex bead agglutination test 100
antimicrobial
- susceptibility testing 24
anti-microphthalmia transcription factor antibody 55
antimitochondrial
- antibody 19
antineutrophil
- cytoplasmic antibodies 19
- cytoplasmic antibodies, perinuclear 127
antinuclear
- antibody 19
- antibody test, fluorescent 73
antiparkinsonian drugs
- anti-cholinergic 21
antiprogesterone used for abortion in early gestation 148
antipyrine 21
antirat
- thymocyte serum 25
antireticular
- cytotoxic serum 13
antiretroviral
- therapy, highly active 83
antirheumatic
- drugs, disease modifying 60
antisense oligonucleotides 24
antiserum
- C-reactive protein 51
- erythrocyte 66
antisheep
- beta-endorphin 9
antishock
- garment, pneumatic 128
- trousers, medical 104
- trousers, military 104
antistreptolysin 24
antitetanus serum 25
antithymocyte serum 25
antitoxin
- tetanus 160
- trivalent botulinic 9
- unit 25
antitrypsin 7
antiviral
- antibody 26
- factor 26
- protein 27
- regulator 27
- repressor regulator 27
antivirin 26
antral peristalsis 21
anxiety 20
- and depression scale, hospital 83
- control training 13
- disorder, generalized 77
- high 83

- index 17
- reaction, intense 22
- reaction, mild 22
- scale, manifest 104
- tension state 25

aorta
- angle of 20
- ascending 6
- dog 56

aortic
- arch syndrome 7
- endothelial cells, murine 103
- first sound 5
- flow 14
- incompetence 17
- insufficiency 17
- occlusions, recurrent 142
- pressure 21
- root, anterior wall 27
- second sound 5
- stenosis 23
- valve 26
- valve area 26
- valve atresia 26
- valve closure 26
- valve defects 26
- valve echocardiogram 26
- valve opening 27
- valve orifice 27
- valve replacement 27
- valve stenosis 27
- valve stroke volume 27
- valve, bicuspid 29
- valvular disease 26
- wall, anterior 8

aortocoronary
- saphenous vein 13
- saphenous vein, bypass graft 13
- venous bypass 13

aorto-pericardial pouch conduit 22

aortopulmonary 21

apalcillin 22

apatite
- and wollastonite containing glass-ceramic 27
- ceramics, porous 127

aperture current setting 13

apex 21
- beat 8

aphasia 22
- primary progressive 135
- test, aachen 7
- test, Halsted 83
- transcortical sensory 165

apheresis
- target value tailored 167

apical
- impulse 17
- membrane vesicles 19
- pulse 21
- rate 22

aplasia
- pure red cell 137

apnea
- and bradycardia 8
- bradycardia, cyanosis 8
- plus-hypopnea index 16

aponeurotic
- system, submuscular 155

apoptosis
- inhibitor 88

apoptotic cells 22

apothecary 21

apparent
- half-life 16
- volume of distribution 26

appearance
- general 77
- rates, normalized protein nitrogen 119

appears 22

appendectomy 21

appendicitis 21

appendix 21, 22

apperception
- test, auditory 7
- test, thematic 160

apple
- mosaic virus 22
- scar skin viroid 24

application
- marketing authorization 109
- new drug 116
- residency, universal 168
- specific integrated circuit 23

appointment 22
- failed 72

appropriate
- for gestational age 15

approved
- code of practice 12
- health plan 16

approximate 22, 180
- lethal concentration 18

approximately
- equal to 180

aptitude
- test, academic 7

apurinic
- acid 21

aqueous
- dextrose solution 62
- vasopressin 27

arachidonic acid 5

arachnodactyly
- congenital contractural 40

arachnoid
- cyst, middle fossa 11

arbitrary unit 25

arched-back nursing 10

architecture
- microvascular 114

area
- affected 5
- anterior hypothalamic preoptic 16
- body surface 34
- catchment 37
- cross section 53
- dorsal medullary depressor 61
- dorsolateral 60
- epidemiological catchment 67
- fractional shortening 76
- health education activity 15
- health education center 15
- health professional shortage 87
- health service 16
- health service development fund 16
- medioventral 114
- medullary ventral 114
- mitral valve 114

- ovarian sectional 125
- postrema 21
- under the "moment" curve 25
- under the curve 25
argentinian
- hemorrhagic fever 16
arginine 22, 141
- codon 15, 44
- glycine-asparagine 143
- hypoxanthine, uracil 17
- tolerance test 25
- vasopressin 27
- vasotocin 27
argon
- ionization detector 17
- laser trabeculoplasty 19
- plasma coagulation 21
Argosy's manhattan II, experimentally modified 104
arithmetic progression 21
arm
- left upper 102
- posterior upper 28
- support, fixed 75
- support, horizontal movable 86
- upper 168
army head nurse 16
Arnold-Chiari malformation 11
around or about 131
arrangements
- multi-institutional 107
array
- superficial linear 153
arrest
- before arrival 8
- cardiac, full 49
arrhythmia
- supraventricular 158
arrhythmic events
- major 103
arrival
- time, hospital 83
arrived to find 24
arrythmogenic right ventricular dysplasia 23
arteria 5
arterial 23
- blood carbon dioxyde partial pressure 127
- blood gases 9
- blood pressure 10
- blood volume effective 67
- conductance superior mesenteric 154
- deep venous 14
- disease extracranial 67
- disease peripheral 127
- end tidal PCO2 difference 127
- hypertension 15, 17
- hypertension, systemic 149
- oxygen saturation 149
- pressure 21
- pressure mean 104
- pressure oscillation, systemic 149
- resistance systemic 146
- trunk brachiocephalic 30
arteries 5
- intrapulmonary 93
arteriography
- ultrasonic 168
arterio-hepatic dysplasia 15
arteriole 5
arteriosclerosis 23, 25
- obliterans 24
arteriosclerotic
- cardiovascular disease 13, 23
- coronary artery disease 23
- disease peripheral 127
- heart disease 23
- occlusive disease 20
- peripheral vascular disease 24
- peripheral vascular occlusive disease 22
- vascular disease 24
arteriovenous 26, 27
- anastomosis 26
- delay 26
- fistula 26
- fistula occlusion bradycardia 29
- haemodialysis continuous 39
- haemofiltration continuous 39
- malformation 22, 27
- oxygen 27
- oxygen difference 26
- oxygen ratio 27
- oxygen saturation difference 26
- oxygen saturation difference, basal 26
- passage time 27
arteritis
- giant cell 78
artery 5, 23
- anterior communicating 12
- blood flow, superior mesenteric 154
- brachial 28
- catheter, umbilical 168
- embolism, superior mesenteric 154
- external carotid 67
- injury, penetrating coronary 128
- internal carotid 89
- middle meningeal 109
- obtuse marginal 123
- posterior descending 129
- posterior interosseous 132
- pressure, brachial 28
- pressure, pulmonary 128
- pulmonary 127
- pulse, posterior tibial 139
- right subclavian 146
- superficial femoral 151
- systolic pressure, pulmonary 128
- umbilical 168
- wedge pressure, pulmonary 128
arthritic 23
arthritis
- collagen-induced 44
- degenerative 55
- juvenile rheumatoid 96
- of unknown diagnosis 25
- rheumatoid 142
arthroplasty
- total shoulder 165
- total toe 166
arthroscopy
- diagnostic 5

- operative 5
arthrotomy
- operative 5
articles
- excess defense 68
articular rheumatism 7
articulation 23
- index 17
artificial 23
- cerebrospinal fluid 13
- chromosome, yeast 177
- circus movement tachycardia 11
- heart energy system 15
- hip joint 16
- insemination 17
- intelligence 17
- intelligence hemostasis consultant system 17
- limb 15
- pneumothorax 21
- respiration 22
- rupture of membranes 23
- ventilation 26
arylhydrocarbon hydroxylase 16
as 180
- desired 14
- directed 170
- evidenced by 14
- much as desired 141
- much as you like 141
- needed 138
- required 138
- soon as possible 23
- tolerated 24
- well as 27
asbestos body 8
ascending 23
- aorta 6
- aorta synchronized pulsation 7
ascites
- carcinoma, Ehrlich 67
ascorbate peroxidase 22
asea brown boveri 8
aseptic
- bone/bone marrow necrosis 10
- meningitis syndrome 19
ash
- Montserrat volcanic 114
ashes
- horticulture waste 88
- incinerator bottom 89
asparagine 23, 114
- codon 5, 7
aspartate aminotransferase 24, 81
aspartic acid 24, 55
- codon 77
aspergillosis
- allergic bronchopulmonary 8, 10
- chronic necrotizing pulmonary 49
- invasive 88
- invasive pulmonary 93
aspergillus
- nidulans 51
aspiration
- biopsy cytology 8
- electric vacuum 71
- fine needle 75
- manual vacuum 113
- meconium 104
- needle biopsy 8
- pneumonia 21
- syndrome 7
- syndrome meconium 104
- transtracheal 166
- uterine 168
aspirin 23
- induced asthma 17
- phenacetin, caffeine 21
- tolerance time 25
aspiryl chloride 11
aspoxicillin 24
assay
- enzyme-linked immunosorbent 69
- estradiol receptor 70
- fluorogenic matrix metalloproteinase substrate 76
- granulocyte agglutination 77
- granulocyte immunofluorescence 79
- immunohistochemical 89
- mouse diaphragm 105
- reverse transcriptase 147
- whole blood acetaldehyde 175
assessment
- and plans 21
- of basic competency 8
- of functioning global 77
- of multiple sclerosis functional 73
- report 22
- score total severity 165
assigned protection factor 22
assist
- contact guard 44
- controlled mechanical ventilation 11
- device, ventricular 172
- system, biventricular 33
- system, left ventricular 102
- system, right ventricular 149
assistance
- mechanical ventricular 114
- refuse/s medical 144
assistant
- head nurse 16
- house physician 16
- house surgeon 16
- occupational therapy 126
- physician 127
assisted
- health insurance plan 16
- respiration 22
- ventilation 26
assistive 24
associate chief of staff 12
associated clonal hematopoietic non-mast cell lineage disorder 16
association
- compressed gas 44
- period 21
associative visual cortex 26
assurance
- quality 140
asthma
- aspirin-induced 17
- bronchial 28
- care training 13

asthmatic bronchitis 8
astigmatism 24
astrocytoma
- anaplastic 5
- with atypical/anaplastic foci 5
asymmetrical
- cortical degeneration syndromes 10
- septal hypertrophy 23
asymptomatic 5
- urinary abnormalities 25
asynchrony
- motion onset 110
at 180
- bedtime 84, 87
- liberty 14
- night 118
- risk 22
- will 141
ataxia
- cerebellar 46
atherectomy
- directional coronary 56
- transluminal extraction 161
atheroembolic
- renal disease 22
atherogenic
- index 17
atherosclerosis
- risk in communities 22
atherosclerotic
- heart disease 15, 23
- plaque 21
athletic trainer 24
atlas 24
atmosphere
- pressure chemical ionization 21
atmospheres
- controlled 37
atomic
- biological and chemical 8
- force microscope 15
- mass unit unified 168
- volume 25
- warfare 27
- weight 25, 27
atopic
- dermatitis 13
atracurium 24
atraumatic
- normocephalic 24
atrazine 24
atresia
- esophageal 66
- extrahepatic biliary 69
atrial
- contraction, premature 127
- enlargement, left 98
- fibrillation 14, 15, 24
- fibrillation, chronic 38
- fibrillation, paroxysmal 127
- fibrillation, rapid 142
- flutter 14, 15, 24
- heart rate 16
- hypertrophy, left 98
- insufficience 17
- natriuretic peptide 20
- pacing 21
- premature beat 21
- premature contraction 21
- pressure, right 142
- septal defect 23
- septostomy, balloon 29
- septum, aneurysm 7
- tachycardia, automatic 7
- tachycardia, multifocal 104
- tachycardia, paroxysmal 128
- triggered pacemaker 7
atrial single-chamber systems
- fixed-rate 5
atrioventricular 26
- block 26
- cana 26
- circumflex branch 26
- conduction system 26
- dissociation 26
- junction 27
- junction rhythm 27
- junctional reentrant 27
- malformations 27
- nodal (conduction) 27
- nodal reentry 27
- node 27
- node dysfunction 27
- node functional refractory period 27
- node reentry tachycardia 27
- opening 27
- pathway 21
- reciprocating tachycardia 27
- reentrant tachycardia 27
- refractory period 27
- septal defect 27
atrium
- left 98
- right 142
atrophy 15, 24
- microvillous 114
- neurogenic muscular 118
- olivopontocerebellar 123
- progressive spinal muscular 139
- x-linked progressive retinal 176
atropine
- coma therapy 13
attach
- defense 56
attaching
- and effacing escherichia coli 14
attachment
- point 20
attack
- grand mal 79
attacks
- sleep 149
attempt
- suicide 149
attending 25
- physician 24
attention
- deficit disorder 14
- deficit disorder, epileptic 67
- deficit hyperactivity disorder 14
attenuation
- broadband ultrasonic 36
- table, harmonic 83
attorney
- malpractice 110
atypical 25
- bronchial epithelium 9

- chronic lymphocytic leukemia 11
- chronic myeloid leukemia 11
- ductal hyperplasia 14
- endometrial hyperplasia 14
- fibroxanthoma 15
- glands, unknown significance 15
- localization of immature precursors 18
- squamous cells 23
- transformation zone 25

audiometry
- brainstem evoked response 35
- evoked response 70

audiovisual 25, 26
audiovisuals on-line (database) 27
auditory 25
- apperception test 7
- brainstem response audiometry 10
- canal, external 67
- evoked potentials, brain stem 34
- evoked response 14
- evoked response, brain stem 28
- field, anterior 5
- vocal sequencing 27

augmentation
- mammoplasty, bilateral 28

augmented
- histamine test 17
- vector 26

Aujeszky's disease virus 14
auric 25
auricle 25
auricular 25
- fibrillation 25

auris
- dextra 13
- sinistra 23
- unitas 25

auscultation 25
- and palpation 21
- and percussion 21, 127

Australia
- antigen 25
- antigen protein 25
- hepatitis-associated antigen 25
- serum hepatitis 25

australia antigen 25
Australian
- pharmacist 21

authorization 25
- application, marketing 109
- marketing 103
- medical 103

autoanalyzer
- sequential multichannel 154
- simultaneous multichannel 154

autoantibodies
- collagen 8
- elastin 9

autoantibody
- antiheart muscle 16

autogenous
- bone graft 9
- hamster tumor 17

autograft
- transfer system, osteochondral 121

autoimmune 17
- complement fixation 17
- deficiency 17
- disease 17
- encephalitis, experimental 67
- hemolytic disease 15
- thrombocytopenic purpura 24
- type chronic active hepatitis 17

autoimmunity 17
autologous
- bone marrow transplant 9

autolymphocyte therapy 19
automated
- external defibrillator 14
- hospital data management system 15
- hospital information system 16
- image analysis 17
- lamella keratoplasty 18
- partial thromboplastin time 22
- volt foot 26
- volt left 27
- volt right 27

automatic
- atrial tachycardia 7
- computerized transverse axial (scanning) 13
- dishwashing detergents, liquid 98
- implantable cardioverter defibrillator 17
- implantable defibrillator 17
- volume controll 26

automobile accident 7
autonomic
- nervous system 20
- neuropathy, diabetic 56

autopsy 5
autoradiography
- in vitro quantitative 95
- quantitative 140

autosensitization
- spongiotic dermatitis 23

autotransfusion
- of UV-irradiated blood 26

auxiliary 26
AV
- block, chronic 39
- sequential (pacemaker) 64

avascular
- necrosis (MRI evaluation) 27
- necrosis of the femoral head 27
- zone 27

average 26
- beta energy 66
- bioequivalence 9
- daily dose 14
- daily dose, highest 83
- daily doses, lifetime 98
- daily gain 14
- diastolic pressure 26
- evoked response 14
- grade point 81
- integrated concentration 17
- interocular difference 17

- reflexes 181
averrhoa
- bilimbi 9
avian
- acute leukemia virus 11
- cell line 63
- herpes virus 17
- infectious bronchitis 17
- laryngotracheitis 19
- myeloblastosis 19
- rho0 cell line 64
- tumor virus 25
aviation
- medicine 26, 27
- medicine technician 27
avidin 26
avidin-biotin complex 8
avoidance reaction 7
avoirdupois 26
avulsion 26
awake 6
award
- performance incentive 132
axial 28
- tomography, computed 38
axilla 27
axillary 27, 28
- count rate 12
- line, anterior 5
- line, middle 104
- line, posterior 127
axio
- buccal 8
- buccocervical 8
- incisal 17
- pulpal 21
axis deviation
- left 98
axonal
- neuropathy, acute motor 19
- neuropathy, acute motor sensory 19
azacycloheptane diphosphonate 15
azauridine 25, 28
azide buffer 127
azidothymidine 28
azobis
- (amidinopropane) dihydrochloride 6
azure B 8

B

B
- cell lines 31, 87
- chain variable 173
- -domain-deleted 32
- symptoms 28
B1-independent rotation phase-cycled 32
B27-arthritis-sacroiliitis-extra-articular features (syndrome) 29
Babinski's sign 28
baboon virus replication 37
baby
- soft diet 34
baby hamster kidney cells 32
Bachelor of Arts 8
bacillary
- meningitis, gram-negative 80
- white diarrhea 37
bacille
- Calmette-Guérin 31
bacilli
- acid fast 14
bacillus
- amyloliquefaciens H, restriction enzyme 28
- cat scratch disease 53
- gram-negative 80
bacitraci
- X 37
bacitracin
- V 36
back 28, 33
- bending, low 99
- board 30
- care 30
- ground noise 10
- ground, interval 32
- pain 33
- pain, chronic low 46
- pain, lower 99
- pressure, urethral 169
- projection, filtered 73
- scatter coefficient, integrated 89
- tenderness, low 99
- to work 36
- upper 169
backscatter
- normalized relative 119
bacteria
- nitrate-reducing 119
bacteria-carrier
- incidence 89
bacterial
- alkaline phosphatase 28
- antigen, undenatured 169
- chlorophyll 31
- endocarditis, acute 9
- endocarditis, subacute 150
- index 32
- nephritis, acute 9
- nosocomial tracheitis 33
- vaginosis 36
bactericidal
- concentration 30
- concentration, minimum 104
- index 32
- permeability increasing protein 34
bacteriological
- warfare 37
bacteriologist 28
bacteriology 28
bacteriorhodopsin 34
bacteriostatic
- water for injection 37
bacterium
- psychophilic marine 9
bacteriuria screening test 35
Bacteroides
- bile esculin 30
baculovirus IAP repeat 32
bad breath 29
bag
- of waters 34
- valve-mask 36
balance
- gate, station 32
- muscle 104

balanced salt solution 35
balanitis xerotica obliterans 37
balkan
- nephropathy, endemic 67
ballistocardiogram 31
ballistocardiography 31
balloon
- assisted endoscopic, retroperitoneal gasless 32
- atrial septostomy 29
- catheter angioplasty 30
- catheter, inoue 89
- pump, intra-aortic 88
balsam 28
bamifylline 28
band 31
- iliotibial 95
- noise, broad 30
Bannayan-Zonana syndrome 37
barb 29
barbital-dependent 31
barbiturate 29
- dependence 31
- nitrous oxide 115
barbituric 29
barely
- noticeable difference 33
bariatrics 29
Barila-Yaguchi-Eveland
- (medium) 37
barium 28
- enema 28, 32
- enema, double-contrast 56
- meal 28
- swallow 29
- swallow test, modified 104
barley
- alkaline protease inhibitor 28
- alpha-amylase/subtilisin inhibitor 29
- yellow dwarf virus 37
Barolet-Biedl syndrome 30
barometer 29
barometric 29
barotrauma
- recurrent sinus 146
barrier
- blood-brain 29
- blood-cerebrospinal fluid 30
Barthel Index 32
Bartholin, Skene, urethral (glands) 35
basal 29
- acid output 28
- acid output to maximal acid output (ratio) 28
- body temperature 30
- cell 30
- cell antigen 30
- cell atypia 30
- cell carcinoma 30
- cell dysplasia 30
- cell epithelioma 31
- cell hyperplasia 31
- energy expenditure 32
- metabolic rate 33
- metabolism 33
- skin resistance 35
- temperature chart 35
base
- blood buffer 29
- budgeting zero 177
- buffer 29
- deficit 31
- excess, actual 9
- in 32
- Mueller Hinton 107
- of natural logarithms, approximately 65
- of prism down 31
- of prism up 36
- of tongue 35
baseline 35
basement membrane
- alveolar wall 27
- collagenase soluble, glomerular 54
- glomerular 77
- zone 33
bashful bladder syndrome 30
basic 28
- aid training 29
- cardiac life support 31
- competency, assessment 8
- cycle length 31
- cycle lengths 31
- fibroblast frowth factor 32
- life support 33
- life support and defibrillation 33
- protein, major 104
- protein, myelin 104
- structural unit 35
- trauma life support 35
basilar 29
- artery migraine 28
- impression 32
basket cell 30
basophil 29
- chemotactic factor 31
- count 8
basophilic 29
- degeneration 31
basophils 29
- leukocytes 29
bath 28
- blanket 29
bathroom 34
- privileges 34
Batten
- disease 31
battered
- woman (or wife) syndrome 37
battery
- neurometric 115
battle
- casualty 30
Bauchinia purpurea alba 34
Baylor Rapid Autologous Transfusion system 34
B-cell 28
- acute lymphoblastic leukemia 28
- chronic lymphoprolipherative disorders 31
- differentiation factor 30
- growth factor 31
- leukemia 31
- lymphoma 31
- lymphoma, nodal marginal zone 118
- lymphoma, primary mediastinal 134
- lymphoma, T-cell-rich 160
- lymphoma, undifferentiated 169

- lymphoproliferative disorder 33
beacons
- molecular 104
bearing
- cast, short-leg non-weight 153
- cells, immunoglobulin 89
- full weight 77
- non-weight 121
- partial weight 140
- toe touch weight 167
beat
- apex 8
- atrial premature 21
- premature ventricular 140
beats 34
because 180
because of 181
Beck
- depression inventory for primary care 32
Becker muscular dystrophies 33
Beckwith-Wiedemann syndrome 37
bed
- bath 29
- board 29
- nucleus of the stria terminalis 33
- rest 34
- rest, complete 39
- wetting 37
bedside
- bag 34
- commode 34
- drainage 34
bedtime 35
beet western yellow virus 37
before 5, 20
- delivery 20, 21
- dinner 20
- meal 10
- noon 19
behavior
- activity profile 28
- alertness 8
- checklist, injury 89
- style questionnaire 35
behavioral
- cues index 31
- disorder 31
- regression or upset in hospitalized medical patients (scale) 36
- risk factor surveillance system 34
- treatment/therapy, cognitive 39
behaviorally anchored rating scale 29
Behçet
- disease 31
- neuro 115
behind the ear (hearing aid) 35
beliefs and behavior
- questionnaire, AIDS 8
belladonna 31
below 179
- knee amputation 33
- the elbow 32
- the knee 33
- waist 37
Bence Jones
- protein 33
Bence Jones (proteinuria) 33
Bender Visual-Motor Gestalt Test 36
bending
- left lateral 100
- low back 99
benefit
- cost (ratio) 30
- maximum hospital 107
benign
- breast disease 30
- breast syndrome 30
- cellular changes (pap smear) 30
- childhood epilepsy 31
- hypertrophic prostate 32
- monoclonal gammopathy 33
- paroxysmal positional vertigo 34
- prostatic hypertrophy 34
- tertian malaria 35
benzamide 29
benzodiazepine 37
- receptor peripheral (type) 37
benzothiazepine 36
benzoyl 37
- arginine methyl ester 28
- ecgonine (cocaine) 32
- thiamine disulfide 35
benzquinamide 37
benzyl
- anti-serotonin 29
- oxycarbonylmethyl 33
Bernard-Soulier syndrome 35
best 124
- available technology 29
Best's macular dystrophy 33
beta
- 1-glycoprotein, pregnancy-specific 156
- adrenergic receptor 29
- adrenergic receptor kinase 29
- adrenergic stimulation 29
- aminoproprionitrile fumarate 28
- amyloid 9
- amyloid peptide 28
- amyloid precursor protein 28
- blockade 29
- blocker 29
- endorphin, antisheep 9
- endorphin-like immunoreactivity 32
- energy, average 66
- hemolytic streptococcus 32
- lipoprotein 33
- particle 181
- peptides, amyloid 24
- thromboglobulin 35
beta-lactamase
- extended-spectrum 71
Bethesda
- unit 36
between
- meals 89
Bezold-type reflex 35
bicarbonate 30, 84
- dialysis 31
- sodium 115
bicaval heart transplantation 31
biceps 32
- jerk 33

- tendon reflex 36
bicinchoninic acid 30
bicolor guaiac test 31
bicuspid aortic valve 29
bidirectional Glenn shunt 32
bifemelane hydrochloride 105
bifocal
- contact lenses 31
bifurcation
- turing-wave 168
bilateral 32
- abductor vocal cord paralysis 29
- acute retinal necrosis 29
- augmentation mammoplasty 28
- breath sounds 30
- bundle-branch block 29
- carotid body resection 30
- facial paralysis 32
- inguinal hernia 32
- lower lung fields 33
- otitis externa 33
- otitis media 33
- salpingo-oophorectomy 35
- tubal ligation 35
- upper dorsal sympathectomy 36
- ureteral occlusion 36
- vas ligation 36
bilaterally, active 8
Bilbao
- Thromboplastin 160
bile
- acids, total serum 165
- duct 31
- duct, common 39, 42
- salts, conjugated 39
- salt-stimulated esterase 35
- salt-stimulated lipase 35
biliary
- atresia, extrahepatic 69
- cholesterol concentration 30
- colic 8, 30
- passages, extrahepatic 69
- tract complication 35
- tract disease 35
- tract pain 35
bilirubin 32
- bisglucuronosyl 32
- concentrations, indirect 89
- monoglucuronosyl 106
- total 160
- unconjugated 169
Billroth I 32
bin 32
binary-coded decimal 30
binding
- capacity 89
- capacity, idiotype 89
- capacity, insulin 89
- capacity, iron 89
- capacity, unsaturated vitamin B 12 169
- globulin, sex hormone 151
- index, thyroid 160
- index, total 160
- inhibition, thyrotropin 160
- inhibitor, diazepam 56
- protein, fatty acid 72
- protein, growth hormone 78
- protein, insulin-like growth factor 91
- protein-5, insulin-like growth factor 91
- ratio, thyroid hormone 162
binocular
- deprivation 31
- interactor, translid 160
- single vision 35
- visual efficiency 36
bioaccumulative
- and toxic, persistent 128
bioassay
- neutral red 119
biobreeding
- rat 29
- Worcester rat 30
bioconcentration factor 31
bioelectrical
- impedance, tetrapolar 160
bioequivalence
- average 9
- individual 89
biofiltration 32
biofragmentable anastomosis ring 29
biological
- effects, relative 142
- false positive 32
- indicator 32
- response modifier 34
- treatment planning 35
- value 36
- warfare 37
- weapon 37
biomechanical ankle platform system 28
biopsy 37
- and curettage 30
- breast 29, 34
- endometrial 69
- fine-needle, aspiration 75
- frozen section, breast 30
- sentinel lymph node 153
- upper gastrointestinal 171
biotechnology
- applied 10
- informatics 32
biotin
- carboxyl carrier protein 30
biotinylated dextran 31
biparietal
- diameter 34
biphasic 32
bipolar 34
- cell 30
BIR-containing proteins 32
Birmingham
- Vasculitis Activity Score 36
birth 180
- center, alternative 8
- cesarean 39
- control 30
- control clinic 30
- control pills 31
- date 31, 61
- living child, term 160
- never gave 121
- weight 37
- weight categories 77
- weight, deficit 56
- weight, low 99
births
- prior 128

bis
- die 32
- in die 32
bisglucuronosyl bilirubin 32
bisphenol-a-glycidyl methacrylate 32
bis-trimethylsilacetylene 35
bis-trimethylsilyltrifluoro-acetamide 35
bitemporal 35
bitrochanteric 35
bivalent 180
biventricular
- assist device 36
- assist system 33
- hypertrophy 36
black 28
- death 31
- female 32
- male 33
- silk suture 35
- widow spider toxin 37
- widow spider venom 37
- woman 37
- women, diabetic 56
bladder 33
- cancer, invasive 89
- carcinoma, antibody against 32
- irrigation, continous 39
- neck obstruction 33
- outlet obstruction 34
- syndrome, bashful 30
- tumor 35
- tumor, transurethral resection 167
- washout 37
Blalock-Taussig (shunt) 35
blanked ventricular sense 37
blanket bath 29
blastic crisis 30
bleeding
- abnormal uterine 25
- breakthrough 29, 35
- dysfunctional uterine 64
- of undetermined origin 36
- postcoital 128
- postmenopausal 134
- third trimester 166
- time 33, 35
- upper gastrointestinal 171
- uterine, functional 77
- vaginal 173
bleomycin, cyclophosphamide, dactinomycin 30
blind
- aid to the 8
block
- atrioventricular 26
- bilateral bundle-branch 29
- bundle branch 29
- complete left bundle branch 46
- design (test) 31
- heart 83
- left bundle branch 99
- paravertebral 140
- right bundle branch 142
blockade
- beta 29
blocker
- beta 29
- calcium channel 40
blocking agent
- neuromuscular 118
blood 33
- activated recalcification time 29
- agar plate 28
- alcohol 28
- alcohol concentration 28
- alcohol level 28
- bank 29
- brain barrier 29
- brain barrier disruption 29
- buffer 29
- buffer base 29
- cell, white 175
- cells, nucleated red 119
- cells, white 175
- cells, whole cord 175
- cerebrospinal fluid barrier 30
- color analyzer 30
- count 30
- count, complete 39
- count, differential 59
- count, full 73
- count, white 175
- culture 30, 33
- culture, umbilical cord 169
- donation, donor-directed 58
- donor 31
- flow 32
- flow, bronchial 30
- flow, cerebral 39
- flow, coronary 39
- flow, coronary sinus 53
- flow, gastric mucosa 79
- flow, hepatic 83
- flow, regional cerebral 142
- flow, renal 142
- flow, tail 160
- flow, thyroid 160
- flow, tissue 160
- flow, tumor 160
- flow, uterine 171
- gas, capillary 39
- gas, venous 173
- gases, arterial 9
- glucose, self monitored 155
- group, AB 8
- grouping system 10
- irradiation, ultraviolett 169
- loss 33
- loss, estimated 67
- monitoring 33
- occult 122
- ova, parasites 34
- oxygenation, level-dependent 33
- peripheral 128
- pressure 34
- pressure cuff 34
- pressure, and pulse 34
- pressure, arterial 10
- pressure, diastolic 56, 179
- pressure, high 83
- pressure, low 99
- pressure, non-invasive 115, 117
- pressure, systemic 150
- pressure, systolic 150, 179
- sedimentation rate 35
- serologic test 35
- stem cell, peripheral 128
- stream infections 35

- sugar 34
- sugar, fasting 73
- sugar, post prandial 128, 136
- temperature monitor 35
- transfusion 36
- transfusion service 36
- type 35
- type, maternal 113
- typing 35
- urea 36
- urea nitrogen 36
- urea nitrogen/creatine ratio 36
- uric acid 36
- vessel 36
- vessel endothelium 36
- vessel invasion 36
- vessel prosthesis 37
- volume 36
- volume expander 36
- volume pulse 37
- volume, central 39
- volume, central circulating 40
- volume, cerebral 39
- volume, circulating 39
- volume, corrected 39
- volume, cortical 39
- Wasserman (reaction) 37
- whole 175
- whole canine 175

blood pressure
- arterial 10

blood transfusion
- autologous 10

Bloomberg syndrome 8

blow
- bottle 29
- on blow 53

blue
- alcian 8
- bloaters (emphysema) 29
- cross 30
- cross (plan) 30
- diaper (syndrome) 31
- shield 30
- tetrazolium 35
- toe syndrome 36
- tongue 35
- tongue, virus 36

blunt
- abdominal trauma 29
- duodenal injury 32
- head trauma 32

board 31
- assembled, printed circuit 128
- back 30
- certified 30

Bodansky 36

bodies
- nuclear 115

bodily
- injury 32

body
- acceleration synchronous with heart rate 29
- centered-cubic 30
- curvilinear 46
- dementia, Lewy 99
- dorsal, medial geniculate 106
- fat, total 160
- impedance, total 160
- iron, total 160
- irradiation, total 160
- mass 33
- mass index 33
- mass, lean 99
- muscle mass, total 160
- obesity, lower 99
- obesity, upper 169
- part 34
- resection, bilateral carotid 30
- substance isolation 34
- surface area 34
- surface area, total 160
- temperature 35
- temperature, basal 30
- temperature, chart 35
- temperature, initial 160
- tomography, computed 39
- ventral, medial geniculate 106
- water 37
- water, total 160
- weight 33, 37
- weight, actual 10
- weight, desirable 56
- weight, dosing 56
- weight, dry 56
- weight, ideal 89, 90
- weight, usual 169

Bolton point 29

bombesin 30

bone 125
- age 28
- and joint 33
- cavity, idiopathic 89
- conduction 8, 30
- density, forearm 73
- density, vertebral 173
- fragment 32
- graft 32
- graft, autogenous 9
- impaction 32
- index, total 160
- index, trabecular 160
- injury 32
- marrow 33
- marrow necrosis 33
- marrow necrosis, aseptic 10
- marrow transplant 33
- marrow transplant, autologous 9
- marrow, microvascular endothelial cells 33
- marrow, plasma cell labeling index 129
- matrix, demineralized 56
- mineral content 33
- mineral content, whole body 175
- mineral density 33
- mineral density, ultradistal radius 170
- morphogenetic protein 33
- necrosis, aseptic 10
- patellar tendon-bone 34
- powder, demineralized 56
- volume fraction, trabecular 160

bones
- joints, extremities 33
- joints, muscles 33

borate-buffered saline 30

border
- brush 29

- disease 31
- membrane vesicle, brush 30
- membrane, brush 30
- right sternal 146
borderline 29
- dull 31
- glucose tolerance test 32
- personality disorder 34
- tuberculoid 35
boric acid solution 29
born 28
- before arrival 29
- on arrival 33
borreliosis
- Lyme 99
Boston Assessment of Severe Aphasia 29
both
- bones 29
- bones, fracture 76, 77
- ears 25
- eyes 127
- lower extremities 33
- lower quadrants 33
- sides 32
- upper extremities 36
- upper quadrants 36
bottle 34
- blow 29
botulinic
- antitoxin, trivalent 9
botulinum toxin 35, 36
botulism toxin pentavalent 9
bound 31
- niacin 33
- niacin, alkali-treated 9
Bovie-assisted uvulopalatoplasty 28
bovine
- albumin, in phosphate buffer 28
- albumin, phosphate saline 28
- alimentary papilloma virus 29
- herpesvirus-1 32
- leucosis, enzootic 67
- neurophysin 33
- orphan virus, enteric cytopathogenic 67
- pleuropneumonia, contagious 39
- respiratory disease (complex) 34
- serum albumin 34, 127
- spongiform encephalopathy 34
- thymus extract 35
- thyroid-stimulating hormone 36
- trypsin 35
- trypsinogen 35
- turbinate (cells) 35
- vaginitis virus 37
- viral diarrhea 36
- viral diarrhea-mucosal disease 36
- virus diarrhea, virus 36
bowel
- congenital short 53
- disease, inflammatory 89
- disorder/distress, functional 73
- large 99
- movement 33
- obstruction, large 99
- signs, active 34
- sounds 34
- sounds normal 35
- sounds regular 35
- sounds, normoactive 115
- syndrome, irritable 89
Bowen disease 31
Bowman-Birk soybean inhibitor 30
brace
- long leg 100
- short-leg 153
brachial 34
- artery 28
- artery, mean (pressure) 28
- artery, output 28
- artery, pressure 28
- index, toe 160
- neuritis, acute 9
- neuropathy, acute 9
brachiocephalic 30
Brachmann-Cornelia de Lange (syndrome) 30
brachytherapy
- computer-assisted frameless stereotactic interstitial 38
bradycardia
- after arteriovenous fistula occlusion 29
- and apnea 8
- tachycardia syndrome 36
brain
- age quotient 29
- computer interface 31
- damage 31
- dead 31
- death 31
- infarction, thrombotic 160
- injury 32
- injury, mild traumatic 113
- injury, traumatic 160
- natriuretic peptide 33
- stem auditory evoked potentials 34
- stem auditory evoked response 28
- stem, evoked response audiometry 35
- stem, response audiometry, auditory 10
- stimulation reinforcement 35
- syndrome, chronic 39, 44
- syndrome, organic 122
- tumor 35
- tumor gene 34
- uptake index 36
branch
- atrioventricular circumflex 26
- bundle 29
- vein occlusion 36
branched
- chain alpha-keto acid dehydrogenase 31
- chain amino acid 30
- chain keto acid 31
branchial cleft anomaly 30
break
- nonrejoining 119
breakpoint
- cluster region 31
- cluster region, minor 104

breakthrough bleeding 29, 35
breast
- biopsy 29, 34
- biopsy/frozen section 30
- cancer 30, 98
- cancer antigen 30
- cancer estrogen-inducible 31
- cancer, advanced 8
- cancer, inflammatory 89
- cancer, interval 89
- cancer, intraductile 89
- cancer, screening-detected 149
- cancers, invasive 89
- conservation surgery 31
- cyst fluid 31
- cyst fluid protein 31
- disease, benign 30
- disease, fibrocystic 73
- meat weight 34
- meat yield 34
- reconstruction, one type of 164
- self examination 34
- syndrome, benign 30
- tumor 35
- tumor frozen section 35
breath
- alcohol on 20
- bad 29
- sounds 34
- sounds, bilateral 30
- sounds, normal 115
breathing
- capacity, indirect maximum 91
- capacity, maximum 104
- difficulty 59
- disorder, functional 73
- disorders, sleep-related 157
- exercise, deep 56
- glossopharyngeal 82
- positive pressure 50
breaths 34
breech presentation 34
brevetoxin 36
brief
- Carroll depression rating scale 30
- pain inventory 34
- psychiatric rating (scale) 34
- stimulus therapy 35
- vestibular disorientation test 36
bright
- red blood 34
- red blood per rectum 34
- signal, unidentified 169
brilliant cresyl blue 30
Briquet disorder 31
brisk and equal 32
British
- standard unit 35
- thermal unit 35, 36
broad
- band noise 30
- sense (L. sensu lato) 152
broadband
- Communications, Trans-European Network-Integrated 161
- ultrasonic attenuation 36
bromcresol green 31
bromo
- benzycyanide 30
- chloro-3-inodolyl phosphate 31
- ethylamine hydrobromide 32
- isovalerylurea 37
- thymol blue lactose 35
- uracil 36
- vinyldeoxyuridine 36
bromodeoxyuridine 36
bromsulphalein (dye) 35
bromthymol blue 35
bronchial
- asthma 28
- blood flow 30
- brushing, transtracheal selective 165
- carcinoma 30
- epithelium, atypical 9
- secretion 34
bronchiolitis
- obliterans with interstitial pneumonia 32
- obliterans-organizing pneumonia 34
bronchitis
- asthmatic 8
- avian infectious 17
- chronic 39
bronchoalveolar
- lavage 28
- lavage fluid 28
- washing 29
bronchodilation 31
bronchodilator 31
bronchoprovocation
- challenge 34
bronchopulmonary
- aspergillosis, allergic 8, 10
- dysplasia 34
bronchoscopy 34
bronchospasm
- airflow-induced 17
bronchovascular markings 36
bronchovesicular 36
bronchus-associated lymphoid tissue 28
broth
- nutrient 115
brought in dead 32
brown
- adipose tissue 29
- bowel syndrome 30
brucellae
- medium, malachite green 106
bruising
- of undetermined origin 36
brush
- border 29
- border, endopeptidase 30
- border, membrane 30
- border, membrane vesicle 30
bubble chamber equipment 31
buccal 36
- cartilage 30
- ganglion 36
- odontoblast layer 33
buccocervical 30
buccodistal 31
budgeting
- zero base 177
buffalo (rat) 36
buffer
- base 29

lx

- blood 29
- Krebs-Hensleit 97
- reticulocyte standard 146
buffered
- salt solution 35
- single substrate 35
buffy coat 30
bulimia
- cognitive distortions scale 30
- nervosa 33
- nervosa, active 9
- test 36
bulla
- osteotomy, lateral 161
bullous pemphigoid 34
bundle 31
- branch 29
- branch block 29
- branch block, bilateral 29
- branch block, incomplete right 94
- branch block, left 99
buoyant density 31
burden
- total worm 167
Burks' Behavior Rating Scale 30
burn
- index 32
- unit 36
burst of ventricular pacing 37
bursting pressure
- colon anastomosis 39
Buruli ulcer 36
Buschke selective reminding (test) 35
bushel 36
busulfan 36
but 36
butanamide 122
Butler-Bloomberg syndrome 8
butyl 36
- methacrylate 33
butylated
- hydroxyanisole 32
- hydroxytoluene 32
butyrate 36
butyric 36
butyrophenone 120
butyrylcholinesterase 31
by 131
- mouth 125, 131, 135
- the way 36
- way of 173
Byler disease 32
bypass
- aortocoronary venous 13
- cardiopulmonary 50
- coronary artery 38
- femoral-below-knee-popliteal 73
- graft, coronary artery 38
- micropouch gastric 106
- saphenofemoral 151
bystander
- cardiac pulmonary resuscitation 37

C

cadaver
- donor 42
cadaveric renal transplant 51
Cadmium 42
café-au-lait spot 47
caffeine 38
calcification
- of ligamentum flavum 46
calcitonin gene-related peptide 44
calcium 37
- carbonate 38
- channel blocker 40
- hydroxyapatite 44
- phosphate cement, fast-setting 76
- pyrophosphate dihydrate 50
- saccharin 38
calculated
- computer 39
calculous cholecystitis
- chronic 40
calendar
- premenstrual experiences 50
calf
- lung surfactant extract 47
- serum 52
calibration curve data 40
California mastitis (test) 47
call for papers 43
called to see patient 54
calmodulin 47
calorie 38, 97
calorimeter
- photo differential scanning 132
calorimetry
- differential scanning 63
calvarial hyperostotic syndrome 44
calvarium and scalp 53
campomelic
- dwarfism 48
- dysplasia 48
- syndrome 52
cana
- atrioventricular 26
canavaninosuccinic acid 53
cancer 37
- breast 30, 98
- cell line, human esophageal epithelial 67
- coagulation factor 41
- colorectal 39
- disseminated peritoneal 62
- family syndrome 53
- inflammatory breast 89
- interval breast 89
- intraductile breast 89
- invasive bladder 89
- invasive breast 89
- lung 98
- multiple synchronous 112
cancer cells
- free, intraperitoneal 90
candela 42
candidiasis
- chronic mucocutaneous 48
canine
- blood, whole 175
- distemper 42
- dose 42
cannabidiol
- abnormal 10
cannabinoids 49
cannula
- nasal 116

capacity
- closing 39
- functional residual 76
- idiotype binding 89
- inspiratory 89
- insulin binding 89
- iodine binding 89
- iron binding 89
- oxygen 121
- timed vital 167
- total volume 167
- vital 173
capillary
- blood cell velocity 39
- blood gas 39
- column gas chromotography 41
- lumen 45
- refill time 51
- wedge, pulmonary 129
capita
- cost, adjusted annual 6
- cost, adjusted average 6
capital
- femoral epiphysis, slipped 150
capitolunate instability pattern 46
capreomycin 47
capsid protein 50
capsule 38
capsules 38
capsulolabral
- reconstruction, anterior 11
carbachol
- cholinergic agonist 41
carbamazepine 39
carbapenem 38
carbohydrate 44
- deficient, glycoprotein syndrome 43
- deficient, transferrin 43
- dehydratase 42
- level, critical 41
carbolic methylene blue 48
carboline carboxylic acid ester 41
CarboMedics 47
carbon
- catabolite repression 51
- coatings, diamond-like 60
- dioxide 42, 49
- dioxide, partial pressure 129
- dioxide, partial pressure in arterial blood 127
- dioxide, tension difference, alveolo-arterial 6
- monoxide 49
- total organic 163
carbonic
- anhydrase 37
- anhydrase, inhibitor 38
carbonyl
- cyanide m-chloro-phenyl-hydrazone 40
- salicylamide 53
carboxy
- methyl 47
- methylcellulose 48
- seminaphthorhodafluor 155
carboxyl
- carrier protein, biotin 30
- esterases 43
- esterases, monomeric 104
- esterases, oligomeric 122
carboxylic
- acid, aminocyclopentane 12
carcinoembryonic antigen 43
carcinogenesis
- endometrial, intraepithelial 69
carcinoid syndrome 52
carcinoma 37
- antigen, squamous cell 150
- basal cell 30
- bronchial 30
- cell line 41
- colorectal 50
- cutaneous squamous cell 53
- differentiated type gastric 59
- early gastric 69
- Ehrlich ascites 67
- hepatocellular 84
- in situ 45
- in situ, ductal 57
- infiltrating, ductal 90
- large cell neuroendocrine 99
- maxillary sinus 112
- metastatic 104
- nasopharyngeal 119
- of the thyroid, warthin-like papillary 176
- oral squamous cell 126
- salivary gland 151
- second thyroid 158
- showing thymus-like differentiation 38
- squamous cell 150
carcinomas
- papillary thyroid 129
card
- medical smart 112
cardiac 38
- arrest 37, 49
- Ca2+ sensitizer 105
- care unit, comprehensive 40
- care, emergency 67
- catheterization 38, 40
- death syndrome, sudden 150
- death, sudden 150
- disease 42
- dullness 42
- dullness, left border 99
- dysrhythmia 42
- failure 43
- failure, congestive 41
- index 44
- insufficiency 44
- intensive care unit 45
- life support, advanced 11
- life support, basic 31
- murmur 47
- muscle 47
- output 49
- output, total 141
- output, ultrasonic 169
- pulmonary resuscitation, bystander 37
- rehabilitation unit 52
- resuscitation team 51
- resuscitation, closed chest 40
- volume 55
cardiogenic shock 52
cardiography
- ultrasonic 169
cardiolipin 45

- complement fixation 41
- fluorescent (antibody) 46
cardiomyopathy 47, 49
- congestive 41
- dilated 57
- hypertrophic 84
- hypertrophic obstructive 86
cardiopathy
- congenital 39
cardioplegia
- terminal warm blood 167
cardiopulmonary
- bypass 50
- exercise testing 50
- resuscitation 50
- syndrome, hantavirus 84
cardiotoxic
- dose, cumulative 40
cardiovascular 55
- disease 42, 55
- disease, acute 13
- disease, arteriosclerotic 13, 23
- disease, clinical 40
- disease, hypertensive 84
- status 55
- surgery 55
- system 55
cardioverter
- defibrillator, automatic implantable 17
care
- clinic, comprehensive 40
- complex, critical 40
- concern, concurrent 40
- coronary intensive 45
- critical 40
- cure coordination 40
- emergency, cardiac 67
- facility, extended 67
- facility, intensive 90
- facility, intermediate 90
- facility, long term 102
- group, preventive 129
- level 101
- level, continuing 41
- long term 102
- management continuity 48
- management continuity across settings 48
- medicine, critical 41
- neonatal intensive 117
- network, community 42
- nursing, coronary 42
- nursing, critical 42
- of 49
- physician, primary 129
- postoperative 135
- table, urological 170
- training, asthma 13
- unit, ambulatory acute 13
- unit, cardiac intensive 45
- unit, coronary/cardiac 42
- unit, intensive 90
- unit, intensive coronary 89
- unit, neonatal intensive 117
- unit, neurointensive 117
- unit, post anesthesia 127
- unit, special 150
- unit, surgical intensive 152
caries
- early childhood 67
- susceptible 52
carmustine 31
carnitine
- free 73
carotid 38
- artery endarterectomy 38
- artery, common 40
- artery, ecternal/extracranial 67
- artery, external 67
- artery, internal 89
- body resection, bilateral 30
- body tumor 39
- cavernous fistula 41
- jugular fistula 45
- sheath 52
- sinus 52
- sinus denervation 53
- sinus hypersensitivity 54
carpal
- instability 45
- instability, non-dissociative 45
- tunnel 54
- tunnel release 54
- tunnel release, endoscopic 68
- tunnel syndrome 54
carpectomy
- proximal row 137
carpometacarpal 47, 48
- joint 48
Carrel-Dakin 42
carrier
- excitatory amino acid 66
- protein, acyl 12
- protein, biotin carboxyl 30
Carroll rating scale for depression 51
cartilage
- buccal 30
- matrix deficiency 48
- matrix protein 51
- midpalatal suture 112
case 52
- conference, consecutive 40
- report forms 51
casein
- hydrolysate-yeast extract-containing medium 42
- kinase 45
cassava latent virus 47
cast
- long arm 98
- long leg 100
- long leg cylinder 100
- short leg 153
- short-leg cylinder 153
- short-leg non weight bearing 153
- short-leg nonwalking 153
- short-leg walking 154
Castleman
- disease 42
castrated male 47
CAT
- scan reconstruction images, three dimensional 57
cat
- domestic shorthaired 63
- scratch 52
- scratch disease 53
- scratch disease bacillus 53
catabolic
- rate, absolute 12

catabolite
- repression, carbon 51
cataract 38
- agent, suckling mouse 155
- anterior polar 21
- congenital 39, 51
- epileptic, fits-mental, retardation, congenital 51
- extraction, extracapsular 67
catarrhal
- colitis, chronic 40
catchment
- area 37
- area, epidemiological 67
catechol
- methyltransferase 42
- O-methyltransferase 49
cathartic
- compound 39
catheter 38
- central venous 55
- drainage, percutaneous 129
- in, urethral 169
- in, urinary 169
- intrauterine 95
- jugular venous 97
- multipurpose silastic 112
- peripherally inserted 132
- related sepsis 51
- urinary 169
catheterization 38
- cardiac 38, 40
- clean intermittent 45
- urethral 169
cathodal
- closure clonus 40
- closure contraction 40
cathode
- ray oscilloscope 51
- ray tube 51
cathodic
- antigen, circulating 40
cationic
- protein, chymotrypsin-like 46
Caucasian 37
caucasian
- adult 37
- adult female 38
- adult male 38
- child 39
- male 47
caudad 42
caudal 42
- central nucleus 42
- part of the medial vestibular nucleus 114
- region of nucleus tractus solitarius 49
- regression syndrome 51
cauliflower
- mosaic virus 47
causa mortis 47
cause
- of death 42, 47, 49
- undetermined 55
- unknown 55
caused by 179, 180
causes 179, 180
cavernous malformation 47
cavity
- idiopathic bone 89
C-cell hyperplasia 41
cefazolin 43
cefoperazone 50
cefotoxin-cycloserine fructose agar 41
ceftiofur free acid equivalent 43
celiac
- disease 42
- disease, childhood 40
celiac sprue 52
cell
- adhesion factor 38
- adhesion molecule, endothelial 173
- adhesion molecule, vascular 173
- atypia 30
- bank, production 128
- bank, working 175
- basal 30
- basket 30
- bipolar 30
- carcinoma antigen, squamous 150
- collector, endocervical 67
- culture infectious dose 50 % 41
- culture, primary 128
- cultures, liver primary 101
- death, programmed 129
- dissociation 42
- dysplasia 30
- glomerular mesangium 112
- line 45
- line, avian 63
- line, avian rho0 64
- line, carcinoma 41
- line, certified 41
- line, minipig kidney 111
- line, mouse Schwann 112
- line, murine fibrosarcoma 76
- lines, B 31
- magnocellular neurosecretory 112
- matrix adhesion regulator 48
- mediated cytolysis or cytotoxicity 48
- mediated cytotoxicity, antibody-dependent 14
- membrane 47
- membrane receptor, plasma 43
- milk somatic 112
- Moloney sarcoma 112
- red blood 142
- sarcoma, reticulum 142
- sickle 150
- sorter, fluorescence-activated 72
- stock, master 105
- surface 52
- surface antigen 53
- surface antigen, tumor-specific 166
- volume, packed 129
- wall protein 55
- whole 175
cellobiose
- quinone oxidoreductase 39
cells
- baby hamster kidney 32
- high frequency 85
- immunoglobulin bearing 89
- interdigitating 90
- irreversibly sickled 94
- mammosomatotroph 112

- mantle storage 112
- marrow stromal 112
- mesangial 112
- mesenchymal stem 112
- mesothelial 112
- miniature squamous 112
- multipotential subserosal 112
- muscle satellite 112
- myelin-forming Schwann 112
- myeloid suppressor 112
- neurosecretory 120
- nonmyelinating Schwann 118
- nonserrated 120
- Spodoptera frugiperda 151
- total viable 167
- undifferentiated 169
- untreated 169
- white 175
- white blood 175
- whole cord blood 175

cellular changes
- benign 30

cellular erythroblastosis
- oncogene 43

cellular oncogene 49

cellularity
- mixed 104
- mixed, classical Hodgkin lymphoma 105

Celsius 37

cement
- fast-setting calcium phosphate 76
- glass ionomer 79

center
- crisis intervention 45
- edge angle 43
- for substance abuse treatment 53
- germinal 77
- of mass 47
- of pressure 49
- regional trauma 147

centers
- for disease control 43
- microtubule organizing 113
- progressively transformed germinal 139

centi
- grade 37
- gram 44
- Gray 44
- liter 45
- meter 44, 47
- morgan 47
- stoke 52

centigrade 37

central
- blood volume 39
- catheter, peripherally inserted 133
- circulating blood volume 40
- conduction time 42
- core disease 40
- hypoventilation syndrome, congenital 41
- midwives' board 48
- mucoepidermoid tumor of the jaws 48
- nervous system 49
- nervous system lymphoma, primary 129
- nucleus, caudal 42
- pontine myelinolysis 50
- public health laboratory 50
- retinal vein 52
- retinal vein occlusion 52
- service 52
- supply 52
- supply room 54
- tegmental field 54
- vein, terminal hepatic venule 162
- venous catheters 55
- venous line 55
- venous pressure 55

centralis lateralis 45

centric relation occlusion 48

centrifugal
- countercurrent chromatography 40

centrifuged
- culture fluid 41

centrilobular emphysema 46

centroblastic
- centrocytic lymphoma 39
- lymphoma 39

centrocytic
- lymphoma 39

centrum medianum 47

cephalin
- cholesterol antigen 40
- cholesterol flocculation 41

cephalopelvic disproportion 50

cerebellar
- artery, anterior inferior 17
- artery, postero-inferior 133
- ataxia 46

cerebral
- amyloid angiopathy 38
- artery infarction, posterior 128
- artery occlusion, middle 104
- blood flow 39
- blood flow, regional 142
- blood volume 39
- hemorrhages, deep 56
- hypoperfusion, critically attained threshold 38
- infarction 44
- ischemia, noncardiac 116
- lymphoma, primary 129
- malaria 47
- mantle 47
- palsy 50
- scintigraphy 52
- subarachnoid venous pressure 53
- thrombosis 54

cerebrocostomandibular 41
- syndrome 42

cerebrospinal 52
- fluid 53
- fluid hypotension 53
- fluid pressure 54
- fluid volume 54
- fluid, artificial 13
- fluid-Wassermann reaction 54
- meningitis, acute 11

cerebrovascular
- accident (stroke) 55
- disease 39, 55

- insufficiency 55
ceroid lipofuscinosis 46
ceroid-lipofuscinosis
- neuronal 100
certainty factor 37
certified 51
- board 30
- cell line 41
- commission 39
- laboratory assistant 46
- laboratory technician 47
- medical assistant 48
- record techniques 51
- registered nurse anesthetist 51
- rehabilitation registered nurse 51
- respiratory therapy technician 52
cervical 37, 43
- collar 30
- compression overloading test 42
- dilation 43
- discectomy and fusion, anterior 10
- discectomy, anterior 10
- fusion, anterior 10
- fusion, posterior 129
- intraepithelial neoplasia 45
- laminectomy 46
- mucosa or mucus 47
- nerve 40
- range of motion 51
- root lesions 51
- spine 52, 54
- spine radiography 51, 54
- sprain, acute 13
- stimulation 52
- strain, acute 13
- thoracic 54
- thoracic, lumbar 54
- traction 54
- traction, intermittent 90
- trauma syndrome, acute 13
- vertebra 55
- vertebrae 40
cervicitis
- mucopurulent 110
cervico
- brachial syndrome 39
- dorsal 42
- dorsal syndrome 43
- linguoaxial 46
cervix 43, 55
cesarean
- birth 39
- delivery 42
- section 52, 53
- vaginal birth after 173
Cesarean section
- low transverse 102
- lower segment 102
cesarean section 52
cesium 52
chain
- reaction, ligase 99
chain reaction
- differential-display polymerase 58
challenge
- bronchoprovocation 34
chamber
- anterior 10
- equipment, bubble 31
chamois contagious ecthyma 41
change 44, 181
- absorbance 181
- decibels 181
- impedance 65
- minimum significant 112
- no significant 120
- pH 181
- pressure 181
changes
- benign cellular 30
channel
- chloride 46
characteristic 44
charcoal
- dextran-coated 56
Charcot
- Leyden crystal 41, 46
- Marie-Tooth 49
charge
- electric 65
- elementary 65
charge-coupled device 40
chart
- basal temperature 35
- body temperature 35
check 45, 180
- list, achievement 11
- out 49
checked 180
checklist
- injury behavior 89
checks with previous results 50
Chediak
- Higashi syndrome 44
- Higashi syndrome gene 44
chemical
- and biological warfare 39
- cleavage of mismatch 41
- dependancy 42
- reaction, reversible 179
- sensitivity, multiple 105
- shift anisotropy 53
chemicals
- endocrine-active 67
chemiluminescence 45
chemistry
- combinatorial 39
- routine admission 154
chemoattractant
- protein, monocyte 105
chemo-embolization
- transcatheter arterial 159
chemokine
- cutaneous T-cell attracting 54
- secondary lymphoid organ 153
chemotactic
- agent, thymus-derived 160
- factor, basophil 31
- factor, crystal-induced 41
- factor, monocyte 104
chemotherapy 44, 54
- adjuvant 14
- high-does 84
- high-dose 84
- intraperitoneal hyperthermic perfusion 93
cherry red spot myoclonus 51
chest 44
- and left arm 45

- back 39
- pain 50
- pain, substernal 157
- physical therapy 50
- radiogram 50
- strap 52
- syndrome, acute 13
- wall 55
- x-ray 55

chick cell agglutination 40
- test 40

Chick-Martin (coefficient) 47
chief 44
- complaint 39, 40
- medical director 48
- of staff 52
- of staff, associate 12

child
- term birth living 160

childbirth without pain 55
childhood
- celiac disease 40
- diseases, usual 169
- epilepsy, benign 31
- illness, unusual 169
- muscular dystrophy 48
- onset 49
- onset growth hormone deficiency 49

children
- of alcoholics screening test 38
- of alcoholics, adult 12
- protective services 50
- social worker 54

chills, fever, night sweats 43
chimpanzee coryza agent 40
Chinese
- medicine, traditional 160
- restaurant syndrome 51

chiropractic
- doctor 56

chirurgiae magister 48
chi-square 181
chitin deacetylases 43
chlamydia 37
chloracetate esterase 43
chlorambucil 46
- vinblastine, procarbazine, and prednisone 44

chloramphenicol 38, 48
- acetyltransferase 38

chloride 45
- channel 46
- diarrhea 46
- hemagglutination, chronic 41

chlorine 45
chloroacetyl 46
chloroethylclonidine 43
chloromercuribenzoate 48
chlorophyll
- bacterial 31

chloroquine
- mepacrine 47
- resistant Plasmodium falciparum 51

chlorphenotane 58
chlorpromazine (thorazine) 50
choice
- model, contextual 41
- reaction time 51

cholangiogram 167
- transhepatic 162
- T-tube 166

cholangiography
- intravenous 95
- percutaneous transhepatic 139

cholangiopancreatography
- endoscopic retrograde 70

cholangitis
- primary sclerosing 138

cholecystectomy 42
- laparoscopic 98, 99

cholecystitis
- chronic calculous 40

cholecystogram 41, 54
- oral 122

cholecystography 41, 54
cholecystokinin 41
- like immunoreactivity 41
- octapeptide 41
- receptor B 41

cholecystokinin-pancreozymin 41
choledocho-jejunostomy
- Roux-Y 149

cholelithiasis 45
cholera
- hog 85
- toxin subunit B 54
- vaccine, whole cell/ recombinant B subunit 175

cholestasis
- total parenteral nutrition-associated 163

cholestatic
- hepatitis, chronic 41

cholesterol
- antigen, cephalin 40
- concentration, biliary 30
- lecithin 45
- lecithin flocculation 46
- low-density lipoprotein 99
- lowering lipid 46
- serum 44
- stone 52

choline dehydrogenase 46
choline phosphate 50
cholinergic
- agonist carbachol 41

cholinesterases 44
cholinomimetic
- effects, observable 122

chondrocalcinosis 131
chondroitin
- 4-sulfate 53
- sulfate 52
- sulfate A 53

chondromalacia 47
chopped meat (medium) 47
chorioamnionic
- hemosiderosis, diffuse 57

choriocarcinoma 40
chorionic
- gonadotropin 44
- gonadotropin, urinary 169
- somatomammotropin 52
- somatomammotropin, A 53
- villous sampling 55

choroidal
- degeneration, senile macular 155

- hemangiomas, circumscribed 41
- hemangiomas, diffuse 57
chromatography
- centrifugal, countercurrent 40
- gas 77, 78
- gas-liquid 79
- gas-solid 82
- gel permeation 82
- head space gas 87
- high pressure (or performance) liquid 87
- thin-layer 162
chromium release test 51
chromogranin A 44
chromosomal
- aberration 37
- in situ hybridization 45
- region, DiGeorge 59
chromosome 52
- abnormality, constitutional 40
- break 53
- female sex 176
- gap 54
- male sex 176
- region, Smith-Magenis 155
- Y 177
- yeast artificial 177
chronic 44
- active hepatitis 38
- active hepatitis, autoimmune-type 17
- airflow obstruction 38
- atrial fibrillation 38
- AV block 39
- brain syndrome 39, 44
- bronchitis 39
- calculous cholecystitis 40
- catarrhal colitis 40
- chloride hemagglutination 41
- cholestatic hepatitis 41
- coronary insufficiency 41
- disease, anemia 10
- fatigue (and immune dysfunction) syndrome 43
- fatigue and immune dysfunction syndrome 43
- fatigue syndrome 43
- granulocytic leukemia 44
- granulomatous disease 44
- heart failure 44
- idiopathic myelofibrosis 45
- inactive cirrhosis 45
- inflammatory demyelinating polyneuropathy 45
- leukemia 45
- liver disease 46
- lobular hepatitis 46
- low back pain 46
- lung disease 46
- lymphocytic leukemia 46
- lymphocytic leukemia, atypical 11
- lymphocytic leukemia/small lymphocytic lymphoma 47
- lymphocytic thyroiditis 47
- lymphoprolipherative disorders, B-cell 31
- lymphosarcoma (cell) leukemia 47
- metabolic acidosis 48
- mucocutaneous candidiasis 48
- myelogenous leukemia 48
- myeloid leukemia, atypical 11
- myelomonocytic leukemia 48
- myeloproliferative disease 48
- necrotizing pulmonary aspergillosis 49
- neutrophilic leukemia 49
- obstructive airways disease 49
- obstructive lung disease 49
- obstructive pulmonary disease 50
- obstructive pulmonary emphysema 50
- peritoneal dialysis 50
- progressive multiple sclerosis 50
- pulmonary emphysema 50
- relapsing pancreatitis 51
- renal failure 51
- renal insufficiency 51
- respiratory disease 51
- restrictive pulmonary disease 51
- schizophrenia 52
- subdural hematoma 54
- superficial keratitis 54
- vascular insufficiency 55
chronological 44
- age 37
Churg-Strauss syndrome 54
chymotrypsin-like
- cationic protein 46
- protein 47
cigarette 45
- consumption 45
- smoker 52
ciliary neurotrophic factor 49
ciliated
- columnar epithelium, pseudostratified 128
cingulate
- cortex, anterior 10
circuit
- application specific integrated 23
circular
- deoxyribonucleic acid, covalently closed 40
- dichroism 42
- muscle 47
circulating
- blood volume 39
- cathodic antigen 40
- immune complexes 45
- monocyte 47
circulation 45
- extracorporeal 67
- motion, sensation 49
- persistent fetal 131
circumference 45
- abdominal 10
- head 83
- occipital-frontal 122
circumferential
- measurement 47
circumflex
- branch, atrioventricular 26
- coronary artery 40
- right 142

Ix

circumscribed
- choroidal hemangiomas 41
cirrhosis
- chronic inactive 45
- of liver 45
- primary biliary 128
cis
- diamminedichloroplatinum 45
cisplatin
- etoposide and bleomycin 130
- methotrexate-vinblastine 49
cistemae
- cylindrical confronting 40
citrate
- phosphate-dextrose 50
- phosphate-double-dextrose adenine 50
- synthase 52
citric acid fermentation 38
clammy and cold 40
clarified 45
class V-like molecule
- Miltenberger 108
classic Kaposi sarcoma 45
classical
- heart transplantation 44
- Hodgkin lymphoma 44
- swine fever 53
classification 46
- after initial multimodal treatment 177
- scheme for leukemia, french american and british 72
clavicle 45, 46
clavicular line
- anterior 11
clean 45
- catch 39
- catch midstream 42
- catch midstream urine 42
- dry, intact 43
- intermittent catheterization 45
- voided specimen (urine) 47
clean catch urine 42
clear 45
- cell endothelioma 41
- to auscultation 54
- to auscultation bilaterally 54
clearance 46
- creatinine 40, 51
- maximum 47
- standard 37
- total body 47
- urea 169
cleft 45
- limb-heart (syndrome) 46
- lip 46
- lip with cleft palate 47
- lip with or without cleft palate 47
- lip without cleft palate 47
- lip/cleft palate 46
cleidocranial
- dysostosis 46
- dysplasia 40
Clerc-Levy-Critesco
- syndrome 46
click
- late systolic murmur syndrome, mid-systolic 112
- mid-systolic 112
client
- interface, common 41
climacteric syndrome 52
clindamycin 48
clinic 45, 46
- birth control 30
- crisis intervention 45
- medical emergency 105
- outpatient 123
- scheduling 52
clinical 37, 45, 46
- and laboratory index, composite 41
- behavioral science 39
- cancer protocols 46
- cardiovascular disease 40
- care management system 42
- data set, uniform 169
- dementia rating 43
- event, major adverse 103
- examination, objective structured 126
- investigation plan 45
- laboratory 46
- laboratory improvement act 46
- laboratory scientist 47, 52
- laboratory technician 47
- materials requisition 49
- medicine 48
- modification 48
- pathology 47
- project manager 50
- records 50
- research unit 52
- social worker, licensed 99
- stage 52
- stage 4 54
- status 52
- supply management 54
- symptom self-evaluation (questionnaire) 53
- target volume 54
- trial 54
- trials exemption 54
- trials of acquired immunodeficiency syndrome drugs 18
- trials office 54
- unit 55
clinically definite multiple sclerosis 43
clinicopathological
- correlation 50
clipping
- infinite amplitude 88
clobazam 46
- n-desmethyl 116
clofibrate 43, 47
clomipramine 46
clonazepam 55
clonidine 37, 47
cloning
- in vitro expression 95
- inhibitory factor 46
clonorchis 47
clonus 45
closed 46
- chest cardiac resuscitation 40
- circle deoxyribonucleic acid 40
- craniocerebral trauma 40
- cup 39

- head injury 44
- reduction 50
- reduction and cast 50
- reduction and percutaneous fixation 51

closing
- capacity 39
- wedge high tibial osteotomy 55

clostridium 45, 47
- difficile 43

closure 45
- aortic valve 26
- clonus, cathodal 40
- contraction, anodal 10
- contraction, cathodal 40
- delayed primary 62
- odor, anodal 12
- pressure, maximum urethral 140
- sound, anodal 13
- tetanus, anodal 13

clot lysis time 47
clothing 47
clotting 45
- time 47
- time, activated 13
- time, Lee-White 103
- time, thrombin 160

cloudy 45, 46
clozapine 47
cluster
- of differentiation 42
- region, breakpoint 31
- region, minor breakpoint 104

clusterin 47
Cmax 48
coagulation 49
- argon plasma 21
- disseminated intravascular 59
- factor, cancer 41
- interstitial laser 91

coagulopathy
- consumptive 39

coal
- workers' pneumoconiosis 55

coat protein 50
coated
- tube radioimmunoassay 54

cobalt 49
cocaine and morphine 48
coccidioidal meningitis 48
coccygeal 42
cochlear
- microphonic 48
- nucleus, anteroventral 26

Cochran
- Mantel-Haenszel test 48

Cockayne syndrome 52
cod liver oil 47
code of practice
- approved 12

codling
- moth 48

codon for alanine
- guanine-cytosine-adenine 78
- guanine-cytosine-cytosine 78
- guanine-cytosine-guanine 78
- guanine-cytosine-uracil 78

codon for arginine 44
- adenine-guanine-adenine 15
- adenine-guanine-guanine 15
- cytosine-guanine-cytosine 44
- cytosine-guanine-guanine 44
- cytosine-guanine-uracil 44

codon for asparagine
- adenine-adenine-cytosine 5
- adenine-adenine-uracil 7

codon for aspartic acid
- guanine-adenine-cytosine 77
- guanine-adenine-uracil 77

codon for glutamic acid
- guanine-adenine-adenine 77
- guanine-adenine-guanine 77

codon for glutamine
- cytosine-adenine-adenine 38
- cytosine-adenine-guanine 38

codon for glycine
- guanine-guanine-adenine 78
- guanine-guanine-cytosine 78
- guanine-guanine-guanine 78
- guanine-guanine-uracil 78

codon for histidine
- cytosine-adenine-cytosine 38
- cytosine-adenine-uracil 38

codon for isoleucine
- adenine-uracil-adenine 25
- adenine-uracil-cytosine 25
- adenine-uracil-uracil 25

codon for leucine
- cytosine-uracil-adenine 55
- cytosine-uracil-cytosine 55
- cytosine-uracil-guanine 55
- cytosine-uracil-uracil 55

codon for lysine
- adenine-adenine-adenine 5
- adenine-adenine-guanine 5

codon for methionine
- adenine-uracil-guanine 25

codon for proline
- cytosine-cytosine-adenine 40
- cytosine-cytosine-cytosine 40
- cytosine-cytosine-guanine 41
- cytosine-cytosine-uracil 42

codon for serine
- adenine-cytosine-cytosine 10
- adenine-guanine-uracil 15

codon for threonine
- adenine-cytosine-adenine 10
- adenine-cytosine-cytosine 10
- adenine-cytosine-guanine 11
- adenine-cytosine-uracil 13

codon for valine
- guanine-uracil-adenine 82
- guanine-uracil-cytosine 82
- guanine-uracil-guanine 82
- guanine-uracil-uracil 83

coefficient
- correlation 181
- integrated backscatter 89
- of thermal expansion 54
- transmission 181

cofactor
- heparin 84

Coffin-Lowry syndrome 47
cognitive
- behavioral treatment/therapy 39
- distortions scale, bulimia 30
- examination, cross-cultural 40

coherence
- magnitude squared 112
coital
- alignment technique 38
colchicine sensitivity 46
cold
- and clammy 40
- hemoglobinuria, paroxysmal 129
- insoluble globulin 45
- stability factor 53
colic
- biliary 30
colistin 45
colitis
- antibiotic-associated pseudo-membranous 6
- antibiotic-associated pseudomembranous 6
- chronic catarrhal 40
- collagenous 39
- Crohn 40
- ulcerative 169
collagen
- autoantibodies 8
- induced arthritis 44
- sponge contraceptive 53
collagenase soluble glomerular basement membrane 54
collagenous colitis 39
collapse
- scapholunate advanced (wrist) 153
collar
- cervical 30
- white 175
collateral
- ligament, lateral 99
- ligament, ulnar 169
- ligament, upper 169
collecting
- system, condom catheter 40
collection
- device, urine 169
collector
- endocervical cell 67
collegiate
- adult children of alcoholics 12
colliculus
- motor layers superior 111
collision
- induced dissociation 45
- motor vehicle 114
colon
- anastomosis bursting pressure 39
- and rectum surgery 51
colonic
- wall stents, endoluminal 68
colony
- count 39
- count, and culture 40
- forming unit, granulocyte and macrophage 79
- forming units 43
- stimulating factor, granulocyte and macrophage 79
colony-forming
- active substance, compact 41
- cells 43
- unit cells 43
- units, generating granulocytes, erythroblasts, macrophages, and megakaryiocytes 44
- units, spleen 44
colony-stimulating
- activity 53
- factor 53
- factor 1 receptor 53
- factor receptor 54
color
- doppler 42
- flow duplex imaging 43
- index 44
- test, flight 75
- vision 55
colorectal
- cancer 39
- carcinoma 50
colored vision 173
columnar
- cells 39
- epithelium, pseudostratified ciliated 128
coma
- hyperosmolar nonketotic 86
- scale, glasgow 78
- therapy, atropine 13
combat support (army) hospital 54
combination 49
- drug 42
combinatorial chemistry 39
combine 49
combined
- mechanical injury 48
- modality 48
- modality therapy 49
- system disease 53
comminuted fracture
- compound 41
commission certified 39
commissurotomy
- percutaneous transvenous mitral 139
common
- acute lymphoblastic leukemia, antigen 38
- all 38
- antigen, enterobacterial 67
- antigen, leukocyte 99
- bile duct 39, 42
- carotid artery 40
- client interface 41
- cold 39
- migraine 48
- toxicity criteria 54
communicable 49
- disease 42
communicating
- artery, anterior 12
- artery, anterior inferior 17
community
- care network 42
- hospital, essential access 67
- mental health centers 48
- rate, adjusted 12
compact
- colony-forming active substance 41
- disk 42

companies
- physician practice management 136
comparative
- genomic hybridization - cytogenetics method 44
- mean dose 48
compare 43
compatibility
- electromagnetic 69
compatible with 55
competitive protein binding 50
complains of 49
complaint
- chief 40
- current 39
- present 128
complaints 49
complement 37
- fixation 17, 43
- fixation, cardiolipin 41
- fixation, lesion on the erythrocyte cell membrane at the site of 66
- guinea pig 82
- lysis inhibitor 46
- receptors, leukocyte 50
- total functional hemolytic 44
complementarity
- determining regions 43
complementary
- and alternative medicine 38
- DNA 43
complementation
- dominant-negative 61
complete
- bed rest 39
- blood count 39
- conversion 39
- left bundle branch block 46
- medium 48
- physical examination 50
- remission 50
- remission, continuous 42
- response 50
- stroke 52
completely
- absent 181
- denaturated 42
complex
- avidin-biotin 8
- critical care 40
- dementia-parkinsonism-amyotrophy 58
- dystrophin-glycoprotein 59
- enzyme-substrate 70
- intervertebral joint 95
- loading 46
- major histocompatibility 107
- major symptom 112
- medial septum 112
- membrane attack 103
- mycobacterium avium 103
- nascent polypeptide associated 115
- protein, dystrophin-associated 56
- pulvinar-posterior-lateral 140
- reaction time 51
- regional pain syndrome (type I and II) 51
complexes
- amygdalohippocampal 15
- migrating spike 112
- synaptonemal 150
compliance
- effective 43
- lung 46
- lung-thorax 47
- of the respiratory system 51
- static respiratory 37
complicating condition 39
complication
- biliary tract 35
- probability, normal tissue 121
complications 48
- major septic 112
component
- extensive, intraductal 69
components
- both 32
composite
- clinical and laboratory index 41
- elements, oct-containing 122
compost stabilization test 50
compound 49
- cathartic 39
- comminuted fracture 41
- muscle (or motor) action potential 48
comprehensive
- cardiac care unit 40
- care clinic 40
- exam 122
- renal scintillation procedure 51
compress 49
compressed
- gas association 44
- spectral assay 53
compression
- antero-posterior 21
- cord 40
- device, sequential 150
- lateral 99
- septal perforator 156
- syndrome 52
- syndrome, uterine 170
computed
- axial tomography 38
- body tomography 39
- tomography, electron-beam 67
- tomography, radiotherapy dedicated 148
- tomography, single photon emission 156
computer
- assisted frameless stereotactic interstitial brachytherapy 38
- assisted minimally invasive surgery 38
- based examination 39
- calculated 39
computerized
- renal tomography 51
- spectral analysis 53
- tomography 54
concavalin A 49
concave 39
- lens 180
concentrate 49
- urine 169
concentrated 49

concentrated strength 52
concentration 37
- approximate lethal 18
- average integrated 17
- bactericidal 30
- biliary cholesterol 30
- blood alcohol 28
- constant initial 45
- maximum allowable 103
- maximum permissible 110
- maximum use 113
- minimal 47
- minimal sporocidal 112
- minimum detectable 105
- minimum spirocheticidal 112
conception
- interval, parturition 129
conceptual
- design 42
concordance 39
concurrent care concern 40
condition
- complicating 39
- critical 40
- general 77
- median 48
- on admission 49
- on discharge 49
- unsatisfactory 169
conditionally streptomycin dependent 53
conditioned
- neurosis ventilation, acute 11
- reflex 50
- stimulus 52
condom
- catheter collecting system 40
conduct
- disorder 42
conductance
- parallel 81
conductances
- end-diastolic 78
- end-systolic 78
conduction
- aberrant ventricular 26
- air 10
- air and bone 8
- air greater than bone 8
- atrioventricular nodal 27
- bone 30
- defect, intraventricular 95
- disorder 42
- pathway, accessory 12
- system disease 53
- system, atrioventricular 26
- time, central 42
- velocities, nerve 117
- ventriculoatrial 172
conductivity 181
conduit
- aorto-pericardial pouch 22
condylion 42
cone-shaped epiphysis 53
conference
- consecutive case 40
confidence
- interval 44
- limit or level 46
- limit, upper 169
confined to bed 54
confocal
- laser scanning microscopy 47
conformity
- european 43
confronting
- cistemae, cylindrical 40
confusional
- state, acute 13
congenital
- cardiopathy 39
- cataract 39
- central hypoventilation syndrome 41
- contractural arachnodactyly 40
- dislocation of the hip 44
- disorders of glycosylation 43
- duodenal obstruction 43
- dyserythropoietic anemia 43
- dysplasia of hip 43
- heart disease 44
- heart disease, cyanotic 41
- hemidysplasia with ichthyosiform erythrodermal and limb defects 44
- hypoplastic anemia 44
- infections with T = toxoplasmosis, O = other, R = rubella, C = cytomegalic inclusion disease, H = hepatitis B a. herpes 163
- limb absence 168
- limb deficiency 46
- lipoid adrenal hyperplasia 46
- localized absence of skin 46
- malformation 48
- muscular dystrophy 48
- rubella syndrome 51
- self-healing reticulohistiocytosis 54
- short bowel 53
- syphilis 52
- talipes equinovarus 54
congestion
- pulmonary venous 140
congestive
- cardiac failure 41
- cardiomyopathy 41
- failure 49
- heart failure 44
- myocardiopathy 48
- right ventricular failure 52
conglutinating
- complement absorption test 40
conjugata
- diagonalis 42
conjugate vaccine
- hemophillus influenzae type B 85
conjugated
- bile salts 39
- equine estrogens, vaginal administration 173
- estrogens, oral 122
conjunctiva
- and sclera 53
conjunctival
- secretion 52
conjunctivitis
- acute hemorrhagic 15
- giant papillary 82
connection
- monosynaptic 112

connections
- modified sampling 112
connective
- tissue disease 54
- tissue disease, mixed 105
- tissue disease, undifferentiated 170
- tissue disease, undifferentiated (unclassifiable) 170
consanguineous
- donor 42
conscious 52
- sedation 52
consciousness 52, 55
- altered level of 18
- level 101
- loss 101
- research and training project 52
consecutive case conference 40
consent
- decree 42
- form, informed 90
conservation
- surgery, breast 31
conservative surgery 52
consistent with 55
constant
- darkness 57
- dielectric 181
- domain of L chain 46
- initial concentration 45
- linear velocity 47
- neutral loss (scanning) 49
- spring 52
constipation 49
constitutional
- chromosome abnormality 40
consultant 49
consultation 49
consultation-liaison (setting) 46
consumer choice health plan 41
consumption
- cigarette 45
- excess post-oxygen 70
consumptive coagulopathy 39
contact
- dermatitis 42
- dermatitis, allergic 10
- dermatitis, eczematous allergic 67
- guard assist 44
- lens 46
- lens, bandage 31
- sensitivity 52
contact lenses
- bifocal 31
contagious
- bovine pleuropneumonia 39
- disease 42
- ecthyma, chamois 41
contaminated
- small bowel 53
- small bowel, syndrome 53
content
- bone mineral 33
- peripheral arterial oxygen 127
- thoracic fluid 161
contershock
- direct current 56
contextual choice model 41
Contin
- morphine sulphate 112
- tablets 112
continue
- same 52
- with 55
continued 49
continuing
- care level 41
- medical education 48
continuity
- care management 48
continuous
- ambulatory peritoneal dialysis 38
- arterio-venous haemodialysis 39
- arterio-venous haemofiltration 39
- bladder irrigation 39
- complete remission 42
- cycling peritoneal dialysis 42
- electronic fetal monitoring 43
- lumbar epidural (anesthesia) 46
- murmur 48
- passive motion machine 50
- positive airway pressure 50
- subcutaneous insulin infusion 54
- tracheal gas insufflation 54
- veno-venous haemofiltration 55
- veno-venous hemodialysis 55
contraceptive
- collagen sponge 53
- device, intrauterine 95
- drugs, steroid 150
- oral 122
- pills, oral 122
- prevalence rate 50
- therapy, oral 122
contracting
- agent, smooth muscle 155
- region, abnormally 12
contraction
- atrial premature 21
- cathodal closure 40
- fetal heart rate-uterine 74
- giant migratory 79
- isovolumic 95
- junctional premature 96
- maximum voluntary 114
- no 181
- premature junctional 133
- premature ventricular 140
- rested state 146
contractions 49
- spontaneous phasic 156
- uterine 169
- ventricular premature 174
contractural
- arachnodactyly, congenital 40
contraindications 44
contralateral
- local anesthesia 46
- renal plasma flow 51
- routing of signals (hearing aid) 51
contrast
- cystogram 39

lx

- medium 48
- sensitivity (test) 52
- sensitivity function 53
- to-noise ratio 49
- ventriculography 55
control
- activity, electrical 67
- center, disease vector 64
- diet 42
- infection, certified 44
- limit, upper 169
- medical ventilation 49
- multidimensional health locus 107
- online medical 123
- protein, nitrogen assimilation 115
- ratio, respiratory 142
- serum 52
- training, anxiety 13
- trial, random 147
controlled
- atmospheres 37
- drug 42
- release infusion system 51
- substances act 53
controller
- oxygen ratio monitor 125
convalescence 52
convalescent 52
conventional
- dialysis 42
- spin-echo 53
conversion complete 39
convex lens 180
convexo-concavc 40
convoluted
- tubule, distal 57
convulsant
- dose, fifty percent 43
convulsive
- disorder 42
- disorder, grand mal 79
- dose 42
cooperative 12
coordination
- care-cure 40
coordinator
- instructor 89
copolymer
- vinyl acetate - maleic acid - vinyl chloride 174
copper reduction test 51
coproporphyrin
- urinary 169
copulatory mechanism 48
cor triatriatum 54
coracoclavicular 40
coralline hydroxyapatite 44
cord
- dysfunction, vocal 173
- spinal 156
- true vocal 167
cord compression 40
cordis standard valves 54
core binding factor (16q22) 39
corn
- gluten feed, dry 56
corneal
- dystrophy 43
- retinal potential 51
Cornelia de Lange syndrome 47
cornu ammonis 38
corona
- lymphocyte 99
coronary
- angiography, quantitative 140
- angioplasty, percutaneous transluminal 139
- artery bypass 38
- artery bypass graft 38
- artery disease 38
- artery disease, arteriosclerotic 23
- artery, circumflex 40
- artery, left 99
- artery, left anterior descending 98
- artery, left circumflex 99
- artery, right 142
- atherectomy (for coronary ostial lesions), directional 56
- atherosclerotic heart disease 38
- blood flow 39
- bypass, minimally invasive directed 108
- cardiac care unit 42
- care nursing 42
- care unit, intensive 89
- care, intensive 89
- disease, multivessel 104
- heart disease 44, 97
- insufficiency 44
- insufficiency, acute 11
- insufficiency, chronic 41
- intensive care 45
- intervention, percutaneous 129
- occlusion, acute 12
- rehabilitation program 51
- sclerosis 52
- sinus 52
- sinus blood flow 53
- sinus flow 53
- treatment, advanced 13
coronary syndrome
- acute 13
corpora cardiaca 40
corporate services administration department 53
corpus
- allatum 38
- callosum 40
- cardiacum peptide, microhodotermes viator 108
- luteum 46
- luteum hormone 46
- luteum insufficiency 46
- luteum stimulating hormone 47
- striatum 52
corpuscular
- cell volume, mean 105
- hemoglobin concentration, mean 105
- hemoglobin, mean 104
corrected 39, 51
- (echo long axis) length 46
- blood volume 39
- count increment 41
- retention time 51
- sinus recovery time 54
correction
- multiplicative scatter 112

correlation
- clinicopathological 50
- coefficient 181
cortex 37
- adrenal 10
- associative visual 26
- motor-sensory 112
- prefrontal 131
cortical
- basal ganglionic degeneration 39
- blood volume 39
- degeneration syndromes, asymmetrical 10
- hyperostosis, human infantile 90
- somatosensory evoked potential 53
- somatosensory evoked response 53
- spreading depression 53
- stromal hyperplasia 54
corticobasal degeneration 39
- syndrome 39
corticoid-sensitive 52
corticosteroid 52
corticosterone 54
- serum 42
- side-chain isomerase 53
corticostriatocerebellar 53
corticotropin
- like intermediate lobe peptide 46
- releasing factor or hormone 51
cortisol
- amniotic fluid 14
- binding globulin 39
- maternal serum 112
- urinary free 170
cortisone
- (compound E) 65
- resistant thymocyte 51
corynebacteria
- leprosy-derived 99
coryza
- agent, chimpanzee 40
cost
- index, geographic practice 82
costal
- artery
- lateral 99
- margin 48
- margin, left 99
- margin, right 142
cost-effectiveness
- ratio, incremental 90
costochondral 40
costovertebral angle 55
Cotrel-Dubousset 43
Coulter counter 40
count 54
- and culture, colony 40
- blood 30
- increment, corrected 41
- median diameter 48
- rate, axillary 12
- red blood 142
- red blood cells 142
- total viable 167
- whire blood 175
- white blood 175
- white cell 175
countercurrent
- chromatography, centrifugal 40
- distribution 40
- electrophoresis 41
counting
- finger 73
counts
- per minute 48, 50
covalently
- closed circular deoxyribonucleic acid 40
cover dressing
- absorbent 10
cow lung lavage 46
cow's
- milk 48
- milk, allergy 48
Coxsackie
- B virus 39
- B3 virus susceptibility 39
C-peptide
- urinary 169
cranial 50
- nerve 37, 49
- nerve number 10 49
- nerve number 5 49
- nerves (2 to 12) 49
- radiation therapy 51
- radiotherapy 51
craniocerebral
- trauma, closed 40
craniocervical 40
- malformation 41
craniospinal defect 53
craniosynostosis 51
- Boston type 53
crash
- motor vehicle 114
C-reactive protein 50, 51
- antiserum 51
- high-sensitivity 87
crease
- distal palmar 62
creatine
- kinase 45
- kinase muscle band 45
- phosphate 51
- phosphokinase 50
creatinine 51
- (ratio), uric acid 168
- clearance 40, 51
- serum 150
crescentic
- glomerulonephritis 44
crest
- left iliac 100
cresyl
- violet 55
Creutzfeldt-Jakob disease 45
cricoid lamina 46
crisis
- blastic 30
- intervention clinic 45
- sickle cell 150
criterion level 46
crithidia luciliae immunofluorescence 46
critical
- carbohydrate level 41
- care 40
- care complex 40
- care medical unit 42
- care medicine 41

- care nursing 42
- closing volume 42
- condition 40
- hematocrit 51
- list 46
- micellar concentration 48
- region, minimal DiGeorge 105
- serum chemistry value 53
- stimulus duration 53

critically
- attained threshold of cerebral hypoperfusion 38

Crohn
- colitis 40
- disease 43

Cronkhite-Canada (syndrome) 40
cross 176
- cultural cognitive examination 40
- reacting protein 51
- section area 53
- sectional echocardiography 53

crossed
- diagonal 43

crowded
- groups, hyperchromatic 84

crown
- crisp experimental index 41
- heel 44
- rump 50

cruciate
- ligament, anterior 11

crus cerebri 40
crush syndrome 52
crutch
- walking 55
- walking, instructions 55

cryoablation
- endometrial 67

cryogenic 52
- storage container 53

cryoglobulin 52
cryoprecipitate 52
cryosurgery 52
cryosurgical iceball gauge 45
cryotherapy 52
cryptidin-related sequence 51
cryst 52
crystal 52
- Charcot-Leyden 41, 46
- induced chemotactic factor 41
- ligand field 46

crystallin
- gene, gamma 52

crystalline 52
c-section 52, 53
c-terminal parathyroid hormone 139
ct-guided needle biopsy 54
cubic 55
- centimeter 39, 47

cues index
- behavioral 31

cuff
- blood pressure 34

culture
- and sensitivity 53
- blood 30, 33
- bound syndrome 39
- fluid, centrifuged 41
- meat starter 112
- mucosal starter 112
- urine 169

cultured macrophages 48
cultures 55
- short-time, unstimulated 172

cum 37
cumulative cardiotoxic dose 40
curative dose 43
curettage
- and biopsy 30
- and dilatation 56

curium 47
current
- alternating 10
- complaint 39
- contents 40
- contershock, direct 56
- densities, scalp 150
- list of medical literature 47
- procedural terminology 50
- smoker 52
- strength 52

currents
- miniature synaptic 112

curriculum vitae 55
curve
- analysis, receiver operating 144

curvilinear body 46
Cushing syndrome 52
customized headholder system 44
cutaneous
- hypersensitivity, delayed 57
- lymphocyte antigen 46
- lymphoid hyperplasia 46
- lymphoma, primary 129
- malignant melanoma 48
- mastocytosis 48
- mastocytosis, maculopapular 110
- squamous cell carcinoma 53
- T-cell attracting chemokine 54

cutdown 43
CVA
- tenderness 55

cyanoacrylate
- methoxypropyl 110

cyanosis 37
- clubbing, edema 41

cyanotic congenital heart disease 41
cycle
- length 46
- length of the idioventricular rhythm 46
- length, basic 31
- length, paced 47
- lengths, basic 31

cycles per second 52
cyclic
- AMP receptor protein 51
- lysine anhydride 46

cyclin-dependent kinases 43
- inhibitors 43

cycling
- peritoneal dialysis, continuous 42

cyclohexyladenosine 44
cyclohexylmethylphosphonofluoridate 49
cyclooxygenase-II 50

cyclophosphamide 50
- adriamycin, and 5-fluorouracil 38
- cisplatin, fluorouracil, and extramustine 41
- methotrexate, 5-fluorouracil 48
cycloserine 52
cyclosporine 52, 54
- A 53
cylinder
- cast, long leg 100
- cast, short-leg 153
cylindrical confronting cistemae 40
cyst
- arachnoid 11
cystadenoma
- macrocystic serous 112
cystathionine beta-synthase 39
cystatin C 42
cysteine 37, 55
cystic
- disease fluid protein 15, gross 78
- duct 43
- fibrosis 43
- fibrosis transmembrane regulator 43
cystine
- lactose-electrolyte-deficient 46
cystitis
- acute hemorrhagic 15
cystogram
- contrast 39
- triple voiding 167
cystoscopic exam 55
cystoscopy 55
cystourethrogram
- voiding 173
cytarabine 22
cytochrome C oxidase 42, 50
cytochrome P450 55
cytokeratin 45
- acidic 45
- neutral to basic 45
cytokine induced-killer cells 45
cytologic smear
- ectocervix 173
- endocervix 173
- vagina 173
cytology
- aspiration biopsy 8
cytolysis or cytotoxicity
- cell-mediated 48
cytomegalovirus 49
- immune globulin 49
cytometry 48
- flow 73
cytopathic effect 50
cytoplasmic
- antibodies, antineutrophil 19
- antibodies, cytoplasmic antineutrophil 38
- antibodies, perinuclear antineutrophil 127
- antineutrophil cytoplasmic antibodies 38
- immunoglobulin 45
- immunoglobulin M 45
- membrane 48
- membrane-associated deoxyribonucleic acid 48
- tail of the amyloid precursor protein 22
cytoplasmic (ratio)
- nuclear 116
cytosine 37
- adenine-adenine codon for glutamine 38
- adenine-cytosine codon for histidine 38
- adenine-guanine codon for glutamine 38
- adenine-uracil codon for histidine 38
- cytosine-adenine codon for proline 40
- cytosine-cytosine codon for proline 40
- cytosine-guanine codon for proline 41
- cytosine-uracil codon for proline 42
- guanine-adenine codon for arginine 44
- guanine-cytosine codon for arginine 44
- guanine-guanine codon for arginine 44
- guanine-uracil codon for arginine 44
- uracil-adenine codon for leucine 55
- uracil-cytosine codon for leucine 55
- uracil-guanine codon for leucine 55
- uracil-uracil codon for leucine 55
cytotoxic
- assay, single-cell liquid 153
- lymphocyte 46
- lymphocyte maturation factor 47
- serum, antireticular 13
- T lymphocytes 54
- T-lymphocyte-associated antigen-4 (CD152) 54
cytotoxicity
- antibody-dependent cell-mediated 14
- monocyte synergistic 112
cytotrophoblast 54
cytoxan
- adriamycin, and vincristine 38
- methotrexate, 5-fluorouracil 48
- plus adriamycin (treatment regimen) 38
- plus epirubicin plus 5 43
- vincristine, prednisone 55

D

inbred strains of rats 55
Dahl
- salt-resistant rats 63
- salt-sensitive 63
daily
- dose 57
- dose, average 14
- dose, highest average 83

- dose, max. recommended 111
- dose, maximum 105
- gain, average 14
- insulin injections, multiple 105
- intake, acceptable 14
- intake, recommended 142
- living, activities 14
- maintenance dose 60
- rumination time 62
- weight 64

D-alanyl-D-alanine peptidase 58

damage
- brain 31
- DNA 58
- glaucomatous optic nerve 81
- non-specific 120
- repair, sublethal 153
- sublethal 153
- target organ 163

danazol 56

dandy-walker
- malformation 65
- syndrome 65

danger
- dog 58

dangerous
- drug 57

Danish
- monitoring trends in cardiovascular diseases study 56
- prostate symptom score 56

dapple
- apple viroid 56

Darier's disease 57

darkness
- constant 57

data
- calibration curve 40
- definition 57
- interchange, electronic 68
- management plan 61
- sheet, material safety 112
- system, uniform 170

database
- drug misuse 61
- mouse genome 106

date
- and time 63
- birth 31
- last seen 60
- of accident 55
- of admission 56
- of birth 56, 61
- of confinement, estimated or expected 68
- of death 61
- of delivery, estimated 68
- of examination 61
- of injury 59, 61
- of surgery 61
- of transfer 62
- of treatment 63

daunorubicin 61
- vincristine and prednisolone 64

daunosamine 61

day 55
- case haemorrhoidectomy 56
- degrees 57
- delivery 57
- of admission 61
- of delivery 57
- postoperative 135
- postovulatory 135

day(s) 55

days
- alternating 13
- of formalin fixation 59
- to first flower 59

D-dimers 57

deacetylases
- chitin 43

deacetylation
- degree of 57

dead 179, 180
- brain 31
- discharged 58
- on arrival 61
- on scene 61

deafness
- nonsyndromic prelingual 120

deamine
- 4-valine-D-arginine vasopressin 64

death 180
- associated protein kinase 56
- black 31
- brain 31
- date 61
- domain 57
- non-sudden 120

death-associated protein kinase 56

debridement and drilling procedure 57

decarboxylase
- amino acid 5
- ornithine 122

decay
- dominance 58

decay-accelerating factor (CD55) - regulates C3 56

deceased 58, 180

decibel 56

decibels
- change 181

deciliter 59, 60

decimal
- binary-coded 30

decision
- support system 63

decomposition
- normal-coordinate structural 120

decompression sickness 57

decrease 58, 179
- apoptotic volume 26
- regulatory volume 149

decreased 180
- sensory perception 63

decreasing 179

decree
- consent 42

decubitus
- dorsal 58
- ulcer 58

decubitus ulcer 63

dedifferentiated 57

deep
- breathing exercise 56
- cerebral hemorrhages 56
- knee bends 60
- pulse 62
- submergence vehicle 63

- tendon reflex(es) 63
- vascular plexus 64
- vastus lateralis 64
- venous insufficiency 64
- venous thrombosis 64
- venous, arterial 14
- x-ray 65
- x-ray therapy 65
defecation 58
defect
- atrial septal 23
- atrioventricular septal 27
- craniospinal 53
- luteal phase 101
- neural tube 121
- no significant 120
- nonsegmental 120
defective viral particles 64
defects
- aortic valve 26
- mitral valve 114
defense
- articles, excess 68
- attach 56
- non-specific 120
defensin
- mediterranean mussel 106
- mytilus galloprovincialis 106
deferred 58
defibrillation
- system, external 68
- systems analyser 63
- threshold 59
defibrillator
- automated external 14
- automatic implantable 17
- automatic implantable cardioverter 17
- implantable-cardioverter 89
defibrillator technician
- automated 14
deficiencies
- digital 57
deficiency 179, 180
- autoimmune 17
- cartilage matrix 48
- childhood-onset, growth hormone 49
- disorders 57
- essential fatty acid 68
- growth hormone 78
- iron 74
- leukocyte adhesion 98
- proximal femoral focal 131
deficient 58
- dopamine 58
deficit 179
- base 31
- birthweight 56
- disorder, attention 14
- functional sensory 76
- neurosensory 120
- prolonged reversible ischemic neurologic 138
definite
- multiple sclerosis, clinically 43
definition
- data 57
deformation
- dielectro 57
deformity
- nasal septal 120
degassed by O2 absorption (lungs) 56
degeneration 58
- acquired hepatocellular 15
- acquired hepatocerebral 15
- basophilic 31
- cortical-basal ganglionic 39
- corticobasal 39
- drusen-related macular 61
- nigrostriatal 120
- olivopontocerebellar 123
- pallido-ponto-nigral 136
- senile macular 155
- senile macular choroidal 155
- striatonigral 155
- syndrome, corticobasal 39
- syndromes, asymmetrical cortical 10
degenerations
- spinocerebellar 150
degenerative
- arthritis 55
- disease 57
- disk disease 58
- joint disease 60
degradation
- endoplasmic-reticulum-associated 70
- products, fibrin(ogen) 75
degree 180
- first 181
- of deacetylation 57
- of dithiocarbamylation 57
- second 181
- third 181
degrees
- day 57
- Fahrenheit 72
dehydratase
- carbohydrate 42
dehydrated 58
dehydroepiandrosterone 59
- sulfate 59
- sulfotransferases 59
dehydrogenase 131
- branched-chain alpha-keto acid 31
- dihydrodiol 57
- isocitrate 89
- malate 105
deionized water 64
Dejerine-Sottas
- syndrome 63
DeKalb Delta 57
delay
- arteriovenous 26
- atrioventricular 26
- pervasive developmental 129
- reduction theory 62
delayed
- cutaneous hypersensitivity 57
- developmentally 57
- excitation 58
- mental development 60
- neuropathy, organophosphorus-induced 123
- nonmatching-to-sample 61
- primary closure 62
- word recall 65
deleted
- domain 58
delirium tremens 63

delivery
- before 20, 21
- cesarean 42
- date, estimated 68
- day 57
- day of 57
- drug 58
- estimated date of 68
- forceps 73
- low forceps 100
- midforceps 106
- normal spontaneous 120
- normal spontaneous vaginal 121
- room 62
- unit, source 151
- uterine 170
delta
- 9-tetrahydrocannabinol 162
- gap 181
- opiate receptor 124
dementia
- (Alzheimer), presenile 129
- complex, AIDS 14
- familial british 73
- frontal lobe 75
- frontotemporal 76
- lacking distinctive histopathology 60
- Lewy body 99
- multi-infarct 108
- of Alzheimer type, pre-senile 129
- of Alzheimer's type 56, 150
- Pick body 128
- pre-senile vascular 140
- vascular 172
- with motor neuron disease 110
demineralized
- bone matrix 56
- bone powder 56
demonstrates 179
demyelinating
- optic neuritis 61
- polyneuropathy, chronic inflammatory 45
- polyradiculoneuropathy 18
denaturated
- completely 42
denaturation
- DNA 58
denaturing
- gradient gel electrophoresis 59
dendritic
- cells 56
- cells, follicular 73
denervation
- carotid sinus 53
dengue
- shock syndrome 63
dense
- cored vesicles 63
- parenchyma 65
densities
- scalp current 150
density
- bone mineral 33
- buoyant 31
- dependence 57
- electric charge 181
- mammary gland 106
- mass 181
- normalized spin 120
- optic 122
dental
- medicine doctor 61
- surgery doctor 58
dentin
- demineralized 57
dentistry
- operative 123
denture
- partial 129
deoxycholate 61
deoxycorticosterone 61
deoxymannojirimycin 110
deoxynojirimycin 61
deoxynucleic
- acid synthesis, unscheduled 170
deoxyribonucleic
- acid 61
- acid, closed circle 40
- acid, covalently closed circular 40
- acid, cytoplasmic membrane-associated 48
deoxyxanthine
- triphosphate 65
department
- emergency 68
- fire 73
- general emergency 78
- outpatient 123
- Social Services 63
dependence
- barbiturate 31
- density 57
- drug 58
dependency
- chemical 42
depersonalisation
- derealization 57
- disorder 57
dephasing
- five dipolar 75
depolarization
- diastolic 57
depolarizing inhibitory postsynaptic potentials 60
depolymerizing
- factor, actin 14
depressed 179
- nonsuicidal 120
depression 179
- and manic depression 60
- Carroll rating scale 51
- cortical spreading 53
- double 58
- inventory for primary care 32
- Leao's spreading 99
- manic 60
- rating scale, brief Carroll 30
- unipolar recurrent 171
depressive
- disorder 57
- disorders, endogenous major 105
depressor
- area, dorsal medullary 61
deprivation
- binocular 31
- no sleep 120
- sleep 150

depth
- dose 57
derealization
- depersonalisation 57
derivations
- ventriculo-peritonial 64
derivative
- glycopeptide moiety modified 80
derived from 179
dermal necrosis
- ulcerative 170
dermatitis
- allergic contact 10
- atopic 13
- autosensitization spongiotic 23
- contact 42
- diaper 57
- generalised exfoliative 78
- herpetiformis 59
- non-specific 120
dermatofibrosarcoma protuberans 59
dermatology 58, 59
dermatophagoides farinae 59
- bodies 59
- faeces 59
dermatosis
- acquired perforating 21
- ulcerative 170
derogatis
- affects balance sheet 56
desaturated phosphatidylcholine 62
descending
- artery, anterior 13
- artery, posterior 129
- necrotizing mediastinitis 61
describe 59
descriptors
- normalized slope 120
desensitization
- and reprocessing, eye movement 69
desferrioxamine 59
desflurane 59
des-g-carboxy prothrombin, specific for HCC 57
design
- conceptual 42
desipramine (norpramin) 61
desirable body weight 56
desktop
- display 57
desmethyl
- diltiazem 60
- doxepin 60
desmoplastic
- neurotropic melanoma 61
desmopressin
- acetate 58
- test for urine osmolality 58
desquamative
- interstitial penumonitis 60
desulfoviridin 63
detection
- early periodic screening 70
- limit 101
- multiple ion 108
detector
- acute ionization 17
- ultrasonic flow 170
detergent
- fiber, neutral 116
-non-soap 120
deteriorated 179
deterioration
- Scale, progressive 130
determine 59
detoxification
- ultrarapid opioid 171
detrusor
- dyssynergia 57
devascularization
- esophagogastric 69
development fund
- area health 16
development(al)
- disorder 57
developmental
- delay, pervasive 129
- dyscalculia 57
- dyslexis 57
- dysplasia of the hip 58
- venous anomaly 64
developmentally
- regulated EPH-related tyrosine kinase gene 62
developmentally delayed 57
deviance
- information criterion 59
deviated 179
deviation 59
- dissociated vertical 64
- left axis 98
- left midline 100
- normalized standard 120
- ratio topography 62
- relative standard 146
- standard 150, 181
- ulnar 170
- units, standard 151
device
- biventricular assist 36
- charge-coupled 40
- esophageal detector 68
- intrauterine 95
- ligament augmentation 98
- positive pressure ventilation 136
- readiness test 62
- related thrombosis 62
dexamethasone 65
- suppression test 63
dexamethasone-resistant thymocytes 62
dexfenfluramine 59
dexter
- oculus 122
dextran 65
- coated charcoal 56
- derivative 57
dextrane
- sulfate sodium 63
dextromethorphan 65
dextrose 65
- 5%, in distilled water 58
- 5%, in normal saline 61
- 5%, with lactated ringers 60
- in distilled water 58
- in normal saline 61
- in water 60, 64
- in water, 50% 65
- solution, 10% aqueous 62

D-glycero-D-manno-heptose 58
di guglielmo's disease 57
diabetes
- insipidus 59
- insipidus nephrotic 116
- insipidus, nephrogenic 116
- insulin dependent 90, 91
- maturity onset 110
- mellitus 60
- mellitus type I, insulin-dependent 90
- mellitus type II, non insulin-dependent 117
- mellitus, adult onset 14, 20
- mellitus, gestational 78
- mellitus, juvenile onset 96
- mellitus, lipoatrophic 99
diabetic
- autonomic neuropathy 56
- black women 56
- ketoacidosis 60
- non-neuropathic 118
- retinopathy 62
- white women 65
diacylglycerol 56
diadinoxanthin 57
diagnosis 59, 65, 181
- admitting 13
- differential 58
- discharge 58
- preliminary anatomic 127
- undetermined 63
diagnostic 59
- and statistical manual 63
- and statistical manual of mental disorders 63
- arthroscopy, operative arthroscopy, and possible operative arthrotomy 5
- peritoneal lavage 62
- radiology 62
- rhyme test 62
- sensitivity 63
- system, massachusetts general hospital's expert 65
- system, single-use 158
diagonal
- crossed 43
diallyl disulfide 57
dialysate
- normal sodium 120
dialysis
- acute peritoneal 21
- automated peritoneal 21
- chronic peritoneal 50
- conventional 42
- peritoneal 129
diameter 59
- antero-posterior 21
- biparietal 34
- count median 48
- disc 57
- internal 90
- minimum lumen 108
- of portal vein 62
- of splenic vein 63
- outer 122
- vascular, changes 57
diameters
- diastolic 57
diametral tensile strength 63
diaminedithiol 57
diaminobenzidine 56
diaminonaphthalene 56
diaminopyridine 56
diamminedichloroplatinum 58
- cis 45
diamond
- like carbon (coatings) 60
diaper dermatitis 57
diaphragm
- urogenital 171
diarrhea
- and vomiting 64
- bacillary white 37
- bovine viral 36
- chloride 46
- constipation 56
diarrheal disease 57
diastolic
- blood pressure 56, 179
- collapse, right ventricle 149
- depolarization 57
- diameters 57
- dysfunction 57
- forward flow 59
- murmur 60
- myocardial dysfunction 60
- peak velocity prosthetic flow 64
- pressure 62
- pressure, average 26
- pressure, pulmonary artery 127
- septal velocity 63
- velocity integral 64
- ventricular pressure 64
diastrophic dysplasia 57
diathermy
- peri-urethral 140
- short wave 159
diatheses
- dyscrasic 58
- psoriatic 129
diazepam 65
- binding inhibitor 56
- binding inhibitor receptor 105
diazobenzene sulfonate 56
dibenzofuran 59
dibenzo-p-dioxin 57
dibutyl
- phthalate 56
dichloro
- 2,2-bis(4-methoxyphenyl)ethene 105
dichotic
- rhyme task 62
- word test 65
dichroism
- circular 42
dicloxacillin 65
dictation 59
dictyostelium STAT 58
dicyano
- hydroquinone 56
did not
- attend (clinic) 61
- keep appointment 60, 61
- show for appointment 61
didanosine 58
dideoxy 57
died 180
- a natural death 61
- from wounds by the action of the enemy 65
- of other causes 61

lx

- with disease 65
dieldrin 57
dielectric
- constant 181
dielectro-deformation 57
diet
- as tolerated 56
- baby, soft 34
- control 42
- free forever 59
- Gln-enriched 78
- low fat 100
- low-protein, animal-based 21
- normal-salt 120
- readiness test 62
dietary
- allowance, recommended 142
- fiber 59
- management of diarrhea 60
dietary fat in feces 59
diethylamine 58
- shift value 63
diethylaminoethyl 58
diethylenetriaminepentaacetic acid 62
diethylstilbestrol 59
diethypyrocarbonate 62
dietician
- registered 142
diff 59
difference 180, 181
- alveolo-arterial carbon dioxide tension 6
- arteriovenous oxygen saturation 26
- average interocular 17
- barely noticeable 33
- dynamic 58
- just noticeable 96
- optical path 123
differences
- no significant 120
differential 59
- blood count 59
- diagnosis 57, 58
- display 57
- metabolic display 60
- RT-PCR 62
- scanning calorimeter, photo 132
- scanning calorimetry 63
- upstream sequence 64
differentially
- methylated domain 60
differentiated
- type gastric carcinoma 59
differentiation
- carcinoma showing thymus-like 38
- factor, B-cell 30
difficulty
- in breathing 59
diffraction
- gas electron 78
- radon transform 62
- x-ray 176
diffuse
- chorioamnionic hemosiderosis 57
- choroidal hemangiomas 57
- duodenitis 57
- histocytic leukemia 59
- idiopathic skeletal hyperostosis 60
- large cell lymphoma 60
- poorly-differentiated lymphocytic lymphomas 129
- proliferative glomerulonephritis 62
- pulmonary disease 62
- rhythmic theta (waves) 62
- sclerosing variant of papillary thyroid carcinomas 63
- well-differentiated lymphocytic lymphoma 65
diffusing
- capacity of the lung for carbon monoxide 60
diffusion
- disc 57
- double 58
diffusional response time 62
diffusion-driven 57
diffusive
- sampler, timed exposure 161
diflufenican 59
difluoromethylornithine 59
DiGeorge
- chromosomal region 59
- critical region, minimal 105
- syndrome 59
digest
- enzymatic ultrafiltrate 71
digestibility
- dry matter 61
digestion
- related thermogenesis 62
- test, high solids anaerobic 87
digestive
- disorder 57
digit
- symbol subtest 63
digital
- deficiencies 57
- imaging microscopy, fluorescence 73
- rectal examination 62
- substraction angiography 63
- subtraction angiography, stepping 150
- subtraction venacavography 63
- subtraction venography 63
- vascular imaging 64
- vascular imaging system 64
- vascular reactivity 64
- video plotter 64
- voltmeter 64
- x-ray prototype 65
- x-ray prototype network 65
digitaria streak virus 63
digitoxigenin
- monodigitoxoside 60
digoxin-like
- substance, endogenous 71
dihydrodiol dehydrogenase 57
diiodothyronine
- total 166
diiodotyrosine 60
diisopropyl
- phosphate 60
dilatation
- and curettage 56
- and evacuation 58
- urethral 170
dilated 59

- cardiomyopathy 57
- fully 73
dilation
- cervical 43
- curettage and biopsy 56
diltiazem 63
dilute 59
dilution
- minimum hemolytic 107
dilutions
- doubling 58
dimensional
- visualization, four 74
dimethadione 60
dimethyl
- aminoazobenzenesulfonyl chloride 56
- aminoazobenzenesulfonyl-amino acid 56
- dioxirane 60
- glycine 61
- sulfamethoxazole 61
- sulfone 61
- sulfoxyde 61
dimethylaminoadamantane 60
diminished 59, 179
diminishing 179
dinner
- before 20
diopter 55
dioxane
- diones, dodecyloxycarbonyl-methyl 60
dioxide
- carbon 42
- titanium 162
dipalmitoyl phosphatidylcholine 62
diphenylhydantoin 62
diphosphate
- adenosie 14
diphosphates
- nucleoside 116
diphosphoglucose
- urine 170
diphtheria
- acellular pertussis, and tetanus toxoids 56
- and tetanus toxoids with pertussis 63
- pertussis, tetanus immunization 62
diplococci
- gram-negative 80
- gram-negative intracellular 80
diploid
- cell vaccine, human 84
- fibroblast, human 84
diploidy
- DNA 58
diploma
- general equivalency 78
- in venereology and dermatology 64
- in veterinary hygiene 64
dipyridamole 62
direct
- antibody testing 56
- current 56
- current contershock 56
- fluorescent antibody test 59
- immunofluorescence 59
- myocardial revascularization 61
- patient care 62
- photometric method 62
- venipuncture 64
- vision internal urethrotomy 64
directed
- coronary bypass, minimally invasive 108
direction
- of flow 179
directional
- coronary atherectomy 56
director
- district 58
disabilities
- developmental 57
disability 56
- permanent partial 136
- permanent total 139
disabled 60
disabling
- not considered 116
disarticulation
- knee 97
- shoulder 150
disaster
- relief nurse 62
- warning system 65
disc 56
- degenerated 57
- diameter 57
- diffusion 57
- displacement 58
- disruption, internal 90
- intervertebral 95
- prolapsed intervertebral 133
discectomy
- and fusion, anterior cervical 10
- anterior cervical 10
discharge 56, 60
- anterior nasal 19
- diagnosis 58
- summary 63
- summary dictated 63
- urethral 170
discharged 56, 65
discharged dead 58
discharges
- generalized epileptiform 78
discoid lupus erythematosus 60
discontinue 56
discontinued 65
discontinuous
- molecular dynamics 60
discrepancy
- leg length 100
discrete wave transform 65
discrimination
- speech-sound 157
- two point 129
discriminative
- reaction time 62
- response task 62
discussed with 64
disease 13, 60, 65
- alpha-chain 181
- atherosclerotic vascular 26
- autoimmune 17
- biliary tract 35

- bovine viral diarrhea-mucosal 36
- cardiac 42
- cardiovascular 42, 55
- Castleman 42
- celiac 42
- central core 40
- cerebrovascular 55
- Charcot-Marie-Tooth 49
- chronic respiratory 51
- communicable 42
- conduction system 53
- connective tissue 54
- contagious 42
- coronary artery 38
- coronary heart 38, 97
- Crohn 43
- Darier's 57
- degenerative 57
- di guglielmo's 57
- diarrheal 57
- disseminated malignant 61
- disseminated mycobacterial 61
- diverticular 58
- Dupuytren's 58
- feather and beak 73
- food-borne 73
- foot and mouth 75
- free interval 59
- free survival 59
- gamma heavy chain 181
- gestational trophoblastic 82
- graft versus host 83
- Graves' eye 78
- hypertensive, arteriosclerotic, cardiovascular 83
- immunoproliferative small intestinal 94
- meibomian gland 106
- Meniere's 105
- modifying antirheumatic drugs 60
- modifying drug 61
- Mulberry heart 107
- multiglandular 106
- multivessel coronary 104
- Nairobi sheep 120
- no active 115
- no acute 115
- organic heart 122
- Osgood-Schlatter 125
- peripheral arterial 127
- peripheral arteriosclerotic 127
- polycystic kidney 22
- polycystic ovarian 129
- questionnaire, Parkinson's 129
- subcortical ischemic vascular 152
- uniglandular 171
- upper respiratory 171
- uremic medullary cystic 171
- valvular heart 173
- vascular, allograft 26
- vector control center 64
- Vogt-Koyanagi-Harada's 174
- von Willebrand 175

disintegrations per minute 62
disjunctive reaction time 62
disk
- compact 42
- disease, degenerative 58

disks
- herniated 84

dislocate 60
dislocation 60
- of hip, congenital 43
- of the hip, congenital 44
- unilateral facet 170

disorder 61
- B-cell chronic lymphoprolipherative 31
- B-cell lymphoproliferative 33
- behavioral 31
- Briquet 31
- conduct 42
- conduction 42
- convulsive 42
- delusional 57
- depressive 57
- development 57
- digestive 57
- dpersonalisation 57
- dysthymic 58
- generalized anxiety 77
- grand mal convulsive 79
- manic-depressive 105
- myeloproliferative 110
- myoproliferative 110
- N-acetylneuraminic acid storage 120
- obsessive-compulsive 122
- of excessive somnolence (narcolepsy) 61
- post-transplant lymphoproliferative 139
- premenstrual dysphoric 134

disorders
- deficiency 57
- dissociative 58
- REM behavioral 142

disorientation
- spatial 150

dispatch
- emergency medical priority 69

dispensary
- outpatient 123

dispense as written 56
dispersion
- optical rotatory 124
- third-order 163

displaced 179
displacement
- disc 58

display
- desktop 57
- differential 57

disposable smoke evacuator 63
disposition 60
disproportion
- cephalopelvic 50

disruption
- blood brain barrier 29
- internal disc 90

dissection
- pelvic lymph node 133

disseminated
- encephalomyelitis, acute 14
- encephalopathy, acute 14
- gonococcal infection 59
- intravascular coagulation 59
- lupus erythematosis 60
- malignant disease 61
- mycobacterial disease 61

- peritoneal cancer 62
dissociated
- vertical deviation 64
dissociation
- atrioventricular 26
- cell 42
- collision-induced 45
- electromechanical 69
dissociative 45
- disorders 58
distal 60, 179
- convoluted tubule 57
- forearm fracture 59
- interphalangeal 60
- interphalangeal joint 60
- interphalangeal joints 60
- palmar crease 62
- pulses 62
- radioulnar joint 63
- radioulnar ligaments 63
- splenorenal shunt 63
- straight tubule 63
- tingling on percussion 63
- tingling on percussion (Tinel's sign) 63
- vein patch 64
distance
- distribution 58
- hearing 84
- pupillary 129
- source-skin 157
- source-surface 157
- visual acuity 64
distant metastasis 103
distemper
- canine 42
distended 60
distension
- duodenal 58
- jugular-venous 97
distilled 60
distilled water 64
distinctive
- histopathology, dementia lacking 60
distortions
- scale, bulimia cognitive 30
distress
- no acute 115
- no apparent 115
- no apparent respiratory 115
- respiratory 142
- syndrome, acute respiratory 22
distributed
- volume pair 64
distribution
- countercurrent 40
- distance 58
- width, red cell 143
district director 58
disuccinimidyl
- suberate 63
dithiobis-succinimidyl-propionate 63
dithiocarbamylation
- degree of 57
dithiothreitol 63
dithranol-2% salicylic acid-white soft vaseline 63
ditto 180
divalent metal transporter 1 61
divalproex sodium 64
divanillylcyclohexane 64
divergent unilateral strabismus 64
diverticular disease 58
diverticulum
- duodenal 58
divide 60
divided 60
- by 180
divided by 180
divinyl
- benzene 64
- porphyrin 64
division
- for the visually handicapped 64
divorced 60
dizygotic 65
dizziness 65
d-limonene 1,2-epoxide 60
DNA
- complementary 43
- damage 58, 77
- damage, single-strand 157
- damage-repair/toleration activities 62
- denaturation 58
- diploidy 58
- fragmentation factor 59
- sequence variations 63
- synthesis phase of a cell cycle 149
do not
- intubate, do not resuscitate 61
- resuscitate 61
docosahexanoic acid 59
doctor
- dental medicine 61
- non surgical 120
- of chiropractic 56
- of dental surgery 58
- of ophthalmology 123
- of osteopathy 61
- of podiatric medicine 62
dodecanedioic acid 58
dodecyloxycarbonyl
- methyl-dioxane-diones 60
dog
- aorta 56
- danger 58
- mesenteric artery 60
- mesenteric vein 61
- pancreas microsomal membranes 62
- saphenous vein 63
doing well 64
domain
- death 57
- deleted 58
- differentially methylated 60
- fibrin binding 73
- Glycosphingolipid-enriched 78
- GTPase effector 78
domestic
- shorthaired cat 63
- violence programs 64
dominance
- decay 58
dominant
- negative complementation 61

- negative mutant 61
done 181
donor
- cadaver 42
- consanguineous 42
- directed blood donation 58
- for bone marrow transplant, matched unrelated 113
- lymphocyte infusion 60
donors
- unrelated 171
dopamine
- deficient 58
dopamine replacement therapy 62
Doppler
- color 42
- flowmetry, laser 99
- sonography, ultrasound 170
- ultrasound 64
- velocity index 64
- velocity profile 64
doppler
- transcranial 160
dorsal 61
- abductors 56
- cervico 42
- decubitus 58
- intercalate segment instability 60
- interosseous (muscle), first 74
- medullary depressor area 61
- metacarpal artery, first 74
- metatarsal veins 61
- motor nucleus 61
- nerve root 61
- outflow 61
- reticular nucleus 62
- root 62
- root entry zone 62
- root ganglion 62
- root terminals 62
- roots 62
- spine 63
- sympathectomy, bilateral upper 36
- vagal nucleus 64
- vein of the penis 64
- vertebrae 55
- zone of membranelle 65
dorsalis
- pedis 62
- pedis pulse 62
dorsi
- flexion 59
- hyperflexion 59
dorsochiasmatic area 56
dorsolateral
- area 60
- outflow 60
dosage
- adjustment in renal failure 56
- indicative 18
dose
- air 65
- canine 42
- convulsive 42
- curative 43
- daily 57
- daily maintenance 60
- dependent 58
- dependent susceptibility 150
- depth 57
- equivalent uniform 71
- fifty percent convulsant 43
- ineffective 90
- lethal 99
- lifetime average daily 98
- limiting toxicity - determined by phase 1 studies 60
- low 99
- maximum permissible 110
- mean hemolytic 107
- mean lung 108
- minimum hemolytic 107
- night shift 120
- nominal standard 120
- radiation absorbed 142
- volume histogram 64
doses
- doubling 58
dosimeters
- thermoluminescent 163
dosing body weight 56
double
- antibody radioimmunoassay 56
- blind placebo controlled food challenge 56
- breath, single cycle 56
- contrast barium enema 56
- crush hypothesis 57
- depression 58
- negative 61
- simultaneous stimulation 63
- valve replacement 64
- ventricular response 64
- vibrations 64
double minutes 61
doubtful 180
down 179
- bilaterally 179
doxorubicin 14, 65
doxorubicin-docetaxel 58
dozen 65
D-Pro2-D-Trp7,9-SP 62
drainage 62
- dependent 57
- of subretinal fluid 63
- percutaneous catheter 129
draining
- vein pressure 64
drains
- Jackson-Pratt 96
dram 62
draw
- a person test 56
- a person, geriatric 78
D-related human leukocyte antigen 86
dressing 62, 63
- dry 58
- dry sterile 63
- emulsion, wound 175
- nitrofurazone soluble 120
dried fat-free 59
dried-droplet 58
driven
- diffusion 57
driver
- designated 57
- programs, designated 58
driving
- under influence 64
- while impaired 65
- while intoxicated 65

lx

driving after drinking 58
drop 82
drops 82
- per minute 82
drosophila s virus 63
drosophila serum response factor 63
Drosophila trithorax
- gene 164
drosophila X virus 65
drospirenone 62
drug 149
- abuse, intravenous 95
- addict, intravenous 95
- anti-cholinergic antiparkinsonian 21
- antihypertensive 15
- combination 42
- controlled 42
- dangerous 57
- delivery 58
- dependence 58
- history 59
- lymphocyte stimulation test 60
- misuse databases 61
- of abuse 20
- reaction, adverse 14
- resistant typhoid fever 62
- safety and surveillance management 63
- use/user, intravenous 95
- users 64
drugs 84
drusen
- related macular degeneration 61
dry
- and intact 59
- body weight 56
- corn gluten feed 56
- dressing 58
- matter digestibility 61
- matter intake 61
- sterile dressing 63
- sterile gauze 63
- weight 64
drying
- loss 101
dual
- energy X-ray absorptiometry 59, 65
- lumen 60
- Switch Valves 63
Duchenne
- and Becker muscular dystrophies 56
- muscular dystrophy 61
Duchenne dystrophy 58
duck virus enteritis 64
duct
- bile 31
- common bile 42
- cystic 43
ductal
- carcinoma in situ - type of breast cancer 57
- carcinoma, infiltrating 90
ductus
- arteriosus, patent 129
Dudley syndrome 15
due to 63, 179, 181
dull
- borderline 31
dullness
- cardiac 42
- submanubrial 155
duodenal
- distension 58
- diverticulum 58
- gastric metaplasia 59
- injury,blunt 32
- obstruction, congenital 43
- ulcer 63
- ulcers 64
duodenitis
- diffuse 57
- non-specific 120
duodenocolonic dissociation and laparoscopic appendectomy 98
duodenogastric
- reflux 59
duodenoplasty
- diamond-shaped anastomosis 57
- excision 68
- side-to side 157
duodenum 58
duplex
- imaging, color flow 43
Duplex Doppler sonography 58
Dupuytren's disease 58
duration
- critical stimulus 53
- gastric emptying 78
- of action 64
- of diabetes 58
- of disease 58
- of voluntary apnea 64
- tetany 63
Durie-Salmon stage 63
during
- (e.g. intraoperative = during surgery) 93
- the day 90
dwarf (mouse) 64
dwarfism
- camptomelic 48
dynamic 65
- difference 58
- hip screw 59
- regional thresholding 62
- velocity 181
dynamics
- discontinuous molecular 60
dynamized system
- anterior 14
dynamometer 65
dyne 65
Dynia
- Majan-Drdlicka factor 61
dysautonomia 65
- familial 73
dyscalculia
- developmental 57
dyscrasic diatheses 58
dyserythropoietic
- anemia, congenital 43
dysfunction
- atrioventricular node 27
- diastolic 57
- diastolic myocardial 60
- neurosecretory 120
- vocal cord 173
dysfunctional uterine bleeding 64

dyskinesis
- tardive 161
dyslexis
- developmental 57
dysostosis
- cleidocranial dysostosis 46
dysphoric
- disorder, late luteal phase 134
- disorder, premenstrual 134
dysplasia
- arterio-hepatic 15
- bronchopulmonary 34
- campomelic 48
- cleidocranial 40
- diastrophic 57
- gastric epithelial 78
- of hip, congenital 43
- of the hip, developmental 58
- otospondylometaphyseal 126
- spondylometaphyseal 155
dyspnea 65
- on exertion 61
- paroxysmal nocturnal 134
dysprosium 65
dysrhythmia
- cardiac 42
dyssynergia
- detrusor 57
dysthymic disorder 58
dystonia
- musculorum deformans 61
dystrophia
- muscularis (mouse) 65
- myotonica-protein kinase (gene on chromosome 19q) 61
dystrophin 61
- associated protein 56
- associated protein complex 56
- glycoprotein complex 59
dystrophy
- Becker, muscular 33
- Best's macular 33
- childhood, muscular 48
- congenital, muscular 48
- corneal 43
- Duchenne 58
- Duchenne and Becker, muscular 56
- gene, myotonic 60
- muscular 105
- reflex sympathetic 146

E

E. coli
- pig enteropathogenic 131
- secreted protein A 71
- secreted protein B 71
- secreted protein D 71
each 65, 66, 140, 141
- eye 127
ear
- bone, conduction threshold 180
- canal ablation, total 161
- inner 90
- left 18, 23
- middle, effusion 105
- nose, and throat 70
- right 13
early
- afterdepolarization 67
- amnion deficit spectrum 67
- amnion deficit syndrome 67
- antigen (in EBV-IM) 66
- antigen, diffuse 67
- childhood caries 67
- detection of alcohol consumption 68
- EBV mRNA 67
- gastric carcinoma 69
- morning urine osmolality 70
- periodic screening detection 70
ears
- both 25
eating 65
EBV
- mRNA, early 67
echo
- contrast agents 67
- contrast, spontaneous 151
- Doppler system, transoesophageal 161
- time 164
- time (MRI) 161
echocardiogram 67
- aortic valve 26
- transesophageal 161
echocardiography
- cross-sectional 53
- stroke volume 158
- transthoracic 166
ecology
- physiological 130
economic
- value added 71
ecternal
- carotid artery 67
ecthyma
- chamois contagious 41
ectopic
- focus 68
- pregnancy 70
ectopy
- supraventricular 159
eczematous
- allergic contact dermatitis 67
edema 65, 68
- factor 68
- four-plus 66
- pulmonary 130
Edinburgh
- Pharmacopoeia 130
edition
- personal 130
education 84
- physical 130
educational age 66
effect 68
- adverse 14
- cytopathic 50
- level, lowest 99
- level, no observable 118
- level, no observable adverse 118
- model, nonlinear mixed 118
- photographic 130
effective
- arterial blood volume 67
- compliance 43
- dose, median 68
- dose, minimum 105

- health benefits, uniform 170
- refractory period 70
effector
- domain, GTPase 78
efficiency
- binocular visual 36
- food conversion 73
- plating 130
effusion
- middle ear 105
- pericardial 130
- persistent otitis media 135
- pleural 130
- radiation related pericardial 145
egg
- albumin 66
- antigen, polysaccharide 130
- phosphatidylcholine 70
- transfer 65
Ehlers-Danlos syndrome 68
Ehrlich ascites carcinoma 67
ehrlichiosis
- human granulocytic 85
Einheit 66
ejection 65
- fraction 68
- fraction, gallbladder 77
- fraction, left ventricular 102
- fraction, ventricular 173
- murmur, systolic 151
- time 71
elastance 65
elastic fibril 68
elastin
- autoantibodies 9
elbow 69
- above the 14
- cast, long above 98
- jerk 69
- under 170
elbow amputation
- above 14
elective abortion 66
electric
- affinity 66
- charge 65
- charge density 181
- field 68
- field vector 65
- stimulation, functional 74
- vacuum aspiration 71
electrical
- activity 66
- activity, pulseless 130
- control activity 67
- muscle stimulation 69
- nerve stimulation, transcutaneus 161
- response activity 70
- stimulation 70
- stimulation, functional 74
- stimulation, transcranial 161
electrically
- detected magnetic resonance 68
electroacupuncture 66, 67
- analgesia 66
electroanes thesia 66
electrocardiogram 67, 69
- fetal 74
electrocardiographic
- complex 147
electroconvulsive therapy 68
Electrocorticograms 68
electrode
- potential 65
- potential, standard 66
electrodiagnosis 68
electrodiagnostic 68
electroencephalogram 68
electrolytes 103
electromagnetic
- compatibility 69
electromechanical
- dissociation 69
electromotive force 65
electromyogram 69
electromyography 69
electron 65
- beam computed tomography 67
- beam, total skin 165
- diffraction, gas 78
- microscope 69
- microscope, universal 170
- microscopy, low-voltage scanning 103
- microscopy, scanning 151
- microscopy, transmission 161
- microscopy, transmission scanning 165
- negative 65
- spin resonance 71
electronic
- data interchange 68
- fetal monitoring, continuous 43
- medical records 69
electronystagmography 70
electrophoresis
- countercurrent 41
- immunofixation 90
- paper 130
- polyacrylamide gel 127
- serum protein 156
- sodium dodecyl sulfate-polyacrylamide gel 151
- urine protein 171
electrophysiological
- abnormality 66
electrosensitive
- protective device 71
electroshock
- therapy 71
electrospray
- ionization 71
electrothermal
- therapy, intradiscal 90
elementary
- charge 65
elements
- mariner-like 108
- oct-containing composite 122
- rare earth 143
elevated 69, 179
elevation 179
eligibility
- presumptive 130
eliptocytosis
- hereditary 84
elixir 69
elongation factor 68
- G 69
- peptide 68
Embden-Meyerhof pathway 69

embolism
- pulmonary 130
embolization
- transarterial 159
embolus
- pulmonary 130
embryo 65
- fetal 68
- fibroblast 68
embryonic antibody 66
emergency
- admission 66
- cardiac care 67
- clinic, medical 105
- department 68
- department, general 78
- drug identification record 68
- facility 68
- medical priority dispatch 69
- medical service 69
- medical technician 69
- Medical Treatment and Active Labor Act 69
- physician 70
- room 70
- ward 72
emergent
- abdominal sonography 67
emission
- tomography, positron 131
emmetropia 65, 69
empathy response task 70
emphysema
- blue bloaters 29
- centrilobular 46
employment 84
emptying
- duration, gastric 78
emulsion
- wound dressing 175
enabled
- VASP homology 71
encephalitis 65
- experimental autoimmune 67
- russian spring-sununer 147
- St. Louis 153
encephalitogenic
- factor 68
encephalography
- ultrasonic 170
encephalomyelitis
- acute disseminated 14
- acute hemorrhagic 15
- experimental allergic 67
encephalopathy
- acute disseminated 14
- acute necrotizing hemorrhagic 19
- bovine spongiform 34
- hypoxic ischemic 85
- subcortical vascular 159
- zoological spongiform 177
end
- airway pressure, positive 130
- arterectomy, carotid artery 38
- diastolic conductances 78
- diastolic pressure, left ventricular 102
- diastolic pressure, pulmonary artery 127
- diastolic velocity 68
- expiratory pressure, zero 177
- stage renal disease 71
- stage renal failure 71
- systolic conductances 78
- tidal CO2 71
endangered (animal) 65
endemic
- balkan nephropathy 67
endo-1,5-alpha-L-arabinase 10
endocardiographic
- amplifier 66
endocarditis
- acute bacterial 9
- subacute bacterial 150
endocervical cell collector 67
endocrine
- active chemicals 67
- adenomatosis, multiple 105
- Disrupter Screening Testing Advisory Committee 68
- neoplasia, multiple 105
endogenous 65
- digoxin-like substance 71
- pyrogens 70
endoluminal
- colonic wall stents 68
endometrial
- biopsy 69
- cryoablation 67
- hyperplasia, atypical 14
- intraepithelial carcinogenesis 69
- scrape 69
- stromal sarcoma 71
endopeptidase
- brush border 30
- neutral 116
endoperoxide
- D-isomerase 131
- E-isomerase 131
- F-isomerase 131
endoplasm 66
endoplasmic
- reticulum 70
- reticulum-associated degradation 70
endorphin
- like immunoreactivity 32
endoscopic
- carpal tunnel release 68
- functional, sinus surgery 74
- gastrostomy, percutaneous 131
- ligation 69
- retrograde cholangiopancreatography 70
- retroperitoneal gasless, balloon-assisted 32
- sclerotherapy 70
- sinus, functional 74
- ultrasound 71
- vein harvest 71
endosseous
- screw implant, narrow-diameter 48
endosteal
- marrow cell, unidentified 170
endo-surgery
- Ethicon 68
endothelial
- cell adhesion molecule 89, 173

- cells 70
- cells, bone marrow microvascular 33
- cells, human umbilical vein 87
- cells, murine aortic 103
- venule(s), high 85
endothelin-1 71
endothelioma
- clear-cell 41
endothelium
- blood vessel 36
- derived relaxing factor 68
endothoracic
- fascia 68
endotracheal 71
- intubation 71
- tube 71, 78
endurance
- athletes 66
- factor 68
- run test 70
enema 66, 70
- barium 28, 32
- double-contrast barium 56
- oil retention 124
- soap suds 157
energy 66
- average beta 66
- expenditure 68
- expenditure, basal 32
- internal 66
- kinetic 66
- potential 130
- X-ray absorptiometry, dual 65
engineer
- professional 130
engineering
- physical 130
- plant 130
enhanced
- green fluorescent protein 69
- structural adjustment facility 70
enlarged 179
enlargement
- left atrial 98
- right atrial 142
enol
- pyruvylshikamate-3-phosphate synthetase 70
enolase
- neuron-specific 120
enoyl
- CoA hydratase 67
ensemble average
- latency corrected 99
entamoeba 66
enteral
- alimentation 66
enteric
- agar, Hektoen 84
- cytopathogenic bovine orphan virus 67
enteritis
- duck virus 64
entero anastomosis 66
enterobacterial
- common antigen 67
enterococcus 66
- vancomycin-resistant 174
enterocolitis
- necrotizing 116
enterohemorrhagic
- Escherichia coli 69
enteropathogenic
- Escherichia coli 70
enteropathogenic Escherichia coli
- verotoxin producing 174
enterotoxin
- B, staphylococcal 151
- staphylococcal 151
entry
- point of 130
- zone, dorsal root 62
environmental
- stress, prenatal 131
- tobacco smoke 71
enzootic
- bovine leucosis 67
enzymatic
- spectrometric method 70
enzymatic ultrafiltrate digest 71
enzymatically active 66
enzyme 66
- immunoassay, microparticle 105
- linked immunosorbent assay 69
- replacement therapy 70
- substrate complex 70
enzymopathy
- urea cycle 169
eosin 70
- methylene blue agar 69
eosinophil 66, 70
eosinophiles 70
eosinophilic
- fasciitis 68
- gastroenteritis 69
- granuloma, unifocal 170
epiadriamycin 67
epiandrosterone 66
epicondyle 66
epidemiological
- catchment area 67
epidermal
- growth factor 69
- proliferative unit 70
epidermis
- uninvolved 170
epidermolysis
- bullosa 67
- bullosa acquisita 67
epidural 68
- steroid injection 71
epilepsy
- benign childhood 31
- myoclonic absence 103
- myoclonic-astatic 103
- partial 130
- severe myoclonic 155
epileptic
- activity, focal 74
- attentional deficit disorder 67
epileptiform discharges
- generalized 78
epinephrine 66, 70
- pilocarpine 130
epiphysis
- cone-shaped 53
- slipped capital femoral 150
episiotomy 70

- left mediolateral 70
- medial 70
- midline 108
- right mediolateral 70
epithelial
- cancer cell line, human esophageal 67
- cells 70
- cells, rat liver 144
- cells, rat lung 144
- dysplasia, gastric 78
- focus 68
- malignant mesotheliomas 69
- tumor with thymus-like differentiation 151
epithelioma
- adenoides cysticum 67
- basal cel 31
epithelium
- iris pigment 93
- pigmented 130
- pseudostratified ciliated columnar 128
- retinal pigment 145
epitope retrieval
- heat induced 85
epitopes
- T- and B-cell, containing immunogen 160
epsilon-aminocaproic acid 67
Epstein-Barr
- nuclear antigen 67
- virus 67, 70
- virus infectious mononucleosis 67
equal 14, 180
- and brisk 32
- to 180
equalization
- pressure 130
- tube, pressure 131
equation
- henderson-hasselbach 85
equilibrium
- acid-base 9
equinovarus
- congenital talipes 54
equipment
- bubble chamber 31
equivalency diploma
- general 78
equivalent
- focus 68
- phenytoin 130
- uniform dose 71
equivocal 180
erection
- penile 130
ergometer
- leg cycle 99
ERP dispersion 145
error 66
- grid analysis 69
- medication administration 103
- probable 130
- proportional 130
- replication 143
eruption
- persistent pigmented purpuric 136
Erwinia
- carotovora subsp. atroseptica 67
erythema
- annulare centrifugum 67
erythroblastopenia
- of childhood, transient 161
erythroblastosis
- fetalis 68
erythrocyte 66
- antibody 66
- antibody, complement 67
- antiserum 66
- fragmentation 68
- protoporphyrin, free 74
- sedimentation rate 71
erythrocytes 70
erythroid 66
erythromycin 66
erythrophagocytic
- lymphohistiocytosis, familial 74
Escherichia coli 66, 67
- attaching and effacing 14
- enterohemorrhagic 69
- enteropathogenic 70
- hemorrhagic 84
- restriction enzyme 68
- verotoxin producing enteropathogenic 174
E-selectin
- adhesion molecule 69
esophageal
- atresia 66
- detector device 68
- epithelial cancer cell line, human 67
- sphincter, lower 99
- sphincter, upper 170
- variceal hemorrhage 71
esophagogastric
- devascularization with splenectomy 69
esophagogastroduodenoscopy 69
esophagus 66
- upper 170
esotropia 71, 158
essential
- access community hospital 67
- amino acid 66
- fatty acid deficiency 68
- fatty acids 68
- thrombocythemia 71
ester 66
esterase
- bile salt-stimulated 35
- D 71
- non-specific 120
estetrol 66
estimated
- blood loss 67
- date of confinement 68
- delivery date 68
- gestational age 69
- lenght of stay 69
- time of arrival 71
- time of departure 71
estivo-autumnal 66
estradiol 66
- bound to albumin 9
- ethinyl 68
- non-protein-bound 119
- receptor assay 70
estriol 66
- unconjugated 170

estrogen 70
- inducible, breast cancer 31
- oral conjugated 122
- receptor 124
- replacement therapy 70
- sulfotransferases 71
estrone 66
ethacrynic acid 66
ethanol 66
- alcohol 71
Ethicon endo-surgery 68
ethinyl
- estradiol 68
ethosuximide 71
ethyl 66
ethylene
- diaminetetraacetic acid 68
- insensitive 69
- oxyde 71
- propylene diene rubber 70
- vinyl, alcohol 71
- vinylacetate 71
etiology 71
- uncertain 170
etoposide 174
- ifosfamide and cisplatin 173
- platinum 130
eucapnic
- voluntary hyperventilation 71
eudistomin M 71
Eudragit 71
eupneic 71
European
- conformity 43
- Society of Paediatric Gastroenterology, Hepatology, and Nutrition 71
eustachian
- tube function 71
- tube(s) 71
evacuation and dilatation 58
evaluate 71
evaluate and advise 66
evaluation 71
- present 130
- program 130
event
- acute life-threatening 19
- adverse 14
- free survival 69
- major arrhythmic 103
- preceding incident 19
every 140, 141
- afternoon 141
- day 141
- four hours 141
- hour 141
- morning 140, 141
- night 141
- night at bedtime 141
- other day 141
- other hour 19
- other night 141
- six hours 141
- two hours 141
- week 141
evidence-based medicine 67
evoked
- potential, right somatosensory 146
- potential, short latent 153
- potentials, somatosensory 157
- response, audiometry 70
- response, audiometry brainstem 35
- response, auditory 14
- response, average 14
- response, brain stem auditory 28
- response, somatosensory 157
exacerbate 72
exacerbation
- chronic bronchitis 9
exam
- comprehensive 122
- cystoscopic 55
examination 66, 72
- and observation 122
- computer-based 39
- cross-cultural cognitive 40
- date 61
- digital rectal 62
- history and physical 87
- mental status 112
- mini-mental state 109
- objective structured clinical 126
- orthopaedic special assessment 125
- orthopedic 122
- pelvic 130
- per vaginam 140
- physical 130, 140
- slit lamp 153
- total skin 165
- under anesthesia 71
- under anesthesia, pelvic 130
- vaginal 173
examiner
- medical 105
example 72
excellent 72
except 72, 176
excess 180
- defense articles 68
- post-oxygen consumption 70
exchange 65, 72
- plasma 130
- sister-chromatid 150
exchanger
- heat and humidity 86
excision 72
- duodenoplasty 68
- wide 175
- wide local 175
excitability
- low, naples 117
excitation
- delayed 58
excitatory
- amino acid 66
- amino acid carrier 66
- postsynaptic potential 70
exemption
- clinical trials 54
exercise 72
- active-resistance 22
- deep breathing 56
- physical 130
- program, home 84
- progressive resistance 137
- reconditioning 143
- test, graded 83
- testing, cardiopulmonary 50
- tolerance test 71
- training 71

exfoliating toxin 72
exfoliative dermatitis
- generalised 78
exhalation 66
exophtalmos-producing substance 70
exosite
- anion-binding 9
exostoses
- osteocartilaginous 122
exotoxin
- Pseudomonas 130
- pyrogenic 130
- toxic shock syndrome 166
exotropia 176
expand 72
expander
- blood volume 36
expectancy (wave) 66
expectation
- mathematical 66
expected
- date of confinement 68
expenditure
- basal energy 32
- energy 68
experiences
- prementrual 50
experiment 66
experimental
- allergic (autoimmune) neuritis 67
- allergic encephalomyelitis 67
- autoimmune encephalitis 67
- index, crown-crisp 41
experimenter 66
expiration 66, 72
- pressure 130
expiratory 72, 90
- flow rate, maximal 105
- flow rate, peak 131
- flow, forced 74
- flow, maximal 105
- flow, maximal mid 109
- flow, peak 131
- volume in one second, forced 74
- volume, forced 74
expired air 66
explain 72
exploratory laparotomy 72
explosive
- limit, upper 170
exposure 66
- factor 68
- limit, permissible 131
- prior to 130
expressed
- antigens, lung carcinoma 99
- sequence tag 71
extend 72
extended
- care facility 67
- field 68
extender
- physician 130
- primary care 138
extensible
- markup language 176
extension 72, 180
- and flexion 74
- extraprostatic 70
extensive
- intraductal component 69
extensor 179
- carpi radialis brevis 68
- carpi radialis longus 68
- carpi ulnaris 68
- digitis minimi 68
- digitorum communis 68
- digitorum longus 68
- hallucis longus 69
- pollicis brevis 70
- pollicis longus 70
- response 179
extent of primary tumor 159
external 72
- auditory canal 67
- carotid artery 67
- defibrillation system 68
- defibrillator, automated 14
- genitalia 72
- radiation therapy 70, 176
- rotation 70
- rotation and extension 72
- rotation in extension 70
- rotation in flexion 70
extinguisher
- tissue-specific 165
extracapsular
- cataract extraction 67
extracardiac
- karyotypic anomalies 67
- structural anomalies 67
extracellular
- fluid 67
- fluid volume 67
- matrix 67
extracorporeal
- circulation 67
- membrane oxygenation 67
- shock wave lithotripsy 71
extracranial
- arterial disease 67
- carotid artery 67
extract 66
- bovine thymus 35
- pancreatic 130
- placental 130
- powdered 130
extracted 66
extraction 66
- atherectomy, transluminal 161
- extracapsular cataract 67
- fraction 66
- microwave-assisted 103
extradomain (the type III unit of fibronectin) 68
extrafine 68
extrahepatic
- biliary atresia 69
- biliary passages 69
extralymphatic 66
extramedullary
- hematopoiesis 69
extranodal
- site, involvement 66
extraocular
- movements 70
- movements intact 70
- muscles 70
extraprostatic extension 70
extrapyramidal
- symptoms 70

extrasystole
- supraventricular 159
extremities 72
- both lower 33
- both upper 36
- lower 99
extremity 72
- left lower 100
- left upper 102
- lower 99, 103
- right lower 144
- right upper 148
- upper 170
extrinsic
- allergic alveolitis 66
- factor 68
exudate
- and hemorrhage 84
- cells, peritoneal 130
- peritoneal 130
eye 66
- each 127
- ear, nose and throat 68
- left 99
- movement desensitization and reprocessing 69
- right 122
- vision 174
eyes
- both 127

F

facet
- dislocation, unilateral 170
facial paralysis
- bilateral 32
facilitation
- proprioceptive neuromuscular 134
facility
- emergency 68
- extended care 67
- intensive care 90
- intermediate care 90
F-actin image
- analysis program 72
factor
- antihemophilic 16
- antihemophilic globulin 16
- basophil chemotactic 31
- bioconcentration 31
- cold stability 53
- colony-stimulating 53
- colony-stimulating, receptor 1 53
- cytotoxic lymphocyte maturation 47
- drosophila serum response 63
- Dynia-Majan-Drdlicka 61
- edema 68
- elongation 68
- encephalitogenic 68
- endurance 68
- exposure 68
- extrinisic 68
- G, elongation 69
- gonadotropin-releasing 80
- granulocyte colony stimulating 78
- guanine releasing 82
- maturation-promoting 111
- or hormone, corticotropin-releasing 51
- osteoclast-activating 121
- osteoclast-stimulating 126
- overgrowth stimulating 126
- peak scatter 138
- peptide elongation 68
- platelet-activating 127
- rheumatoid 143
- stem cell 150
- thyroid transcription 166
- vascular permeability 174
- VII 77
- VII antigen 77
- VII coagulant activity 77
- VII gene on chromosome 72
- von Willebrand 175
factors
- serum inhibition 152
Fahrenheit degrees 72
failed
- appointment 72
- to keep appointment 77
failure
- acute hypoxemic respiratory 16
- acute left ventricular 19
- acute renal 22
- acute respiratory 22
- cardiac 43
- congestive 49
- congestive right ventricular 52
- free survival 74
- heart 85
- left ventricular 103
- multiple organ 110
- multiple organ system 110
- organ system 126
- righr heart 143
- to thrive 77
failure to descend 76
fall down - go boom 73
falling 179
Fallot, tetralogy 163
false positive
- biological 32
familial
- adenomatous polyposis 73
- british dementia 73
- dysautonomia 73
- erythrophagocytic lymphohistiocytosis 74
- histiocytic lymphohistiocytosis 74
family
- Adaptability and Cohesion Evaluation Scales 72
- centered maternity care 73
- history 74
- medical doctor 75
- members and significant others 76
- nurse practitioner 75
Fanconi's anemia 72
farnesyl
- protein transferase 76
- transferase inhibitor 76
fascia
- endothoracic 68
fascicular block
- left anterior 98

- left posterior 101
fasciculation 15
fasciculus
- medial longitudinal 108
fasciitis
- eosinophilic 68
fast blue
- Luxol 100
fasting
- blood sugar 73
- glucose, impaired 91
fast-setting
- calcium phosphate cement 76
fast-spin
- echo 76
fast-twitch
- red (skeletal muscle) 77
- white (skeletal muscle) 77
fat
- area, ratio 143
- bodies, urinary 170
- weight 77
- yield 77
fatal
- dose, minimum 106
fat-free mass 74
father 72
- of child 75
fatigue
- syndrome, chronic 43
fatty
- acid activation protein(s) 72
- acid binding protein 72
- acid cis 9 110
- acid enriched, odd-carbon 122
- acid, unesterified 170
- acids, essential 68
- acids, non-esterified 116
- acids, polyunsaturated 140
- acids, saturated 151
- liver, pregnancy 15
feather and beak disease 73
fecal
- occult blood testing 75
- output 75
feed
- dry corn gluten 56
feeder
- universal 170
fee-for-service 74
felbamate 73
feline
- sarcoma proto-oncogene 74
feline leukemia virus 74
feline sarcoma
- vaccine-associated 172
- viral oncogene 173
feline sarcoma A tumor 76
fellow
- post-sophomore 138
female 72
- adult 14
- black 32
- sex chromosome 176
- white 175
- worm burden 77
femoral 74
- artery, superficial 151
- below-knee-popliteal bypasses 73
- epiphysis, slipped capital 150
- focal deficiency, proximal 131
- head, avascular necrosis 27
- head, osteonecrosis 123
- popliteal 74
femur
- neck 118
fentanyl self-administration 76
fermentation
- citric acid 38
fertilization
- in vitro 95
fetal 74
- calf serum 73
- circulation, persistent 131
- death, intrauterine 95
- electrocardiogram 74
- heart rate 74
- heart rate-uterine contraction 74
- heart sounds 74
- heart tones 74
- hemoglobin, hereditary persistence 87
- maternal hemorrhage 75
- monitoring, continuous electronic 43
- sialoglycoprotein 76
- sulfoglycoprotein antigen 76
- weight 77
fever 74
- argentinian hemorrhagic 16
- drug resistant typhoid 62
- due to infection 74
- hay 85
- of undetermined origin 77
- of unknown origin 77
- rheumatic 143
- Rocky Mountain spotted 144
fiber
- dietary 59
- neutral detergent 116
- outer spiral 126
fibril
- elastic 68
fibrillary
- acidic protein, glial 78
fibrillation
- atrial 14, 15, 24
- auricular 25
- paroxysmal atrial 127
- rapid atrial 142
- ventricular 173
fibrin
- binding domain 73
- degradation products 74
fibrinogen
- degradation products 75
fibrinopeptide
- A 75
- B 75
fibroblast 74
- embryo 68
- growth factor 74
- growth factor, acidic 15
- human diploid 84
- human lung 86
- specific antigen 76
fibroblastic
- reticulum cells 76
fibrocartilage
- complex, triangular 161
fibrocystic
- breast disease 73

lx

fibrodysplasia
- ossificans progressiva 75
fibromyalgia
- syndrome 75
fibronectin 75
fibroplasia
- retrolental 144
fibrosarcoma 76
fibrosis
- cystic 43
- marrow 106
fibroxanthoma
- atypical 15
field
- central tegmental 54
- crystal ligand 46
- extended 68
- low power 101
- of vision 173
- vector, electric 65
figure
- of Merit 75
filamentous actin 72
film unshapness 170
filtered
- back-projection 73
filtration
- rate, glomerular 78
- rate, urine 170
- tangential flow 161
filum
- terminale, tight 161
finasteride 75
findings
- no significant 120
fine-needle
- aspiration 75
- aspiration biopsy 75
finger 72
- index 90
- middle 106
- movement 75
- stick 76
finger counting 73
fingerbreadth 73
fingertips to toes
- forward flexion 74
fire
- department 73
first
- degree 181
- dorsal interosseous (muscle) 74
- dorsal interosseus (muscle of the hand) 73
- dorsal metacarpal artery 74
- meiotic anaphase 17
- menstrual period 75
- pregnancy 138
- responder, medical 106
- time wheezing 77
first aid 72
fiscal year 77
fistula
- arteriovenous 26
- carotid-cavernous 41
- carotid-jugular 45
- tracheoesophageal 161
five
- dipolar dephasing 75
- factor Model of personality 74
- factors score 74
fixation
- autoimmune complement 17
- closed reduction and percutaneous 51
fixed
- arm support 75
- rate ventricular single-chamber systems 175
- scheduled access 76
flaccid 75
- paralysis, acute 15
flame
- ionization detectors 74
flammable
- limit, upper 170
flank 75
flap
- low 99
- reconstruction, latissimus dorsi 99
flavin adenine dinucleotide 72
flexible
- spending account 76
flexion 75, 179, 180
- adduction and internal rotation 73
- adduction, internal rotation and extension 73
- and extension 74
- angle of greatest 15
- extension, rotation 74
- forward 74
- left lateral 100
flexor 75, 179
- carpi radialis 73
- carpi ulnaris 73
- digitorum profundus 74
- digitorum superficialis 74
- pollicis brevis 75
- pollicis longus 75
flight of colors test 75
flocculation
- cephalin-cholesterol 41
- cholesterol-lecithin 46
floor
- of mouth 75
flow
- aortic 14
- BOLD (blood oxygenation level-dependent) - Dependence 73
- coronary sinus 53
- cytometric immunophenotyping 73
- cytometry 73
- detector, ultrasonic 170
- diastolic forward 59
- diastolic peak velocity prosthetic 64
- filtration, direct 59
- filtration, tangential 161
- maximal inspiratory 108
- maximal mid expiratory 109
- maximal midexpiratory 109
- peak expiratory 131
- rate, inspiratory 91
- rate, maximal expiratory 105
- rate, maximal inspiratory 108
- rate, maximal midexpiratory 109
- rate, maximum mid expiratory 109

- velocities, maximum 106
fluency
- word 175
fluid 75
- amniotic 14
- breast cyst 31
- Carrel-Dakin 42
- content, thoracic 161
- extracellular 67
- force 74
- hyperalimentation 83
- intravenous 95
- ounce 75
- protein, breast cyst 31
- protein, gross cystic disease 78
- spinal 156
- subretinal, drainage of 63
- Wassermann reaction, cerebrospinal 54
fluids 75
- push 131
fluorapatite 72
fluorescein
- isothiocyanate 75
fluorescence
- activated cell sorter 72
- digital imaging microscopy 73
- in situ hybridization 75
- polarization immunoassay 75
- resonance energy transfer 76
fluorescent
- antibody test, direct 59
- antinuclear antibody test 73
- focus inhibition test, rapid 143
- treponemal antibody absorption test 76
fluorogenic matrix metalloproteinase substrate assay 76
fluorouracil
- treatment regimen 77
fluticasone propionate 75
flutter
- atrial 14, 15, 24
- ventricular 173
FMRP-interacting
- protein, nuclear 121
foaminess 181
focal
- deficiency, proximal femoral 131
- epileptic activity 74
- lymphocitic sialadenitis 76
- nodular hyperplasia 75
- suprabasal acantholysis 76
focus
- ectopic 68
- epithelial 68
- equivalent 68
focused
- ultrasound, high intensity 85
follicle
- associated lymphoid tissue 73
- stimulating hormone 76
- stimulating hormone, urinary 170
follicular
- dendritic cells 73
- hyperplasia 74
- lymphoma 75
- lymphoma large cell 75
- lymphoma mixed small cleaved and large 75
- lymphoma small cleaved 75
- small cleaved cell lymphomas 76
follow
- through series, small bowel 150
- through, small bowel 155
- up 77
- up, medical 106
followed by 179
food
- borne diseases 73
- challenge, double-blind placebo controlled 56
- conversion efficiency 73
- scrap ashes 76
foot 180
- and mounth disease 75
- angle, standing 151
- compression, intermittent pneumatic 93
- feet (measure) 76
- left 99
- shock aggression 76
for
- (duration) 176
- further appointment 74
- your information 77
foramen
- mental 107
- ovale, patent 131
force
- electromotive 65
- fluid 74
- horizontal ground reaction 74
- negative inspiratory 117
- zero insertion 177
forced
- expiratory flow 74
- expiratory volume 74
- expiratory volume in one second 74
- vital capacity 77
forceps
- delivery, low 100
- elective low 69
- low 99
forceps delivery 73
forearm 72
- bone density 73
- distal fracture 59
- left 100
foreign
- body 73
- body, intraocular 93
form
- informed consent 90
formal
- college approved, postgraduate meeting 73
formaldehyd
- urinary 170
formaldehyde-treated albumin 76
formalin fixed paraffin embedded tissues 74
formation
- volume, hippocampal 85

forming unit
- granulocyte and macrophage colony 79
forward
- angle light scatter 76
- flexion 74
- flexion,fingertips to toes 74
fosamax international trial 75
fosfomycin 75
four
- dimensional visualization 74
- plus edema 66
- times a day 141
- times a week 141
Fourier
- transform infrared 77
- transform infrared, spectroscopy 77
fowl adenovirus serotype 8 174
fowled
- up beyond all recognition 77
fractal signature analysis 76
fraction 180
- ejection 68
- extraction 66
- free 74
- of inspired oxygen 75
- shunt 141
fractional 76
- excretion of sodium 74
- shortening area 76
fracture 76, 77, 180
- complete, angulated 73
- complete, comminuted, compound 73
- complete, deviated 73
- complete/compound, comminuted 73
- distal forearm 59
- healing system, sonic accelerated 149
- intervention trial 75
- intracapsular 90
- linear 99
- of both bones 76, 77
- open 122
- open reduction jaw 125
- probability, remaining lifetime 144
- simple comminuted 76
- simple, complete, comminuted 76
fragile
- mental retardation 75
- X syndrome 77
fragment
- amino-terminal 24
- bone 32
- wounds, multiple 106
fragmentation
- erythrocyte 68
frameless
- stereotactic interstitial brachytherapy, computer-assisted 38
framework 76
free
- amino acid pool 72
- carnitine 73
- erythrocyte protoporphyrin 74
- fraction 74
- from disability 74
- radical scavenger 105
- survival, progression 131
- thyroxin 76
- thyroxin (T4) index 77
free testosterone 161
French
- American and british classification scheme for leukemia 72
french
- standardization institute 15
French Society of Arthroscopy score 151
frequency 181
- activity, spindle 151
- adaptation, spike 151
- angular 181
- expected, in a cell of a contingency table 66
- following response 74
- low 99
- of respiration 76
- ultra high 171
- ultrasonic 170
frequently asked questions 73
fresh frozen plasma 74
Friend
- leukemia integration 1 gene 75
friend
- derived murine immunosuppressive virus 74
frontal
- lobe dementia 75
frontoanterior
- left 100
frontotemporal dementia 76
frontotransverse
- left 100
frozen
- section 76
- section analysis 76
- section, breast tumor 35
- shoulder syndrome 76
fructose
- 1,6-diphosphate 74
- six phosphate aldolase gene 76
fructose-six phosphate aldolase 76
full
- blood count 73
- free range of motion 74
- joint range of motion 75
- passive movements 76
- range 76
- range of joint movement 76
- range of motion 76
- range of movement 76
- term 76
- term normal delivery 77
- thickness skin graft 77
- weight bearing 77
full-spectrum data analysis 76
fully
- lactating 75
fully dilated 73
function
- associated antigen 1, lymphocyte 100
- associatedantigen, lymphocyte 100
- contrast sensitivity 53
- eustachian tube 71

- test, kidney 97
- test, muscle 106
- tests, liver 100
- tests, pulmonary 131

functional
- activity of plasminogen activators in plasma 72
- activity of plasminogen activators in urine 72
- assessment of multiple sclerosis 73
- bowel disorder 73
- bowel distress 73
- breathing disorder 73
- electric stimulation 74
- electrical stimulation 74
- endoscopic sinus 74
- endoscopic sinus surgery 74
- hemolytic complement, total 44
- independence measures 75
- profile length 75
- refractory period, atrioventricular node 27
- residual capacity 76
- sensory deficit 76
- uterine bleeding 77

fundal height 74
fungal strain 75
fusion
- posterior cervical 129
- posterolateral interbody 133

fuzzy logical model of perception 75

G

G-6-Pase glucose-6-phosphatase 81
G-6-PD 82
gain
- average daily 14

gait
- disorder, autoantibody, late-age, onset, polyneuropathy 77
- orthosis, reciprocating 143
- training 82

gallbladder 77
- disease 77
- ejection fraction 77
- series 77

gallon 77
gallop
- murmurs, rubs 80
- rub, murmur 82

galloprovincialis defensin 1
- mytilus 106

gallops 106
galveston orientation and amnesia test 81
gamete
- intrafallopian transfer 79

gamma
- crystallin gene 52
- globulin 78
- globulin, aggregated human 16
- globulin, antihuman 16
- glutamyltransferase 78
- glutamyltranspeptidase 78
- heavy chain disease 181
- hydroxy-beta-aminobutyric acid 81

gammopathy
- benign monoclonal 33

gangliocytic paraganglioma 81
ganglion
- buccal 36
- dorsal root 62
- paracervical 129

ganglionectomy
- superior cervical 150

ganglioneuroblastoma 80
ganglionic
- degeneration, cortical-basal 39

gangrenosum
- peristomal pyoderma 136

gap 77
- 0 77
- 1 77
- 2 77
- anion 15, 181
- delta 181
- detection, modulation 106

garment
- pneumatic anti-shock 128

gas 179
- and oxygen 81
- association, compressed 44
- chromatography 77, 78
- chromatography, head space 87
- chromatography, vacuum distillation 173
- chromatography/mass spectrometry 78
- chromotography, capillary column 41
- electron diffraction 78
- liquid chromatography 79
- oxygen, and ether 81
- solid chromatography 82
- venous blood 173
- volume, thoracic 161

gasless
- balloon-assisted, endoscopic retroperitoneal 32

gastric
- analysis 77
- bypass, micropouch 106
- carcinoma, differentiated type 59
- carcinoma, early 69
- emptying duration 78
- epithelial dysplasia 78
- foveolar mucin 113
- inhibitory peptide 79
- metaplasia, duodenal 59
- mucin, human 85
- mucosa 79
- mucosa blood flow 79
- mucosal barrier 79
- parietal cell 82
- pneumatosis 81
- resection 82
- type 82
- ulcer 82

gastro-(o)esophageal 80
gastrocnemius 77
gastroenteritis 78
- eosinophilic 69
- transmissible 161

gastroenterology 78

gastroesophageal 78
- reflux 81
- reflux disease 78
gastrointestinal 79
- biopsy, upper 171
- bleeding, upper 171
- hemorrhage, acute upper 25
- hemorrhage, upper 171
- hormone 79
- series, upper 171
- tract 79
- tract, lower 100
- tract, upper 171
- upper 171
gastroparesis diabeticorum 78
gastroplasty 81
gastrostomy
- percutaneous endoscopic 131
- tube 82
gated magnetic resonance imaging 80
gauge 180
- cryosurgical iceball 45
gauze
- dry sterile 63
gay-related
- immunodeficiency 82
gaze
- left lateral 100
gaze nystagmus 80
GDP-mannose pyrophosphorylases 80
Geiger-Muller (counter) 79
gel
- electrophoresis, denaturing gradient 59
- electrophoresis, polyacrylamide 127
- electrophoresis-derived enzyme-linked immunosorbent assay 78
- permeation chromatography 82
gemderma osteodysplastica hereditaria 81
gene
- brain tumor 34
- Chediak Higashi syndrome 44
- coiled-coils 42
- homeobox 86
- occludin-related 125
- phosphoenolpyruvate synthase 136
- product 81
- recognition and analysis internet link 82
- von Hippel-Lindau disease 173
- Wilms tumor 176
general 78
- accounting office 77
- anaesthetic/anesthesia 77
- appearance 77
- assistance medical care 77
- by endotracheal tube 78
- condition 77
- emergency department 78
- equivalency diploma 78
- health 78
- medical clinic 79
- medical council 79
- medical service 80
- medicine 79
- medicine and surgery 80
- nursing care 80
- operating room 81
- paralysis 81
- paralysis, progressive 132
- paresis 81
- physic 81
- practice 81
- practitioner 81
generalized
- anxiety disorder 77
- epileptiform discharges 78
- exfoliative dermatitis 78
- lymphadenopathy, persistent 132
- osteoarthritis 81
gene-related
- peptide, calcitonin 44
genes
- encoding response regulators 145
- hordein 86
genetic
- manipulation 79
- prediabetes 81
geniculate
- body dorsal, medial 106
- body ventral, medial 106
- body, lateral 100
- body, medial 106
geniculo-hypothalamic tract 79
genitalia
- external 72
genitourinary 82
- system 83
genomic
- hybridization, comparative 44
genotype
- ZZ (deficiency of a 1-antitrypsin) 177
geographic
- practice cost index 82
geometric
- mean 79
- mean diameter 80
- mean titer 80
- progression 81
- unsharpness 170
geriatric
- draw-a-person 78
- mental state 80
- nurse clinician 80
- nurse practitioner 80
germ
- cell tumor 78
- cell, primordial 131
German
- Hodgkin lymphoma study group 79
germinal
- center 77
- centers, progressively transformed 139
- matrix hemorrhage 80
- matrix related hemorrhage 80
geroderma osteodysplastica 80
gerontologic
- nurse practitioner 80
Gerstmann-Sträussler
- syndrome 82
gestalt test
- Bender visual-motor 36

gestation 78
gestational
- age 77
- age, appropriate for 15
- age, estimated 69
- age, large 100
- age/birthweight categories 77
- diabetes mellitus 78
- trophoblastic disease 82
gestationis
- herpes 85
get
- out of my examination room 81
giant
- cell arteritis 78
- cell, interstitial pneumonia 79
- melanosome 79
- migratory contraction 79
- papillary conjunctivitis 82
gibbon ape
- leukemia virus 79
- leukemia virus receptor 79
gigaohm 83
Gilbert-Meulengracht syndrome 80
gingival
- margin trimmer 80
- stomatitis, acute herpetic 16
gingivitis
- acute necrotizing ulcerative 20
- acute ulcerative 25
gland
- disease, meibomian 106
- of unknown significance, atypical 15
glandular
- dose, mean 106
Glasgow
- Coma Scale 78
- outcome score 81
glass
- ceramic apatite and wollastonite containing 27
- ionomer cement 79
glasses
- or corrective lenses, without 157
glaucomatous
- optic nerve damage 81
Glenn
- shunt, bidirectional 32
glial
- cytoplasmic inclusions 78
- fibrillary acidic protein 78
- growth factor 78
gliosis
- progressive subcortical 138
gln-enriched diet 78
global
- amnesia, transient 161
- assessment of functioning 77
- information system 79
globe
- temperature, wet bulb 175
globulin 181
- aggregated human 16
- antihemophilic 16
- antihuman 16
- antihuman lymphocyte 16
- antihuman thymocyte 17
- cold insoluble 45
- cortisol binding 39
- factor, antihemophilic 16
- thyroid binding 160
globus pallidus 81
glomerular
- basement membrane 77
- basement membrane, collagenase soluble 54
- filtration rate 78
- mesangium cell 112
glomerulonephritis 80
- acute 15
- crescentic 44
- diffuse proliferative 62
- membranoproliferative 111
- post streptococcal 138
- rapidly progressive 145
glomerulosclerosis
- focal and segmental 76
glossopharyngeal
- breathing 82
glucathione peroxydase 82
glucose 79
- 1-phosphate 81
- 3-phosphate dehydrogenase 82
- 6-phosphatase 81
- 6-phosphate 81
- 6-phosphate dehydrogenase 81, 82
- dependent insulinotropic peptide 79
- impaired fasting 91
- in normal saline (solution) 79
- monophosphate 80
- nitrogen (ratio) 80
- nitrogen ratio 79
- output, hepatic 85
- oxidase 80
- oxidase test 81
- oxidation quotient 81
- pentaacetate 81
- phosphate 81
- phosphate yeast 131
- saline solution 82
- tolerance test 82
- tolerance test, abnormal 15
- tolerance test, borderline 32
- tolerance, impaired 91, 94
- transporter 79
glucosidase 79
glutamate
- (ammonia) ligase 79
- dehydrogenase 79
- dehydrogenase pseudogene 79
- oxaloacetate transaminase 81
- receptor 79
glutamic
- acid 66, 79
- acid, codon 77
- acid, diethyl ester 78
- oxaloacetic transaminase, mitochondrial 81
- pyruvic transaminase 82
glutamic acid
- codon 77
glutamine 79, 140
- codon 38
glutathione
- oxidized 82

- peroxidase 81
- reduced 82
- reductase 82
- S-transferase 82
gluten
- feed, dry corn 56
glyceral
- dehyde-3-phosphate 81
- methacrylate 79
glyceride 79
glycerol
- 3-phosphate 81
- 3-phosphate dehydrogenase 81
- phosphate dehydrogenase 82
glycerophosphate 81
glycerophosphorylcholine 82
glyceryl
- monostearate 80
glycine 77, 79
- codon 78
glycogen
- phosphorylase 81
- phosphorylase, dephosphorylated low-activity form 82
- synthase 82
glycolic acid 133
glycopeptide 81
- moiety, modified derivative 80
glycophorin 81
- B 82
- C 82
glycophosphatidilinositol 82
glycoprotein 81, 162
- myelin-associated 103
- syndrome, carbohydrate-deficient 43
- tumor-specific 165
glycosphingolipid
- enriched domains 78
glycosylation
- congenital disorder 43
glycosylphosphatidylinositol 82
glyphosate
- oxydoreductase 81
gnathion 80
gnotobiote 80
goal of treatment 81
goblet cell mucin 113
god only knows 81
goiter
- toxic multinodular 163
gold 25
Gomori methenamine silver stain 80
gonadal
- dysgenesis, mixed 106
- tissue cells, rainbow trout 148
gonadotropin 80
- chorionic 44
- human chorionic 84
- human menopausal 86
- primate chorionic 129
- releasing factor 80
- releasing hormone 80
- releasing hormone receptor 80
gone on arrival 81
goniodysgenesis
- menta1 retardation-short stature 80
gonion 79, 80
gonococcal 78
- infection, disseminated 59
- ophthalmia neonatorum 81
gonococcus 78
gonorrhea 78, 80
gonorrheal
- invasive peritonitis 79
good
- clinical practice (guidelines) 78
- clinical research practice 78
- laboratory practice 79
- manufacturing practice 80
- partial remission 82
- pharmacy practices 82
Goodpasture
- antigen 81
- syndrome 9, 81
grade point average 81
graded exercise test 83
gradient
- alveolar 5
- arterial 5
- echo 82
- echo (MRI) 78
- moment nulling 80
- motion rephasing 80
- portosystemic pressure 136
grading
- histopathological 77
graduate
- medical education 80
- nurse 80
graft
- bone 32
- coronary artery bypass 38
- iliac bone 89
- iliac crest bone 89
- vein 173
- versus host disease 83
- vs. host reaction 83
grain 82
gram 44, 77, 78, 79, 80
- meter 79, 80
- molecular volume 80
- molecular weight 80
- molecule 80
- negative 79, 80
- negative bacillary meningitis 80
- negative bacillus 80
- negative diplococci 80
- negative intracellular diplococci 80
- negative rods 80
- positive 79, 81
grams
- per cubic centimeter 79
- per liter 80
- per milliliter 80
- per square meter 82
grand
- mal (epilepsy) 79
- mal convulsive disorder 79
- multiparity 79
- old man of the emergency room 81
grand mal
- attack 79
grandfather
- maternal 106
- maternal, great 106
- paternal 131

grandmother 79
- maternal 106
- paternal 132
granular
- cell tumor, malignant 106
- cell, nerve sheath tumor 78
- progenitor cell 82
granule membrane protein 80
granulocyte
- agglutination assay 77
- and macrophage colony forming unit 79
- and macrophage colony stimulating factor 79
- colony stimulating factor 78
- immature 91
- immunofluorescence assay 79
- macrophage 79
granulocytes 82
granulocytic
- ehrlichiosis, human 85
- leukemia, acute 15
- leukemia, chronic 44
granuloma
- unifocal eosinophilic 170
granulomatosis
- Wegener's 175
granulomatous
- disease, chronic 44
granulomembranous body 79
granulosa
- cell tumor, adult 15
graphic
- amplifier, endocardio 66
Graves' eye disease 78
gravida 77, 82
- para 81
gravity
- specific 156
gray matter 79
Grays 83
great 82
- grandfather, maternal 106
greater 82
- than 179, 180
- than or equal to 180
greater than 179
green
- fluorescent protein 78
- fluorescent protein, enhanced 69
- monkey kidney (cells) 80
grid
- analysis, error 69
grifolafrondosa 78
grivet monkey cell 79
groove
- binder, minor 106
gross 82
- cystic disease fluid protein 15 78
- domestic product 78
- leukemia virus 79
- motor 79
- motor activity 79
- product 81
grossly 82
group 81, 82
- high mobility 86
- IX pollen allergen from barley (Hordeum vulgare) 86
groups
- diagnosis-related 62
- hyperchromatic crowded 84
growth
- arrest 77
- associated protein-43 77
- defect, monolayer 106
- factor, acidic fibroblast 15
- factor, basic fibroblast 32
- factor, B-cell 31
- factor, epidermal 69
- factor, fibroblast 74
- factor, insulin-like 91
- factor, insulin-like (somatomedin) 91
- factor, platelet derived 129
- factor, unidentified 171
- factor, vascular endothelial cell 173
- factor,glial 78
- factors, transforming 161
- hormone (somatotropin) 78
- hormone binding protein 78
- hormone deficiency 78
- hormone deficiency type IB, isolated 91
- hormone deficiency, childhood-onset 49
- hormone releasing factor 79
- hormone therapy 79
- hormone, human 85
- hormone, pituitary 132
- hormone-releasing hormone (somatocrinin) 82
- medium 79
- post-exponential 130
- promoting activity 81
- retardation, intrauterine 95
- standard, life-death 99
growth hormone 78
GTPase effector domain 78
GTPase-activating proteins 77
guaiac
- test, bicolor 31
guanidino
- ethyldisulphide 78
- propionic acid 81
guanine 77
- adenine-adenine codon for glutamic acid 77
- adenine-cytosine codon for aspartic acid 77
- adenine-guanine codon for glutamic acid 77
- adenine-uracil codon for aspartic acid 77
- cytosine-adenine codon for alanine 78
- cytosine-cytosine codon for alanine 78
- cytosine-guanine codon for alanine 78
- cytosine-uracil codon for alanine 78
- guanine-adenine codon for glycine 78
- guanine-cytosine codon for glycine 78
- guanine-guanine codon for glycine 78
- guanine-uracil codon for glycine 78
- monophosphate reductase 80
- nucleotide 80

- nucleotide-binding (protein) 80
- nucleotide-binding protein, alpha-transducing 80
- nucleotide-binding protein, beta transducing 80
- releasing factor 82
- uracil-adenine codon for valine 82
- uracil-cytosine codon for valine 82
- uracil-guanine codon for valine 82
- uracil-uracil codon for valine 83

guanosine
- 3' 5'-cyclic phosphate 80
- monophosphate 80
- nucleotide-binding alpha Z polypeptide 80

guard
- assist, contact 44

Guillian-Barre syndrome 77
guinea
- pig 81
- pig albumin 81
- pig anti-insulin serum 81
- pig complement 82

Guizhi-Fuling-Wan 78
gun
- shot wound 82

gut
- mucosa lymphocyte 80

gutta percha 81
gyn 83
gynecology 83
- and obstetrics 122

H

H. pylori outer membrane protein 86
haemodialysis
- continuous arterio-venous 39

haemofiltration
- continuous arterio-venous 39
- continuous veno-venous 55

haemophilus
- aegyptius, restriction enzyme 83
- influenzae 85
- influenzae Rd, restriction enzyme 85
- influenzae type B 85

haemorrhoidectomy
- day-case 56

Hagedorn
- neutral protamine 119

hairy cell leukemia 84
half
- life 181
- life, apparent 16
- time, aggregation 17
- upper 168
- value 88
- value, layer 88

hallucinations
- sleep-related 157

Halobacterium
- halobium 85

haloperidol 86
Halsted aphasia test 83
hamartoma
- mutiple 107

hamster
- tumor, autogenous 17

hand
- grip, left 100
- motion 86
- side, left 100

handicapped
- multiply 106

Hank
- balanced salt solution 107

hantavirus cardiopulmonary syndrome 84
haptoglobin 86
hard of hearing 85, 86
harmonic attenuation table 83
harvest
- endoscopic vein 71

has
- been drinking 83
- not voided 86

Hassal's corpuscles 83
hay fever 85
hazard
- analysis and critical control point 83

hazardous
- events (database), acute 15
- waste incinerator 88
- waste index 88

hazardous materials 83
Hb 85
head 84
- arm, trunk 83
- circumference 83
- ears, eyes, nose, and throat 84
- holder system, customized 44
- holder, Vogele-Bale-Hohner 173
- injury 85
- injury, closed 44
- injury, minimal 107
- nurse, army 16
- of bed 86
- out water immersion 88
- position, natural 117
- space gas chromatography 87
- trauma, blunt 32
- ultrasound 87

headache 83
- medication-induced 108

headphone 132
healing well 88
health
- benefits, uniform effective 170
- care maintenance 84
- care, academic 15
- center, academic 15
- education activity, area 15
- education center, area 15
- general 78
- information administrator, registered 143
- information technician, registered 143
- insurance plan 16
- locus of control, multidimensional 107
- mental 106
- outcomes research 86
- plan, accountable 16

- plan, approved 16
- plan, consumer choice 41
- professional shortage area 87
- related quality of life 87
- service development fund 16
- service, area 16

healthy
- volunteers 88
- way of life 88

hearing
- distance 84
- loss 85
- loss, occupational noise-induced 123

heart 50, 87, 180
- and lungs 85
- block 83
- disease 84
- disease, acquired valvular 26
- disease, acute 15
- disease, arteriosclerotic 23
- disease, atherosclerotic 15, 23
- disease, atherosclerotic coronary 38
- disease, congenital 44
- disease, coronary 44, 97
- disease, cyanotic congenital 41
- disease, ischemic 91
- disease, Mulberry 107
- disease, organic 122
- disease, rheumatic 143
- disease, valvular 173
- disease, ventricular 173
- energy system, artificial 15
- failure 85
- failure, acute 15
- failure, chronic 44
- failure, congestive 44
- failure, right 143
- liver, kidney 86
- lungs, abdomen 86
- murmur 86
- rate 87
- rate, atrial 16
- rate, fetal 74
- rate, intrinsic 91
- rate, maximal 107
- regular rate and rhythm 87
- sound, second pulmonic 127
- sounds 87
- sounds, 1st to 4th 149
- sounds, fetal 74
- syndrome, acquired valvular 26
- tones, fetal 74
- transplantation, bicaval 31
- transplantation, classical 44
- weight index 88
- work index 88
- worm infection 88

heat 181
- and humidity exchanger 86
- humidity index 85
- induced epitope retrieval 85
- load stimulator, metabolic 107
- loss, evaporative 69
- withdrawal latency 88

heat, reddening, swelling, tenderness 87

heavy
- chain disease 181

height 87
- fundal 74
- midparental 111
- width index 88
- width-length 88

Hektoen enteric agar 84

helical computed tomographic 84

helicobacter pylori 86

helper-dependent (e.g. adenoviral vectors) 84

hemagglutination
- chronic chloride 41
- inhibition 85, 91

hemangiomas
- circumscribed choroidal 41
- diffuse choroidal 57

hematocrit 51, 84
- and hemoglobin 84
- critical 51

hematology 84
- profile 84

hematoma
- chronic subdural 54
- necessitans, pelvic 132
- retroperitoneal 145
- subdural 150

hematopoiesis
- extramedullary 69

hematopoietic
- progenitor cells 87
- stem cell, pluripotential 132

hematoxylin
- and eosin stain 84
- phosphotungstic acid 139

heme
- oxygenase, microsomal 107

hemeselect 87

hemiblock
- left anterior 98
- left posterior 101

hemiglobin
- cyanide 85
- methemoglobin 85

hemipelvectomy 86

hemiplegic
- migraine, mercury-hydroxypropane 107

hemoccult
- rehydrated 86
- sensa 86

hemochromatosis
- hereditary 85

hemodialysis 84
- (high dependency) unit 84
- continuous veno-venous 55
- maintenance 107
- optimal 124

hemodynamically
- weighted 88
- weighted imaging 88

hemoglobin 83, 85
- A1c - used for monitoring blood glucose 83
- and hematocrit 84
- concentration, mean corpuscular 105
- mean corpuscular 104
- saturation, mixed venous 159

hemoglobin/hematocrit 85

hemoglobinuria
- paroxysmal cold 129
- paroxysmal nocturnal 134

hemolysis, elevated liver enzymes, low platelets syndrome 84
hemolytic
- anemia 83
- anemia, microangiopathic 103
- complement, total functional 44
- dilution, minimal 107
- disease of the newborn 84
- disease, autoimmune 15
- dose, mean 107
- dose, minimum 107
- uremic (syndrome), acute 17
- uremic syndrome 87
hemophagocytic
- lymphohistiocytosis, infection-associated 88
- syndrome, infection-associated 88
- syndrome, virus-associated 172
hemophillus
- influenzae type B conjugate vaccine 85
- influenzae type B polysaccharide vaccine 83
hemorrhage
- acute upper gastrointestinal 25
- and exudate 84
- deep cerebral 56
- esophageal variceal 71
- fetal-maternal 75
- germinal matrix 80
- germinal matrix related 80
- intracerebral 90
- intraventricular 95
- post-partum 136
- subarachnoid 149
- upper gastrointestinal 171
hemorrhagic
- conjunctivitis, acute 15
- cystitis, acute 15
- encephalomyelitis, acute 15
- encephalopathy, acute necrotizing 19
- escherichia coli 84
- fever, argentinian 16
- leukoencephalitis, acute 16
- pancreatitis, acute 16
hemosiderosis
- diffuse chorioamnionic 57
hemostasis
- consultant system, artificial intelligence 17
henderson-hasselbach equation 85
Henoch-Schönlein purpura 87
heparin
- assosiated thrombocytopenia 83
- cofactor 84
- induced thrombocytopenia 85
- lock 84
- low molecular weight 101
- unfractionated 171
hepatic
- artery thrombosis 83
- artery, right 143
- blood flow 83
- cell adenomas 84
- glucose output 85
- iminodiacetic acid (imaging or scanning) 85
- insufficiency 85
- necrosis, massive 107
- vein 88
- venule, terminal 162
- weight index 88
hepatitis
- A virus 83
- acute 15
- acute viral 26
- associated antibodies 83
- australia serum 25
- autoimmune-type chronic active 17
- B immune globuline 83
- B surface antigen 83
- B virus 83
- C virus 84
- C, posttransfusion 139
- chronic active 38
- chronic cholestatic 41
- chronic lobular 46
- infectious 91
- serum 151
hepatobiliary scan 85
hepatocellular
- carcinoma 84
- degeneration, acquired 15
hepatocerebral
- degeneration, acquired 15
hepatojugular 85
- reflux 85
hepatosplenomegaly 87
heptane carboxamide (an H1 receptor antagonist) 87
heptose
- D-glycero-D́-manno 58
hereditary 16
- eliptocytosis 84
- hemochromatosis 85
- motor and sensory neuropathies 86
- neuropathy with liability to pressure palsies 86
- nonpolyposis colon cancer syndrome 86
- osteodystrophy, albright 16
- persistence of fetal hemoglobin 87
- pyropoikilocytosis 87
- spherocytosis 87
Herndon-Dudley syndrome 15
hernia 84
- bilateral inguinal 32
- hiatal 85
- left inguinal 100
herniated
- disc syndrome 84
- disks 84
- nucleus pulposus 86
herpes
- gestationis 85
- like virus 86
- simplex 87
- simplex virus 87
- virus 88
- virus, avian 17
- virus, human 85
- virus-1, bovine 32
- zoster virus 88
herpetic gingival stomatitis 16

Hertz 88
heterophil
- antibody titer 83
heterotopic
- ossification 86
heterozygosity
- loss 101
hexamethyl
- propyleneamine oxime 86
hexose
- monophosphate (oxidative shunt) 86
Heymann
- nephritis, passive 132
HGB 85
hiatal
- hernia 85
hierarchy
- process, analytic 16
high 179
- albumin transport 83
- alcohol-drinking 83
- and intermittent doses of calcitriol, intravenous administration 96
- anxiety 83
- blood pressure 83
- brooding temperature 85
- density lipoprotein 84
- density polyethylene 84
- dose 84
- dose chemotherapy 84
- efficiency particulate air/ adsorption 84
- endothelial venule(s) 85
- frequency cells 85
- frequency oscillatory ventilation 85
- grade squamous intraepithelial lesion 85
- intensity focused ultrasound 85
- mobility group 86
- molecular weight kininogen 85, 86
- outlet resistance 86
- power field 87
- pressure (or performance) liquid chromatography 87
- pressure neurologic syndrome 87
- pressure, air at 16
- risk 87
- sensitivity C-reactive protein 87
- solids anaerobic digestion test 87
- squamous intraepithelial lesion 87
- throughput screening 87
- tibial osteotomy, closing wedge 55
- water intake 88
- zone tolerance 88
high-dose
- chemotherapy 84
higher
- order repeat 86
highest
- average daily dose 83
highly
- active antiretroviral therapy 83
hindpaw withdrawal latency 88
Hinton
- Base 107
hip
- arthroplasty, total 162
- joint, artificail 16
- knee-ankle-foot orthosis 85
- prosthesis, total 162
- replacement, total 162
- revision, total 162
- screw, dynamic 59
- waist index 88
hippocampal
- formation volume 85
histamine
- test, augmented 17
histidine 83, 85
- alpha-hydrazine analog of 16
- codon 38
histiocytic
- leukemia, diffuse 59
- lymphohistiocytosis 86
histiocytocis
- Langerhans cell 99
histiocytosis
- intestine, malignant 107
- like B-cell lymphoma 107
- malignant 106
histocompatibility
- locus antigen 86
- major complex 107
histogram
- dose volume 64
- poststimulus time 139
histology 85
histone acetyltransferase 83
histopathological grading 77
histopathology
- dementia lacking distinctive 60
history 85, 88
- and physical (examination) 86
- and physical examination 87
- drug 59
- family 74
- marital 106
- medical 106
- medical eye 105
- neurologic 117
- of 86
- of present illness 87
- past medical 134
- past pertinent 136
HIV virus
- specific viral protein 81
- viral protein specific 127
HLA
- antigens inherited paternal 93
- DR antigen 62
Hochu-ekki-to 162
Hodgkin
- and Reed-Sternberg cells 87
- lymphoma, classical 44
- lymphoma, mixed cellularity 105
- lymphoma, nodular lymphocyte predominant 118
- lymphoma, nodular sclerosis classical 120
- lymphoma,B symptoms 28
- morbus 106
Hodgkin lymphoma 99

lx

- lymphocyte predominant 101
- lymphocyte-rich classical 101
Hodgkin's
- disease (lymphoma) 84
- disease, nodular sclerosing 120
Hoehn and Yahr (scale) 88
hog
- cholera 85
- cholera virus 84
holosystolic murmer 87
holter
- monitor, ambulatory 16
Holtzman inkblot technique 85
home 84
- exercise program 84
- visit 88
homeobox gene 86
homing receptor 86
homocysteic acid 84
homocysteine
- adenosyl 15
homogeneous staining regions 87
homologous
- restriction factor 87
homologue of rap 86
homology
- enabled/VASP 71
- pleckstrin 132
homosexuality 181
homovanillic acid 88
homozygous
- familial hypercholesterolaemia 86
hora somni 87
hordein genes 86
hordeum vulgare 86
horizontal 86
- ground reaction force 74
- movable arm support 86
hormone
- (somatocrinin), growth hormone-releasing 82
- anterior pituitary 22
- antidiuretic 14
- bovine thyroid-stimulating 36
- corpus luteum 46
- follicle stimulating 76
- gastrointestinal 79
- gonadotropin-releasing 80
- luteinizing 100
- luteinizing hormone-releasing 100
- luteotropic 100
- maturation-inducing 108
- melanocyte-stimulating 112
- molt-inhibiting 108
- parathyroid 139
- pigment-dispersing 129
- prolactin release inhibiting 138
- receptor, adrenocorticotropic 13
- receptor, thyroid-stimulating 165
- releasing factor, thyroid-stimulating 165
- releasing hormone, thyroid-stimulating 165
- replacement therapy 87
- thyroid stimulating 165
- thyrotropic 167
- urinary follicle-stimulating 170
horse
- sickness, african 16
horseradish peroxidase 87
horticulture waste ashes 88
hospital
- admission 83
- anxiety and depression scale 83
- arrival time 83
- benefit, maximum 107
- combat support 54
- data management system, automated 15
- day 84
- essential access community 67
- information system, automated 16
- municipal 106
- neuropsychiatric 117
- record 87
- treatment 87
- visit 88
hospitalization 88
hospitalized
- medical patients, behavioral regression or upset 36
hostility
- index, active 16
hot
- moist packs 86
- pack 86
- plate 86
- water irrigation 88
- wet pack 88
hot and cold 83
hour 83, 87, 180
- of sleep 87
- one 181
- three 181
- two 181
hours
- alternate 19
house
- officer 86
- physician, assistant 16
- surgeon, assistant 16
HTN
- pulmonary 132
human
- alveolar macrophage 83
- bladder carcinoma, antibody 32
- bone morphogenetic protein, recombinant 143
- chorionic gonadotropin 84
- diploid cell vaccine 84
- diploid fibroblast 84
- esophageal epithelial cancer cell line 67
- gammaglobulin, aggregated 16
- gastric mucin 85
- globulin, aggregated 16
- granulocytic ehrlichiosis 85
- growth hormone 85
- herpes virus 85
- herpes virus 8 85
- IgG, aggregated 17
- immuno-deficiency virus 85

- infantile cortical hyperostosis 90
- leukocyte antigen 86
- leukocyte antigen, D-related 86
- leukocytea associated antigens (HL-A matching for BMT) 86
- lung fibroblasts 86
- lymphotropic virus 87
- menopausal gonadotropin 86
- oestrogen receptor 86
- oxidoreductase 86
- papilloma virus 87
- performance laboratory 87
- placental lactogen 87
- rabies immunoglobin 87
- resources management systems 87
- serum albumine 87
- T-cell lymphotropic virus, types I 87
- umbilical vein endothelial cells 87

humidity
- relative 143

Hurthle
- cell neoplasms 132

H-wave therapy 88
hyaline membrane disease 86
hybrid white leghorn 88
hybridization
- comparative genomic 44
- in situ 94

hydratase
- enoyl CoA 67

hydrazide
- maleic 106

hydrazine 120
- analog, histidine 16

hydrocarbon
- polycyclic aromatic 127

hydrocephalus
- normal pressure 119

hydrochloric acid 84
hydrochloride 84
hydrochlorothiazide 84
hydrodynamics
- magneto 107

hydrogen 83
- ion concentration 132
- peroxide 86
- sulfide 87

hydroperoxyeicosatetraenoic acid 87
hydroxy
- apatite coated porous alumni 83
- butyrate dehydrogenase 83
- corticosteroids 122
- dinitrophenyl 118
- eicosatetraenoic acid 84
- eicosatetraenoic acids 85
- ethyl methacrylate-methyl methacrylate 84
- ethylmethacrylate 84
- indoleacetic acid 85
- lapatite 83
- lapatite ceramic 83
- nonanoate, poly-3- 132
- propyl methylcellulose 87
- steroid oxidoreductase 86

hydroxylase
- arylhydrocarbon 16

hydroxynefazodone 132
hydroxynorephedrine 132
hyperactivity
- disorder, attention deficit 14

hyperalimenation 88
hyperalimentation
- fluid 83
- intravenous 95

hypercholesterolaemia
- homozygous familial 86

hyperchromatic
- crowded groups 84

hyperfractionated
- radiotherapy 85

hyperglycemic
- hyperosmolar non-ketotic 85

hyperglycinaemia
- nonketotic 117

hyperintensities
- white matter signal 176

hyperosmolar
- nonketotic coma 86
- syndrome, non-ketotic 117

hyperosmolarity-responsive 86
hyperostosis
- diffuse idiopathic skeletal 60
- human infantile cortical 90

hyperostotic
- syndrome, calvarial 44

hyperparathyroidism 87
- primary 132

hyperplasia
- atypical ductal 14
- basal cell 31
- C-cell 41
- cortical stromal 54
- cutaneous lymphoid 46
- focal nodular 75
- follicular 74
- myointimal 108
- plasmactytic 132
- usual ductal 170

hyperpneic 88
hyperpolarization
- after 16

hypersensitivity
- carotid sinus 54
- delayed cutaneous 57
- syndrome, phenytoin 132

hypertension 87
- arterial 15, 17
- isolated systolic 94
- obliterative pulmonary 123
- portal 132
- pregnancy-induced 133
- primary pulmonary 136
- pulmonary 132
- systemic arterial 149

hypertensive
- arteriosclerotic cardiovascular disease 83
- cardiovascular disease 84
- disease, renal 143
- rats, spontaneously 151
- vascular disease 88

hyperthermia
- malignant 106

hyperthermic
- perfusion chemotherapy, intraperitoneal 93

hyperthyroidism 87
hypertrichosis lanuginosa, acquired 16

hypertrophia
- left 100
- right 143
hypertrophic
- cardiomyopathy 84
- obstructive cardiomyopathy 86
- osteoarthropathy 86
- prostate, benign 32
- subaortic stenosis, idiopathic 91
hypertrophy
- asymmetrical septal 23
- biventricular 36
- left atrial 98
- left ventricular 103
- right ventricular 149
hyperventilation 88
- eucapnic voluntary 71
hypocellular acute leukemia 83
hypodermic 83, 88
hypodermically 88
hypogonadism
- hypogonadotropic 16
hypogonadotropic
- hypogonadism 16
hypophospbatemic
- rickets, sex-linked 153
hypoplastic
- anemia, congenital 44
hypopospadias
- pseudovaginal perineoscrotal 136
hypotension
- cerebrospinal fluid 53
hypothalami
- periventricularis 132
hypothalamic
- lesion, medial 107
- nucleus, paraventricular 132
- preoptic area, anterior 16
hypothalamo
- pituitary-adrenocortical 87
hypothalamus
- ventrolateral 174
hypothermia
- accidental 15
hypothesis
- double-crush 57
hypoventilation
- syndrome, alveolar 16
- syndrome, congenital central 41
hypoxanthine
- aminopterin and thymidine 83
- azaserine and thymidine 83
- guanine phosphoribosyl transferase 85
- phosphoribosyltransferase 87
hypoxemic
- respiratory failure, acute 16
hypoxia
- mild 106
hypoxic
- ischemic encephalopathy 85
- training, intermittent 91
hysterectomy
- intrafascial vaginal 95
- laparoscopic assisted vaginal 99
- total abdominal 159
- total vaginal 167
- vaginal 173
- with bilateral salpingo-oophorectomy, total 162
hysterosalpingography 87

I

i 92
iap
- repeat, baculovirus 32
ibuprofen 89
ICD-O
- morphologic rubric 90
- topographic rubric 90
iceball
- gauge, cryosurgical 45
ictus
- lacunar 100
ideal
- body weight 89, 90
identical 180
- with 180
identification 90
- record, emergency drug 68
idiopathic
- amyloidosis 18
- bone cavity 89
- hypertrophic subaortic stenosis 91
- myelofibrosis, chronic 45
- premature adrenarche 93
- skeletal hyperostosis, diffuse 60
- thrombocythemia 95
- thrombocytopenic purpura 95
idiotype
- binding capacity 89
idioventricular
- rhythm 95
- rhythm, cycle length 46
if necessary 156
Ig superfamily 91
IgG antibody
- indirect immunofluorescent 90
IL-1 receptor related protein 91
iliac
- bone graft 89
- crest bone graft 89
- crest, left 100
- spine, anterior inferior 18
- spine, anterior superior 23
- spine, posterior superior 139
- vascular resistance 95
ilio
- lumbar 91
- tibial band 95
ill defined 90
illness
- mental 107
- past medical 134
illnesses
- previous 19
illusion
- oculoparalytic 123
- somatogravic 151
image
- analysis program, F-actin 72
- analysis, automated 17
imaging
- gated magnetic resonance 80

- hemodynamically weighted 88
- magnetic resonance 111
- microscopy, fluorescence digital 73
- post-radiosurgical 137
- power motion 134
- system, digital vascular 64

imipramine (Tofranil) 92

immature
- granulocyte 91
- precursors, atypical localization 18

immediate 92
- postsurgical prosthetics 93

immediately (L. statim) 158

immersion
- head-out water 88

immersive
- virtual reality 95

immigration
- and naturalization service 92

immobilization
- test, treponema pallidum 163

immobilize 92

immobilizing
- viscosity, minimum 108

immune
- complexes, circulating 45
- deficiency syndrome, acquired 85
- globulin, cytomegalo virus 49
- globulin, varicella-zoster 175
- globulin, zoster 177
- globuline, hepatitis B 83
- plasma, zoster 177
- serum globulin 94

immunglobulin 181

immunization
- diphtheria, pertussis, tetanus 62

immunize 92

immunizing unit 95

immuno magnetic particles 92

immunoadjuvant 141

immunoassay
- fluorescence polarization 75
- microparticle enzyme 105
- optical 122

immunodeficiency
- disease, acquired 17
- disease, severe combined 150
- gay-related 82
- syndrome 18
- virus, human 85

immunofixation electrophoresis 90

immunofluorescence
- assay, granulocyte 79
- crithidia luciliae 46
- direct 59
- indirect 91

immunofluorescent
- IgG antibody, indirect 90

immunogen
- T- and B-cell epitopes containing 160

immunoglobins 79

immunoglobulin 91
- A 91
- bearing cells 89
- cytoplasmic 45
- D 91
- E 91
- G 91
- intravenous 95
- M 91
- M, cytoplasmic 45
- surface 152
- thyroid stimulating 165
- variable region gene 91

immunohistochemical
- assay 89

immunohistochemistry 91

immunology
- and allergy 17

immunomagnetic separation 92

immunoperoxidase 92, 94
- stain, using an antibody against CD 138 43

immunophenotyping
- flow cytometric 73

immunoprecipitation assay 93

immunoproliferative
- small intestinal disease 94

immunoreactive 94
- insulin 94

immunoreactivity
- adrenocorticotropin-like 13
- beta-endorphin-like 32
- cholecystokinin-like 41
- neurotensin-like 121
- somatostatin-like 153

immunosorbent
- assay, enzyme-linked 69

immunotherapy
- specific 23

immunotoxins 95

impaction
- bone 32

impaired
- fasting glucose 91
- glucose tolerance 91, 94

impedance
- change 65
- tetrapolar bioelectrical 160
- thoracic 162
- total body 160

implant
- bridge, osseointegrated 122
- narrow-diameter endosseous screw 48

implantable
- cardioverter defibrillator 89
- defibrillator, automatic 17
- permanently 132

implantation
- pacemaker 134

importable drug delivery system 90

important 92

impression 92
- basilar 32
- material, vinyl polysiloxane putty 174

improved 92, 179

improvement
- continuous quality 50
- maximum medical 109

impulse
- apical 17

impurities and volatile matter 108

impurity
- phenol red 137

in
- electrocardiography, an undulating deflection that follows the T wave 168
- my humble opinion 92
- my opinion 92
- situ 94
- situ hybridization 94
- situ hybridization, chromosomal 45
- situ hybridization, fluorescence 75
- situ keratomileusis, laser 98
- situ, carcinoma 45
- situ, melanoma 108
- vitro 95
- vitro expression cloning 95
- vitro fertilization 95
- vitro quantitative autoradiography 95
- vitro released 95
- vivo 95
- vivo recovery 95
inactivated poliovirus vaccine 94
inactivator
- anaphylatoxin 17
inappropriate
- antidiuretic hormone secretion, syndrome 152
- secretion of antidiuretic hormone 88
- secretion of antidiuretic hormone, syndrome 88
inbred strains of rats 20
inch 180
inches 92
incidence of bacteria-carrier 89
incidence rate
- age-adjusted 5
incident
- mass casualty 105
- report 94
incident command 89
incinerator
- hazardous waste 88
incinerator bottom ashes 89
incision
- and drainage 90
- of the prostate, transurethral 167
incisors
- maxillary primary 134
inclusion
- bodies, osmiophilic 122
- neuronal intranuclear 117
inclusions
- glial cytoplasmic 78
incompetence
- aortic 17
incomplete 92
- abortion 92
- combustion products 133
- right bundle-branch block 94
inconclusive 92
incontinence
- urinary stress 172
increase 92, 179
- value, maximum 108
- volume regulatory 174
increased 92, 179, 180
increasing 179
increment 181
incremental
- cost-effectiveness ratio 90
incurred
- accidentally 17, 88
indefinite 180
independence
- premarital residential 137
independent 92
- medical examiner 91
- power producers 93
Index
- Barthel 32
index
- active hostility 16
- adiposity 17
- aggregation 17
- air velocity 26
- amniotic fluid 15
- ankle to brachial 9
- anxiety 17
- apnea-plus-hypopnea 16
- articulation 17
- atherogenic 17
- bacterial 32
- bactericidal 32
- behavioral cues 31
- body mass 33
- burn 32
- color 44
- finger 90
- free thyroxin (T4) 77
- hazardous waste 88
- heart weight 88
- heart work 88
- heat-humidity 85
- height-width 88
- hepatic weight 88
- hip-waist 88
- left ventricular end-diastolic volume 102
- left ventricular end-systolic volume 102
- mandibular cortical 105
- mental health 107
- obliteration prediction 123
- osteoblastic proliferation 123
- pain management 134
- pain rating 137
- Pediatric Risk 137
- phosphate reabsorption 137
- photochemical reflectance 137
- plasma cell apoptotic 128
- platelet reactivity 137
- power ratio 137
- pressure relief 137
- proliferation rate 137
- proliferative 156
- Psychopathy Resemblance 137
- relative fluorescence 143
- resistive 143
- respiratory control 142
- respiratory disturbance 142
- stroke 151
- systolic delay time 151
- thyroid binding 160
- thyroxine binding 160
- toe brachial 160
- total binding 160
- total bone 160
- total thromboplastin 167
- trabecular bone 160
- ultraviolet 172

- unequal ventilation 172
- vascular resistance 174
- venous reflux 174
- vocational rehabilitation 174
- volume 173
indicates 179
indication 92
indicative
- dosage 18
- radiation dose 60
indicator
- biological 32
indices of platelet activation 93
indirect
- bilirubin concentrations 89
- immunofluorescence 91
- immunofluorescent IgG antibody 90
- maximum breathing capacity 91
individual
- bioequivalence 89
- therapy 95
indole
- 3-propionic acid 93
- 3-pyruvic acid 93
indolent
- systemic mastocytosis 94
indomethacin 92
indophenyl acetate esterase 93
induced systemic resistance 95
induction
- post recurrence 137
- rapid sequence 146
ineffective dose 90
infant 92
- respiratory distress syndrome 94
infarction 92
- acute myocardial 19
- anterior lateral myocardial 18
- cerebral 44
- inferior myocardial 92
- myocardial 107
- non-Q-wave myocardial 119
- painless myocardial 134
- perioperative myocardial 134
- posterior cerebral artery 128
- posterior myocardial 134
- previous myocardial 134
- Q-wave myocardial 141
- right ventricle myocardial 149
- rule-out myocardial 144
- thrombolysis in myocardial 162
- thrombotic brain 160
- transmural perioperative myocardial 163
- weight 96
infected 92
infection
- acute viral respiratory 27
- associated hemophagocytic lymphohistiocytosis 88
- associated hemophagocytic syndrome 88
- bloodstream 35
- control, certified 44
- disseminated gonococcal 59
- heartworm 88
- inflammation, no sign 120
- lower respiratory tract 102
- no acute 115
- opportunistic in AIDS 18
- overwhelming postsplenectomy 124
- respiratory tract 148
- soft tissue 158
- upper respiratory tract 172
- urinary tract 172
- viral respiratory 174
infections
- opportunistic 122
infectious
- disease 17, 90
- hepatitis 91
- hypodermal and hematopoietic necrosis virus 91
- mononucleosis 91
- mononucleosis, Epstein-Barr virus 67
- mononucleosis-like 92
- particle, proteinaceous 138
infective
- dose, minimum 108
- vector, mean number 108
inferior 92, 179
- colliculus 89
- myocardial infarction 92
- oblique 93
- phrenic artery 93
- vena cava 95
infiltrating
- ductal carcinoma 90
- pancreatic ductal adenocarcinoma 93
infiltration
- with eosinophilia, pulmonary 133
infinite amplitude clipping 88
inflammation
- placental membrane 134
inflammatory
- bowel disease 89
- breast cancer 89
- demyelinating polyneuropathy, chronic 45
- disease, pelvic 133
influenza
- vaccine, multivalent 108
informatics
- biotechnology 32
information
- mental health 107
- processing ability 93
- processing, rapid 144
informed consent form 90
infostructure
- tissue microarray 163
infrared 94
- near 117
infusion 92
- intravenous piggyback 95
- nitroprusside 121
- system, controlled-release 51
ingredient
- activbe 17
inguinal
- hernia, left 100
inguinal hernia
- right 144
inhalation 92
- therapy 95
inhaled nitric oxide 92

inhaler
- dry powder 62
- metered-dose 105
inherited
- paternal HLA antigens 93
inhibiting
- hormone, mullerian 108
- pattern, reflex 144
inhibition
- hemagglutination 85
- of hemagglutination 91
- overproduction 123
- reverse transcriptase 148
- test, rapid fluorescent focus 143
- thyrotropin binding 160
inhibitor
- angiogenesis 17
- angiotensin-converting enzyme 10
- Bowman-Birk soybean 30
- carbonic anhydrase 38
- complement lysis 46
- diazepam binding 56
- farnesyl transferase 76
- monoamine oxidase 104
- of apoptosis 88
- of virus replication 95
- placental ribonuclease 137
- placental RNase 137
- protease 137
- tissue factor pathway 161
inhibitors
- serin protease 151
inhibitory
- concentration, minimal 108
- dilution, maximum 108
- dose, minimum 108
- factor, cloning 46
- factors, lymphocyte E-rosette 144
- peptide, gastric 79
- postsynaptic potential 94
- postsynaptic potentials, depolarizing 60
- volumes, minimal 108
initial
- body temperature 160
- multimodal treatment, classification 177
- patient survey 93
initial(ly) 92
initiation factor
- in the translational step of viral replication 68
inject 92
injection 92
- drug users 90
- epidural steroid 71
- intracytoplasmic sperm 90
- intramuscular 92
- intravenous 95
- multiple vitamin 114
- multi-syringe time-based 113
- percutaneous ethanol 131
- time-based 160
- transbronchial 160
- transbullar 160
injured 92
injuries
- multiple soft tissue 113
- violence-related 174
injury 92
- behavior checklist 89
- blunt duodenal 32
- bodily 32
- bone 32
- brain 32
- combined mechanical 48
- date 59, 61
- minimal head 107
- no bone 115
- nonaccidental 115
- not known 92
- pelvic vascular 140
- penetrating coronary artery 128
- personal 132
- preservation-reperfusion 137
- severe torso 158
- traumatic brain 160
- vector, major 108
inkblot
- technique, Holtzman 85
inner
- ear 90
- quadrant, left 100
inorganic orthophosphate 132
inosine
- 5'-monophosphate 92
inositol
- 1,4,5,-triphsophate 93
inoue balloon catheter 89
inpatient 93
in-process control 93
insemination
- artificial 17
insertion
- force, zero 177
inside (e.g. intracavitary) 93
insignificant 180
inspection
- palpation, percussion, auscultation 93
- unaided visual 172
inspiration 92
- prolonged mechanical 134
inspiratory 90, 92
- capacity 89
- flow rate 91
- force, negative 117
- Rrs 94
inspired
- oxygen, fraction 75
instability
- carpal 45
- dorsal intercalate segment 60
- pattern, capitolunate 46
- volar intercalary wrist 174
institutional review board 94
instruction
- tooth brushing 160
instructions
- crutch walking 55
- or directions 152
instructor coordinator 89
instrument
- patient review 137
- quality control 94
- standardization and calibration 94
instruments
- ProFile Ni-Ti rotary 137
insufficiency
- aortic 17
- atrial 17

- cardiac 44
- cerebrovascular 55
- chronic vascular 55
- corpus luteum 46
- deep venous 64
- hepatic 85
- Leydig cell 99
- mitral 107, 108
- primary chronic adrenal 128
- progressive renal 137
- pulmonic 132
- tricuspid 162
- vertebrobasilar 173

insufflation
- continuous tracheal gas 54
- transtracheal 167

insulation
- urea formaldehyde foam 170

insulin
- binding capacity 89
- coma therapy 90
- dependent diabetes 90, 91
- dependent diabetes mellitus, type I 90
- immunoreactive 94
- infusion, continuous subcutaneous 54
- injections, multiple daily 105
- lente 98
- like growth factor 155
- like growth factor (somatomedin) 91
- like growth factor, binding protein 91
- like growth factor-binding protein-5 91
- likegrowth factor 91
- promoter, rat 144
- protamine zinc 140
- shock therapy 95

insulinotropic
- peptide, glucose-dependent 79

insurance 92
- no 117
- plan, assisted health 16

intact
- extraocular movements 70

intake
- acceptable daily 14
- and output (as for fluids) 93
- dry matter 61
- high water 88
- protein 137

integral
- diastolic velocity 64

integrated
- backscatter coefficient 89
- circuit, application specific 23
- concentration 17
- pulse amperometry 93
- summary of safety 95
- voltage, mean 108

integrity
- plasma membrane 134

intelligence
- artificial 17
- quotient 94
- scale for children, Wechsler 175

intensification
- post-remission 137

intensity-modulated radiotherapy 92

intensive
- care 89
- care facility 90
- care nursery 90
- care unit 90
- care unit, cardiac 45
- care unit, mobile 108
- care unit, neonatal 117
- care unit, pediatric 133
- care unit, pulmonary 133
- care unit, spinal cord 150
- care unit, surgical 152
- coronary care 89
- coronary care unit 89
- therapy 95
- therapy observation unit 93
- therapy unit 95

interactive
- voice response 95

interactor
- translid binocular 160

interagency
- testing committee 95

interbody
- fusion, posterolateral 133
- spacers, titanium 162

intercalate
- segment instability, dorsal 60
- segment instability,dorsal 60

intercellular
- adhesion molecule 1 89
- adhesion molecules 89

interchange
- electronic data 68

interclass
- variance, maximization 108

interconnection
- open systems 126

intercostal
- margin 90
- space 90, 94
- space, left 100

interdigestive
- migratory motor complex 92

interdigitating cells 90

interface
- brain-computer 31
- common client 41
- membrane, synovial-like 153
- protocol, serial line 153

interference pattern analysis 93

interferon 91

interleukine 91
- 2 91

intermediate 91
- care facility 90
- lobe peptide, corticotropin-like 46
- lymphocytic lymphoma 91
- tectobulbar pathway 160
- trophoblast 95
- view reprojection 95

intermittent 92
- cervical traction 90
- hypoxic training 91
- mandatory ventilation 92
- pneumatic foot compression 93
- positive pressure breathing 93
- positive pressure respiration 93

- positive pressure ventilation 93
- positive-pressure inflation with oxygen 93
internal 92, 93
- acoustic canal 88
- and external 90
- carotid artery 89
- derangement of the knee 90
- diameter 90
- disc disruption 90
- energy 66, 168
- mammary artery, left 100
- medicine 91
- rotation 94
- rotation in extension 94
- rotation in flexion 94
- tibial torsion 95
- urethrotomy, direct-vision 64
international
- neuroblastoma staging system 92
- normalized ratio 92
- prognostic index 93
- sensitivity index 94
- system of units 151
- unit 95
- unit of enzyme activity 168
- units 95
internet
- link, gene recognition and analysis 82
interocular difference 17
interosseous
- artery, posterior 132
- ligament, scapholunate 153
- membrane 93
- nerve, anterior 18
- nerve, posterior 133
interphalangeal 93
- distal 60
- joint, distal 60
- joint, proximal 133
- proximal 133
interphalangeal joint 93
interruption
- of pregnancy, voluntary 173
interscapular line 94
interstitial
- brachytherapy, computer-assisted frameless stereotactic 38
- laser coagulation 91
- lung disease, respiratory bronchiolotis 142
- penumonitis, desquamative 60
- pneumonia, acute 18
- pneumonia, giant cell 79
- pneumonia, usual 171
- pneumonitis, lymphoid 100
- tumor therapy 95
interthecal 95
interval 92
- background 32
- breast cancer 89
- confidence 44
- disease free 59
- history 91
- postmortem 134
- postpartum resumption 137
- pre-response 137
- time 181
- ventricular response 174
intervascular
- ridging 95
intervention
- percutaneous coronary 129
interventional
- magnetic resonance imaging 92
- radiology 95
- vascular radiology 95
interventricular
- septal defect 96
intervertebral 95
- disc 95
- disc, prolapsed 133
- joint complex 95
intestinal
- obstruction 93
- obstruction from peritoneal bands, syndrome 98
- peptide, vasoactive 173
- submucosa (hernia repair), small 152
- type 95
- vascular resistance 95
intimate partner abuse 93
intraaortic
- balloon pump 88
intraarterial 88
intracapsular
- fracture 90
intracellular
- Ca2+ concentration 128
- diplococci, gram-negative 80
- fluid 90
- receptor 94
intracerebral 89
- hemorrhage 90
intracranial
- mass lesion 92
- pressure 90
intracutaneous 89
intracytoplasmic
- sperm injection 90
intradermal 90
intradiscal
- electrothermal therapy 90
intraductal
- component, extensive 69
intraductile
- breast cancer 89
intraepithelial
- carcinogenesis, endometrial 69
- lesion, high squamous 87
- lesion, high-grade squamous 85
- lesion, low grade squamous 102
- lesions, squamous 152
- neoplasia (grades I, II, III), cervical 45
- neoplasia, mammary 108
intrafallopian
- transfer, gamete 79
- transfer, zygote 177
intrafascial
- vaginal hysterectomy 95
intrahepatic
- portosystemic shunt, transjugular 162
- portosystemic stent shunts, transjugular 162

intralobar
- pulmonary arteries 93
intramedullary 91
- rod 92
intramolecular
- vibrational energy redistribution 95
intramuscular 91
- injection 92
intranuclear
- inclusion, neuronal 117
intraocular
- foreign body 93
- lens 93
- lens, posterior chamber 129
- pressure 93
- silicone prosthesis 94
intraoperative
- radiotherapy 93
intraosseous 93
intraperitoneal 93
- free cancer cells 90
- hyperthermic perfusion chemotherapy 93
intrapulmonary
- arteries 93
intrarenal
- vascular resistance 96
intraretinal
- microvascular abnormalities 94
intrathecally 93
intrauterine 95
- catheter 95
- contraceptive device 95
- device 95
- fetal death 95
- growth retardation 95
- pregnancy 95
- term pregnancy 95
- transfusion 95
intravaginal
- ring 96
intravascular 95
- coagulation, disseminated 59
- ultrasonography 96
intravenous 95
- administration of high and intermittent doses of calcitriol 96
- administration, maternal 108
- cholangiography 95
- drug abuse 95
- drug addict 95
- drug use/user 95
- fluids 95
- hyperalimentation 95
- immunoglobulin 95
- injection 95
- line 95
- line, peripheral 133
- peripheral 133
- piggyback infusion 95
- push 95
- pyelogram 95
- pyelography, rapid-sequence 146
- regimen 96
- regional anesthesia 96
- urogram 96
- urography 96
intraventricular
- conduction defect 95
- hemorrhage 95
- reentry 96
intrinsic
- heart rate 91
- sympathomimetic activity 94
intubation
- endotracheal 71
- rapid sequence 146
invasion
- blood vessel 36
- lymphatic 98
- plasmid antigens proteins 93
- venous 172
invasive
- aspergillosis 88
- bladder cancer 89
- breast cancers 89
- peritonitis, gonorrheal 79
- pulmonary aspergillosis 93
inventory
- Beck depression 32
- brief pain 34
- mental health 107
- Personal Reaction 137
inventory/nursing
- home, neuropsychiatric 119
inversion
- point respiratory 137
inverted
- repeat outer domain 96
- repeats 96
investigation
- plan, clinical 45
investigational
- new drug 92
investigative site support center 95
in-vitro-retinae 96
involvement
- single extranodal site 66
iodine
- binding capacity 89
- protein bound 128
iodo-l-phenylalanine 93
ion
- channels, mechanosensitive 112
- transport peptide 95
ionization
- chamber, scanning liquid 153
- detector 17
- detector, argon 17
- detectors (chromatography), flame 74
- electrospray 71
ionophore of bivalent cations 89
ipamorelin 93
iridium 94
iris
- neovascularization 121
- pigment epithelium 93
iron 74
- binding capacity 89
- binding capacity, total 162
- deficiency 74
- deficiency anemia 90
- serum 151
- total body 160
irradiation
- dose, minimum 108
- total body 160

- total needed 163
- total nodal 163
- ultraviolet 172
- ultraviolett blood 169
irregular 94
irrigation 94
- continuous bladder 39
- hot-water 88
- pipe-associated 93
- vaginal 173
irritable bowel syndrome 89
irritation
- acute nerve root 20
is to 180
ischemia
- noncardiac cerebral 116
ischemic
- attacks, transient 162
- heart disease 91
- neurologic deficit, prolonged reversible 138
- neurologic deficit, reversible 144
- optic neuropathy, anterior 18
isobutyl
- cyanoacrylate 89
- ichloroformate 89
isocapnic
- ventilation, maximal 108
isocitrate
- dehydrogenase 89
isoflurane 94
isolated
- growth hormone deficiency type IB 91
- limb perfusion 91
- perfused rat kidney 93
- systolic hypertension 94
isolation
- body substance 34
isolectin 101
isoleucine 88, 91
- codon 25
- peptide histidine 132
isoleucyl-tRNA synthetase 123
isomerase
- corticosterone side-chain 53
- phosphoribose 137
isometric
- strength, maximal 108
isoniazid 92
isoprenoid
- phytane 132
- pristane 137
isopropanol 137
isopropyl
- alcohol 93
- amine 93
- antipyrine 93
isoproterenol
- hydrochloride 93
isoproylthiogalactoside 94
isovolumetric regulation 96
isovolumic
- contraction 95
- relaxation 96
ivermectin 96

J

Jackson-Pratt drains 96
Jakob-Creutzfeldt disease 96
Janus kinase(s) 96
jaundice
- obstructive 123
jaw
- fracture, open reduction 125
- jerk 96
jejunostomy
- tube 96
jerk
- ankle 18
- biceps 33
- elbow 69
- jaw 96
job
- disability, transient 162
joint 96
- acromioclavicular 10, 11
- arthroplasty, total 162
- carpometacarpal 48
- complex, intervertebral 95
- disease, degenerative 60
- disease, traumatic 162
- distal interphalangeal 60
- intraphalangeal 93
- metacarpophalangeal 105
- metatarsalphalangeal 110
- movement, full range 76
- patellofemoral 131
- proximal interphalangeal 133
- proximal radioulnar 138
- range of motion, full 75
- sacroiliac 151
- space narrowing 96
joints
- distal interphalangeal 60
jugular
- vein 96
- venous catheter 97
- venous distension 97
- venous pressure 97
- venous pulse 97
jugulovenous 97
jump
- vertical 174
junction 96
- atrioventricular 27
- myoneural 110
- neuromuscular 118
- squamocolumnar 150
- uretero-bladder 169
junctional
- premature contraction 96
- reentrant, atrioventricular 27
just noticeable difference 96
juvenile 96
- onset diabetes mellitus 96
- osteochrondritis dissecans 96
- rheumatoid arthritis 96
Juzen-taiho-to
- a kampo medicine 162

K

Kaneda
- anterior spinal/scoliosis system 97
Kaposi
- sarcoma 18, 97
- sarcoma herpes virus 97
- sarcoma, classic 45
kappa
- opiate receptor 124

Karnofsky performance status 97
keep
- open 97
- veins open 97
keep open rate 97
keratinocytes 97
keratitis
- chronic superficial 54
- ichthyosis, and deafness 97
keratoconjunctivitis
- sicca 97
- superior limbic 153
keratomileusis
- laser in-situ 98
keratoplasty
- automated lamellar 18
keratosis
- lichen planus-like 101
keto
- acid, branched-chain 31
- acidosis 97
- acidosis, diabetic 60
- genic steroids 97
- steroids 97
ketoacidosis
- alcoholic 18
ketoconazole 97
Ketohexokinase 97
kick
- knee 97
kidney 97
- cells, baby hamster 32
- cells, green monkey 80
- disease, polycystic 22, 129, 133
- function test 97
- left 100
- liver, spleen 97
- stone 97
- ureters, bladder (x-ray) 97
Kikuchi-Fujimoto disease 97
killed
- vaccine, measles 108
killer
- cells, cytokine induced 45
- cells, natural 117
killifish 97
kilo
- bases 97
- calorie 97
- gram 97
kilocalorie 97
kinase
- beta-adrenergic receptor 29
- casein 45
- creatine 45
kinases
- cyclin-dependent 43
- inhibitors, cyclin-dependent 43
- uridine-cytidine 169
kinetic
- energy 66
- energy of alpha particles 66
kininogen
- high molecular weight 85
- high-molecular weight 86
Kirschner wire 97
Kjeldahl
- nitrogen, total 162
Kliger iron agar 97
knee
- arthroplasty 22
- arthroplasty with metal-backed patellar components 104
- arthroplasty, total 162
- bearing amputation 97
- bends, deep 60
- disarticulation 97
- extension, total 162
- internal derangement 90
- jerk 97
- kick 97
- replacement, total 162
- revision, total 162
Koch's
- old tuberculin 126
- original tuberculin 126
Krebs-Hensleit buffer 97

L

L
- chain, constant domain 46
l,2-bis (aminophenoxy) ethane-N,N,N,N'-tetraacetic acid 29
L. monocytogenes
- detection system 100
- plating medium 101
labeling
- index, bone marrow plasma cell 129
labor
- and delivery 99
- delivery recovery postpartum 99
- room 101
laboratory 98
- assistant, certified 46
- information system 100
- practice, good 79
- scientist, clinical 47, 52
- technician, certified 47
- technician, clinical 47
laceration 98
lacking
- distinctive histopathology, dementia 60
lacrimal
- gland, nictitans 117
lactate
- dehydrogenase 99
lactated Ringer's solution 101
lactating
- fully 75
- late 100
lactic 98
lactobacillus 97
lactogen
- human placental 87
lacunar ictus 100
lambda 97
Lambertville/Maybee/Raisinville 101
lamina
- cricoid 46
laminectomy 98
- cervical 46
lamotrigine 102

Langerhans
- cell histiocytocis 99
- cells 99
language
- extensible markup 176
laparoscopic
- appendectomy and duodenocolonic dissociation 98
- cholecystectomy 98, 99
laparoscopy 98
- under local anesthesia 102
laparotomy 98
- exploratory 72
large 100
- bowel 99
- bowel obstruction 99
- cell lymphoma, diffuse 60
- cell neuroendocrine carcinoma 99
- cell, anaplastic 18
- cell, follicular lymphoma 75
- for gestational age 100
- white (pig) 103
laryngeal
- nerve, superior 153
- resistance 144
laryngoscopy
- and abdominal thrusts, simultaneous 153
laryngotracheitis
- avian 19
laryngotracheobronchitis
- acute 19
laser
- acoustic microscope, scanning 153
- coagulation, interstitial 91
- Doppler flowmetry 99
- in-situ keratomileusis 98
- scanning microscopy 47
- therapy, ultraviolet 172
- thermokeratoplasty 102
- trabeculoplasty 19
- yttrium-aluminum-garnet 177
last
- menstrual period 101
late
- transplant generation 102
late luteal phase dysphoric disorder 134
late-lactating 100
latency
- corrected ensemble average 99
- heat-withdrawal 88
- hindpaw withdrawal 88
- step-down 150
- test, multiple sleep 112
lateral 98
- (view in x-rays) 99
- bending, left 100
- bulla osteotomy 161
- collateral ligament 99
- compression 99
- costal artery 99
- flexion, left 100
- geniculate body 100
- neck, soft tissue 158
- pulvinar, ventral part 140
- rectus 101
- right 144
- sacrum anterior 102
- spinal nucleus 102
- spread of freeze (of a cryosurgical iceball) 102
- tegmental tract 102
latex 97
- agglutination, slide 153
- bead agglutination test, antilactoferrin 100
- gloves, natural 117
Lathyrus ochrus 101
latin 98
latissimus
- dorsi, flap reconstruction 99
lavage
- bronchoalveolar 28
- diagnostic peritoneal 62
- fluid, broncho-alveolar 28
laxative 99
- of choice 101
layer
- buccal odontoblast 33
- half-value 88
- outer, plexiform 123
lead 128
- on the left arm in electrocardiography, unipolar limb 27
- on the left leg in electrocardiography, unipolar limb 26
- on the right arm in electrocardiography, unipolar limb 27
leads to 179
lean body mass 99
lean tissue growth 102
Leao's spreading depression 99
learning
- lecture-based 99
- problem-based 128
lecithin/shingomyelin ratio 102
lecture-based learning 99
Lee-White clotting time 103
left 98, 102
- anterior descending (coronary artery) 98
- anterior fascicular block 98
- anterior hemiblock 98
- anterior oblique 98
- atrial enlargement 98
- atrial hypertrophy 98
- atrial pressure 98
- atrium 98
- axis deviation 98
- border of cardiac dullness 99
- bundle branch block 99
- bundle branch block, complete 46
- circumflex coronary artery 99
- coronary artery 99
- costal margin 99
- ear 18, 23
- ear-bone conduction threshold 180
- eye 99, 125
- eye, vision 174
- foot 99
- forearm 100
- frontoanterior 100
- frontotransverse 100
- hand grip 100
- hand side 100

- hypertrophia 100
- iliac crest 100
- iliac region 100
- inguinal hernia 100
- inner quadrant 100
- intercostal space 100
- internal mammary artery 100
- lateral 100
- lateral bending 100
- lateral flexion 100
- lateral gaze 100
- leg 100
- little finger 100
- lower 100
- lower extremity 100
- lower leg 100
- lower lid 100
- lower lobe (lung) 100
- lower quadrant 179
- lower quadrant (abdomen) 100
- lumbar region 100
- lung 100
- mediolateral 100
- mentoanterior 100
- mentoposterior 101
- mentotransverse 101
- midline deviation 100
- occipital posterior 101
- occipitoanterior 101
- occipitolateral 101
- occiput transverse 101
- otitis media 101
- outer quadrant 101
- posterior fascicular block 101
- posterior hemiblock 101
- pulmonary artery 101
- quadrant, upper 171
- sacroanterior (fetal position) (Lat.sacrolaeva anterior) 152
- sacroposterior (fetal position) (Lat. sacrolaeva posterior) 153
- sacrotransverse (fetal position) (Lat.sacrolaeva transversa) 154
- sacrum anterior 102
- sacrum posterior 102
- sacrum transverse 102
- salpingo-oophorectomy 102
- side 102
- sternal border 102
- upper arm 102
- upper extremity 102
- upper lobe (lung) 102
- upper outer quadrant 102
- upper quadrant 179
- upper quadrant (abdomen) 102
- ventricle 102
- ventricle centers of gravity at end-diastole 78
- ventricular assist system 102
- ventricular ejection fraction 102
- ventricular end-diastolic pressure 102
- ventricular end-diastolic volume index 102
- ventricular end-systolic volume index 102
- ventricular failure 103
- ventricular failure, acute 19
- ventricular hypertrophy 103
- ventricular pressure, time derivative 62
- ventricular shortening fraction 103

leg 100
- cycle ergometer 99
- cycle ergometer (LCE), functional electrical stimulation (FES)-induced 74
- cycle ergometer, induced 74
- left 100
- left lower 100
- length discrepancy 100
- right 144

legionella 98

leishmania 98

length 98
- functional profile 75
- of stay 101
- of stay, estimated 69
- polymorphism, restriction-fragment 143

lengths
- basic cycle 31

lens
- bandage contact 31
- concave 180
- intraocular 93
- posterior chamber, intraocular 129
- reflex, single 153

lenses
- contact, bifocal 31

lente insulin 98

lentigo
- maligna 100
- maligna melanoma 100

lesion
- high squamous intraepithelial 87
- intracranial mass 92
- low grade squamous intraepithelial 102
- medial hypothalamic 107
- on the erythrocyte cell membrane at the site of complement fixation 66

lesions
- cervical root 51

less
- severe than 180
- than 179, 180
- than or equal to 180

less than 179

lethal 98
- concentration 50% 99
- concentration, approximate 18
- concentration, minimum 108
- dose 99
- dose 100 % 99
- dose, minimum 108

leucine 98, 99
- codon 55

leucinol 101

leucosis
- enzootic bovine 67

leukemia
- acute granulocytic 15
- acute lymphoblastic 5, 18
- acute lymphocytic 18
- acute myeloblastic 19
- acute myelogenous 19

- acute non-lymphocytic 20
- acute undifferentiated 25
- adult T-cell 24
- atypical chronic lymphocytic 11
- atypical chronic myeloid 11
- B-cell 31
- B-cell acute lymphoblastic 28
- chronic 45
- chronic granulocytic 44
- chronic lymphocytic 46, 47
- chronic lymphosarcoma (cell) 47
- chronic myelogenous 48
- chronic myelomonocytic 48
- chronic neutrophilic 49
- diffuse histocytic 59
- french american and british classification scheme 72
- hairy cell 84
- hypocellular acute 83
- integration 1 gene, Friend 75
- mast cell 105
- prolymphocytic 133
- promyelocytic 134
- seconary 152
- virus receptor, gibbon ape 79
- virus, avian acute 11
- virus, feline 74
- virus, gibbon ape 79
- virus, gross 79
- virus, murine 109

leukocyte
- adhesion deficiency 98
- alkaline phosphatase 98
- antigen, D-related human 86
- antigen, human 86
- basophils 29
- common antigen 99
- complement receptors 50
- polymorphonuclear 134
- protease inhibitor, secretory 153
- thermostable alpha-glycoprotein 102

leukocytes 99
- polymorphonuclear 135

leukoencephalitis
- acute hemorrhagic 16

leukoencephalopathy
- sclerosing 152

leukotriene B4 102

level
- blood alcohol 28
- criterion 46
- mouse potency 111
- of care 101
- of care, alternative 18
- of consciousness (in Glasgow Coma Scale) 101
- of consciousness, altered 18

level-dose 99

levo- 98

Lewy
- body 99
- body, dementia 99

Leydig cell insufficiency 99

liability
- other party 123

licensed
- clinical social worker 99
- practical nurse 101

lichen planus-like keratosis 101

licking
- grooming and arched-back nursing 100

lid
- left lower 100
- lower 100
- upper 171

lidocaine 98, 99, 100

life 181
- death growth standard 99
- health-related quality of 87
- mean 181
- support (basic) and defibrillation 33
- support, advanced 19
- support, advanced cardiac 11
- support, advanced pediatric 22
- support, advanced trauma 24
- support, basic 33
- support, basic cardiac 31
- support, basic trauma 35
- support, pediatric advanced 127
- support, prehospital trauma 132
- threatening event, acute 19
- time average daily doses 98
- year, quality-adjusted 140
- years saved 103

ligament 98, 100
- augmentation device 98
- of Treitz 101
- periodontal 129
- posterior cruciate 129
- proximal radioulnar 138
- radioscapholunate 146
- reconstruction tendon interposition (procedure) 102

ligamentum
- flavum, calcification 46

ligand-mimetic
- antibody, novel monovalent 176

ligase
- glutamate (ammonia) 79

ligation
- bilateral tubal 35
- endoscopic 69
- postpartum tubal 136

light 98, 102
- and accommodation 98
- fragment sleep 100
- illumination, ultraviolet 172
- perception 101
- perception, normal 118
- reflex 101
- reflex, pupillary 133
- scatter, forward angle 76
- ultraviolet 172

limb
- absence, congenital 168
- artificial 15
- deficiency, congenital 46
- heart (syndrome), cleft 46
- lead on the left arm in electrocardiography, unipolar 27
- lead on the left leg in electrocardiography, unipolar 26

- lead on the right arm in electrocardiography, unipolar 27
- medullary thick ascending 113
- perfusion, isolated 91
- support, single 153
limbal
- epithelial, rabbit 144
limbic
- keratoconjunctivitis, superior 153
limit
- of detection 101
- of quantification 101
- or level, confidence 46
- permissible exposure 131
- values, threshold 163
limitation of liability 101
limitation of movement 101
limited 102
- contact dynamic compression plate 99
limits
- maximum residual 111
- normal 117
- of linearity 101
- of normal, upper 171
line
- anterior axillary 5
- B cell 31
- central venous 55
- interface protokoll, serial 153
- interscapular 94
linear
- array, superficial 153
- fracture 99
- velocity, constant 47
lingual 98
- odontoblast layer 101
linoleic
- acid 98
- acid-deficient 98
- acid-rich 98
lip
- cleft 46
lipase
- bile salt-stimulated 35
lipid
- cholesterol-lowering 46
lipoatrophic diabetes mellitus 99
lipofuscinosis
- ceroid 46
lipoid
- adrenal hyperplasia, congenital 46
lipooligosaccaride (endotoxin virulence factor of N. gonorrhoeae) 101
lipopolysaccharide 101
- (LPS) core AB cluster genes 101
- (LPS) core C gene 101
lipoprotein
- beta 33
- cholesterol, low-density 99
- high density 84
- lipase 101
- low-density 99
- very low density 174
liposclerosing
- myxofibrous tumor 102
liposomes
- stabilized 152
liquid 100
- automatic dishwashing detergents 98
- chromatography, high pressure (or performance) 87
- cytotoxic assay, single cell 153
- ionization chamber, scanning 153
- membrane, permeation 133
list 37
listeria 98
liter 97, 98
- per minute 100
lithotripsy
- extracorporeal shock wave 71
little
- finger, left 100
Liu-Jun-Zi-Tang, a herbal medicine exerting gastroprotective action 162
liver 98
- and spleen 102
- antigen, soluble 153
- cirrhosis 45
- cirrhosis, postnecrotic 134
- disease, alcoholic 18
- disease, chronic 46
- esterase, rabbit 144
- function tests 100
- kidney, spleen 100
- primary cell cultures 101
- spleen, kidney 102
- triglycerides 102
- X receptors 103
living
- and well 103
- facility, adult congregate 11
load on the sacrum 101
loading
- complex 46
lobe
- peptide, corticotropin-like intermediate 46
lobe (lung)
- left lower 100
- left upper 102
- right middle 144
- right upper 148
lobular 101
- carcinoma in situ 99
- hepatitis, chronic 46
local
- anesthesia 98
- anesthesia, contralateral 46
- medical officer 101
localization
- index, splenic 153
- signal, nuclear 118
localized
- absence of skin, congenital 46
locomotion
- amphetamine-induced 18
locus
- of control, multidimensional health 107
- of enterocyte effacement 99
loline alkaloid 101
lolium perenne
- allergen 101

long
- above elbow (cast) 98
- acting thyroid stimulator 99
- arm cast 98
- arm navicular cast 98
- leg brace 100
- leg cast 100
- leg cylinder cast 100
- leg splint 100
- leg walking cast 100
- QT syndrome 101
- spacing segment 153
- term care 102
- term care facility 102
- terminal repeats 102
- TRPC 102
long term
- goal 102
long-latency response 100
long-term
- gentamicin 102
- glioblastoma multiforme survivor 102
- group 102
- potentiation 102
long-time
- (72-96 hours) stimulated cultures 102
loose 102
loss
- evaporative heat 69
- hearing 85
- of consciousness 101
- of heterozygosity 101
- of movement 101
- of sight 101
- on drying 101
Lotus tetragonolobus 102
low 98
- alcohol-drinking 98
- back bending 99
- back pain, chronic 46
- back tenderness 99
- birth weight 99
- blood pressure 99
- contact dynamic compression plate 99
- density lipoprotein 99
- density lipoprotein cholesterol 99
- dose 99
- dose warfarin 99
- fat diet 100
- flap 99
- forceps 99
- forceps delivery 100
- frequency 99
- grade squamous intraepithelial lesion 102
- iodine thyroglobulin 102
- molecular polypeptide factors of thymus 76
- molecular weight heparin 101
- outlet resistance 101
- power field 101
- temperature group 102
- tension glaucoma 102
- transcript gene 102
- transport group 102
- viscosity silicone rubber 103
- voltage scanning electron microscopy 103
- zone tolerance 103
lower 98, 179
- back pain 99
- body obesity 99
- esophageal sphincter 99
- extremities 99
- extremities, both 33
- extremity 99, 103
- extremity, left 100
- gastro-intestinal tract 100
- leg, left 100
- lid 100
- lid, left 100
- limit of normal 100
- lobe (lung), left 100
- lung fields, bilateral 33
- motor neuron (signs) 101
- quadrant 101
- quadrant (abdomen), left 100
- quadrants, both 33
- respiratory tract 102
- respiratory tract infection 102
- right quadrant 101
- trunk rotation 102
lowered 179
lowering 179
lowest effect level 99
low-protein diet
- animal-based 21
L-selectin
- adhesion molecule 98
lumbar 98
- epidural (anesthesia), continuous 46
- fusion, posterior 133
- puncture 101
- region, left 100
- spinal stenosis 102
- spine 102
- strain, acute 19
- trauma syndrome, acute 19
- vertebra, second 98
- vertebra, third 98
- vertebrae 1 - 5 98
- vertebrae, load 101
lumbarization 98
lumbo
- dorsal pain 99
- sacral 102
lumen
- capillary 45
- diameter, reference 144
- dual 60
luminance 98
- defined 99
lung
- cancer 98
- cancer, non-small cell 120
- cancer, small cell 150
- capacity, total 162
- carcinoma expressed antigens 99
- compliance 46
- disease, chronic 46
- disease, chronic obstructive 49
- disease, respiratory bronchiolitis interstitial 142
- dose, mean 108
- fibroblasts, human 86
- fields, bilateral lower 33
- lavage, cow 46
- left 100

- right 144
- right lower lobe 144
- thorax compliance 47
- transplantation, single 154

lungs
- and heart 100
- clear to auscultation 99

lunotriquetral 102
lupus
- erythematosis 99
- erythematosus (systemic) activity measure 153
- erythematosus (systemic), disease activity index 153
- erythematosus, discoid 60
- erythematosus, systemic 153
- nephritis 101

lupus erythematosis
- disseminated 60

luteal
- phase defect 101
- phase, short 153

luteinizing
- hormone 100

luteinizing hormone-releasing hormone 100
luteotropic hormone 100
Luxol fast blue 100
Lyme borreliosis 99
lymph 98
- node 101
- node biopsy, sentinel 153
- node dissection, pelvic 133
- node T cell mutation, paucity 133
- node, sentinel 153
- nodes, peripheral 133

lymphadeno(nodal)-dysplasia 98
lymphadeno(nodal)dysplasia 98
lymphadenomegaly 98
lymphadenopathy 98
- angioimmunoblastic 18
- persistent generalized 132

lymphangiodysplasias 98
lymphatic invasion 98
lymphoblastic
- leukemia, acute 18
- leukemia, B-cell, acute 28
- lymphoma 99

lymphoblastic leukemia
- acute 5

lymphocyte 98, 103
- antigen, cutaneous 46
- corona 99
- cytotoxic 46
- E-rosette inhibitory factors 144
- function-associated antigen 100
- function-associated antigen 1 100
- globulin, antihuman 16
- gut mucosa 80
- infusion, donor 60
- maturation factor, cytotoxic 47
- mediated cytotoxicity, spontaneous 153
- mononuclear 110
- nodular poorly differentiated 119
- predominant 101
- reaction, mixed 109
- serum, antihuman 16
- sheath, periarteriolar 127
- small 152
- stimulation test, drug 60
- tests, primed 133
- tumor-infiltrating 162

lymphocytes 103
lymphocytic
- leukemia, acute 18
- leukemia, atypical chronic 11
- leukemia, chronic 46, 47
- lymphoma, diffuse well-differentiated 65
- lymphoma, intermediate 91
- lymphomas, diffuse poorly-differentiated 129
- lymphomas, nodular poorly-differentiated 129
- thyroiditis, chronic 47

lymphogranuloma venereum 100
lymphohistiocytosis
- familial erythrophagocytic 74
- familial histiocytic 74
- histiocytic 86
- infection-associated hemophagocytic 88

lymphoid
- hyperplasia, cutaneous 46
- interstitial pneumonitis 100
- irradiation, selective 153
- irradiation, total 163
- organ chemokine, secondary 153
- tissue, bronchus-associated 28
- tissue, follicle-associated 73
- tissue, mucosa associated 104

lymphoma
- adult T-cell 24
- B-cell 31
- classical Hodgkin 44
- diffuse large cell 60
- diffuse poorly-differentiated lymphocytic 129
- diffuse well-differentiated lymphocytic 65
- follicular 75
- follicular small cleaved cell 76
- Hodgkin 99
- Hodgkin, B symptoms 28
- intermediate lymphocytic 91
- kinase, anaplastic 18
- large cell, follicular 75
- lymphoblastic 99
- malignant histiocytosis-like B-cell 107
- mantle cell 105
- mantle zone 114
- mixed small cleaved and large follicular 75
- nodal marginal zone b-cell 118
- nodular lymphocyte predominant Hodgkin 118
- nodular poorly-differentiated lymphocytic 129
- nodular sclerosis classical Hodgkin 120
- non-Hodgkin's 117
- primary brain 128
- primary central nervous system 129

lx

- primary cerebral 129
- primary cutaneous 129
- primary effusion 131
- primary lymphoplasmacytic 133
- small cleaved follicular 75
- small lymphocytic 47, 153
lymphomatoid
- papulosis 103
lymphoplasmacytic
- lymphoma, primary 133
lymphoproliferative
- disorder B-cell, chronic 31
- disorder, post-transplant 139
lymphosarcoma
- (cell) leukemia, chronic 47
lymphotropic
- virus types I, human T-cell 87
lympohocyte
- culture, mixed 108
lysergic acid diethylamide 102
lysine 97, 103
- codon 5
lysis
- inhibitor, complement 46
- time, clot 47
LysoTracker Green DND-26 102
lysyl oxidase 101
lysyl oxidase-like protein 101

M

M protein
- type-specific 165
macerated 103
maclura pomifera 111
macrocystic
- serous cystadenoma 112
macrocytic 103
macrodactyly
- simplex congenita 112
macroglobulinemia
- Waldenström's 176
macromolecul 109
macrophage
- alveolar 19
- arming factor, specific 154
- cultured 48
- human alveolar 83
- splenic 154
macroscopic 103
macular
- choroidal degeneration, senile 155
- degeneration, drusen-related 61
- degeneration, senile 155
- dystrophy, Best's 33
maculopapular
- cutaneous mastocytosis 110
Maelzels metronome 109
magnesia
- milk 110
magnesium 106
- chloride 106
- deficient 106
magnetic
- resonance (analysis), protonic 134
- resonance angiography 111
- resonance angiography, three-dimensional 61
- resonance imaging 111
- resonance imaging, gated 80
- resonance imaging, interventional 92
- resonance neurography 111
- resonance tomography 111
- resonance venography 111
- resonance, electrically detected 68
- stimulation, repetitive transcranial 148
- stimulation, transcranial 163
- susceptibility 181
magnetization
- decay curve, transverse 163
- transfer ratio 113
magneto
- hydrodynamics 107
magnitude
- squared coherence 112
magnocellular
- neurosecretory cell 112
maintenance
- dose, daily 60
- hemodialysis 107
- methadone 109
- of certification 110
- pre-installation 133
- routine 144
major 104
- adverse clinical event 103
- arrhythmic events 103
- basic protein 104
- depressive disorders, endogenous 105
- histocompatibility complex 107
- injury vector 108
- interspecific variant 108
- medical 109
- septic complications 112
- symptom complex 112
majority 104
malachite green brucellae medium 106
malaria
- cerebral 47
malate
- dehydrogenase 105
male 103
- adult 19
- black 33
- castrated 47
- caucasian 47
- sex chromosome 176
- white 176
maleic
- hydrazide 106
malformation
- arteriovenous 22
- cavernous 47
- congenital 48
- craniocervical 41
- Dandy-Walker 65
malformations
- arteriovenous 27
- atrio-ventricular 27
maligna
- lentigo 100
- melanoma, lentigo 100
malignancy
- index, prostate 134
- occult primary 124
malignant 104

- disease, disseminated 61
- granular cell tumor 106
- histiocytosis 106, 107
- histiocytosis of intestine 107
- hyperthermia 106
- melanoma 109
- melanoma, cutaneous 48
- melanoma, prognostically high-risk sites 28
- mesothelioma 109
- mesothelioma, mixed 109
- mesotheliomas, epithelial 69
- mixed mesodermal tumor 109
- neoplasm 110
- oligoastrocytomas 110
- spindle-shaped cells 112
- syndrome, neuroleptic 118
- ventricular arrhythmias 113

malleolus
- medial 109

malleus
- manubrium to 109

Mallory
- bodies 104
- Weiss syndrome 113

malnutrition
- protein-energy 131

malpractice attorney 110

mammalian
- homologue of the Drosophila trithorax gene 164

mammary
- artery, left internal 100
- gland density 106
- intraepithelial neoplasia 108

mammogram 104, 109

mammoplasty
- bilateral augmentation 28

mammosomatotroph
- cells 112

managed
- Health Care Associates 107

management
- companies, physician practice 136
- diarrhea, dietary 60
- drug safety and surveillance 63
- indicator, pressure 134
- system, clinical care 42
- systems, human resources 87

mandatory
- ventilation, intermitt. 92

mandibular
- cortical index 105
- index, panoramic 134
- lingual vertical releasing incisions 109

manganese 109

manic
- depression 60
- depressive disorder 105

manifest anxiety scale 104

manipulation
- genetic 79
- osteopathic 123
- under anaesthesia 113

Mannheimia
- haemolytica 106

Mann-Whitney rank sum statistic 168

Mantel-Haenszel
- test 106

mantle
- cell lymphoma 105
- cerebral 47
- storage cells 112
- zone lymphoma 114

manual
- diagnostic and statistical 63
- diagnostic and statistical of mental disorders 63
- function score 106
- muscle test 109
- traction 113
- vacuum aspiration 113

manubrium to malleus 109

manufacturing
- practice, good 80

Marasmius oreades agglutinin 110

Marek disease virus 105

margin
- intercostal 90

marginal
- artery, obtuse 123
- vascular arcade 113
- zone 114

Marie-Bamberger
- syndrome 104

mariner-like elements 108

marital history 106

marked 108

market
- value added 113

marketing
- authorization 103
- authorization application 109
- initiative, prevention 134

markings
- bronchovascular 36

married 103, 104

marrow
- cell, unidentified endosteal 170
- fibrosis 106
- stromal cells 112

Marshall Marchetti 109

mask
- non-rebreather 119

mass 103
- casualty incident 105
- density 181
- fat-free 74
- lesion, intracranial 92
- mediastinal 109
- spectrometry 78, 111

Massachusetts
- general hospital's expert diagnostic system 65

massage 104, 113

masses, tenderness, rebound 113

masses, tenderness, rebound, guarding 113

massive 104
- hepatic necrosis 107
- volume administration 113

mast
- cell disease, systemic 155
- cell leukemia 105
- cell sarcoma 105
- cells 104

mastectomy
- modified, radical 111
- simple 154

master
- cell stock 105

lx

- in social work 113
- of arts 103
- of Science 112
- of science 154
- of surgery 48
- seed virus 113
mastitis, metritis, agalactia 109
mastocytosis
- aggressive systemic 23
- cutaneous 48
- indolent systemic 94
- maculopapular cutaneous 110
- systemic 154
matched
- unrelated donor - for bone marrow transplant 113
material
- other regulated 125
- safety data sheet 112
materials
- hazardous 83
- Services Center 112
maternal 104
- blood type 113
- derived antibodies 103, 105
- grandfather 106
- grandmother 106
- great grandfather 106
- Health Program 107
- intravenous administration 108
- serum a-fetoprotein 111
- serum cortisol 112
maternity
- care, family-centered 73
mathematical expectation 66
matrix
- attachment region 104
- extracellular 67
- metalloproteinase 109
matter
- gray 79
maturation
- inducing hormone 108
- promoting factor 111
mature intermediate villi 108
matured in vitro 108
maturity onset diabetes 110
maxilla 104
maxillary 104
- sinus carcinoma 112
maxillary primary incisors 134
maximal 104
- acid output 104
- expiratory flow 105
- expiratory flow rate 105
- heart rate 107
- inspiratory flow 108
- inspiratory flow rate 108
- isocapnic ventilation 108
- isometric strength 108
- mid expiratory flow 109
- midexpiratory flow 109
- midexpiratory flow rate 109
- recommended daily dose 111
- therapy 113
- voluntary activation 113
maximization
- of interclass variance 108
- ordered subset expectation 126
maximum 104
- allowable concentration 103
- benefit from hospitalization 104
- breathing capacity 104
- breathing capacity, indirect 91
- clearance 47
- concentration 48
- daily dose 105
- flow velocities 106
- hospital benefit 107
- increase value 108
- inhibitory dilution 108
- intensity projection 108
- mean total score 109
- medical improvement 109
- mid expiratory flow rate 109
- permissible concentration 110
- permissible dose 110
- residual limits 111
- to left 108
- to right 111
- tolerated dose - phase 1 studies 113
- urethral closure pressure 140
- urethral pressure 113
- use concentration 113
- volume ventilation 114
- voluntary contraction 114
- voluntary ventilation 114
- Volunteer Activity 114
May
- Grünwald-Giemsa stain 106
- Hegglin anomaly 107
Mayer-Rokitansky-Kuster-Hauser syndrome 111
Mayfield
- skull pin head holder 106
McMaster
- Health Index Questionnaire 107
Meadowlands
- Sports Complex 112
meal
- barium 28
- last 19
mean
- arterial pressure 104
- corpuscular hemoglobin 104
- corpuscular hemoglobin concentration 105
- corpuscular/cell volume 105
- diameter, geometric 80
- dose, comparative 48
- geometric 79
- glandular dose 106
- hemolytic dose 107
- integrated voltage 108
- length of utterance 109
- life 181
- lung dose 108
- number of infective vector 108
- orthostatic acceleration 110
- peripheral temperature 111
- platelet volume 111
- residence time 111
- statistical 181
- survival time 113
- titer, geometric 80
- velocity 113
measles
- killed vaccine 108

- mumps, rubella 109
measurement
- circumferential 47
measures
- independence, functional 75
meat
- starter culture 112
mechanical
- injury, cmbined 48
- inspiration, prolonged 134
- pain threshold 111
- pressure therapy 111
- ventricular assistance 114
mechanism
- copulatory 48
- of action 103, 110
- of injury 110
mechanomyography 109
mechanosensitive
- ion channels 112
meconium
- aspiration 104
- aspiration syndrome 104
medial 105
- amygdala 103
- geniculate body 106
- geniculate body, dorsal 106
- geniculate body, ventral 106
- hypothalamic lesion 107
- longitudinal fasciculus 108
- malleolus 109
- orbital 110
- preoptic area 111
- pulvinar 140
- rectus 111
- septum cholinergic neurons 112
- septum complex 112
- tibial stress syndrome 113
- vestibular nucleus 113
- vestibular nucleus, caudal part 114
medialis dorsalis 105
median
- absolute error 103
- condition 48
- diameter, count 48
- effective dose 68
- survival times 113
mediastinal
- B-cell lymphoma, primary 134
mediastinal mass 109
mediastinitis
- descending necrotizing 61
mediastinoscopy 112
medical
- advice, against 19
- advisor 103
- air evacuation 103
- antishock trousers 104
- assistant, certified 48
- authorization 103
- care utilization 105
- care, general assistance 77
- Center Health Plan 107
- clinic, general 79
- control, online 123
- council, general 79
- device communication, standards 155
- director, chief 48
- doctor 105
- doctor, family 75
- doctor, local 100
- doctor, private 134
- education, continuing 48
- education, graduate 80
- emergency clinic 105
- examiner 105
- examiner, independent 91
- eye history 105
- first responder 106
- follow up 106
- history 106
- insurance claim examiner 108
- literature analysis and retrieval system 105
- literature, current list 47
- major 109
- management analysis 109
- materials account 109
- office audit 110
- officer of day 110
- officer, local 101
- officer, visiting 174
- record, problem oriented 135
- Records Department 111
- records, electronic 69
- Sciences Campus 112
- Service Corps 112
- service, emergency 69
- smart card 112
- student 111
- technician, emergency 69
- unit, critical care 42
- ventilation, control 49
medically
- indigent adults 107
- underserved area 113
medication 19, 105
- administration errors 103
- induced headache 108
- sustained 154
medications
- no regular 119
medicine 105
- aerospace 19
- and surgery, general 80
- clinical 48
- complementary and alternative 38
- critical care 41
- evidence-based 67
- internal 91
- technician, aviation 27
- traditional Chinese 160
medicine + science in sports + exercise 113
mediolateral
- left 100
- oblique 109
- right 144
medioventral
- area 114
mediterranean mussel defensin 106
medium
- casein hydrolysate-yeast extract-containing 42
- malachite green brucellae 106
- minimal 109
- Mueller-Hinton agar 107
medroxyprogesterone acetate 110
medulla 103

- rostral ventrolateral 149
medullary
- depressor area, dorsal 61
- thick ascending limb 113
- velum 19
- ventral areas 114
medulloblastomas 104
megabalanus
- volcano 114
megakaryocyte 108
megamitochondria 109
megawatt 114
Meibomian
- gland disease 106
meiosis I
- paternal 134
meiotic
- anaphase, first 17
- sister-chromatid recombination 111
melanoblastoma 104
melanocyte-stimulating hormone 112
melanoma 105
- antigen 104
- assessment 9
- desmoplastic neurotropic 61
- in situ 108
- lentigo maligna 100
- malignant 48, 109
- metastatic 109
- nodular 118
- superficial spreading 157
melanosome
- giant 79
melatonin 105
membrane
- alveolar capillary 11
- anaerobic system 104
- attack complex 103
- attack complex, soluble 154
- brush border 30
- cytoplasmic 48
- disease, hyaline 86
- glomerular basement 77
- inhibitor of reactive lysis (CD59) 108
- interosseous 93
- mucous 109
- ovalbumin under the control of the rat insulin promoter 144
- oxygenation, extracorporeal 67
- permeability, alveolar-capillary 11
- premature rupture 138
- protein, granule 80
- rupture 144
- secretory component 111
- vesicle, brush border 30
- vesicles, apical 19
- vestibular 174
membranelle
- dorsal zone 65
membranoproliferative glomerulonephritis 111
memorandum of agreement 110
Meniere
- disease 105
meningeal
- artery, middle 109
meningitis
- acute cerebrospinal 11
- coccidioidal 48
- gram-negative bacillary 80
- meningococcal 109
- syndrome, aseptic 19
meningococcal
- disease, systemic 155
- meningitis 109
menstrual
- period 110
- period, first 75
- period, last 101
- period, last normal 101
- period, previous 134
menstrually related migraine 109
mental
- age 103
- attitude, positive 134
- development, delayed 60
- foramen 107
- health 106
- Health Act Commission 107
- Health Association 107
- Health Care 107
- health care unit 107
- health centers, community 48
- Health Demographic Profile System 107
- health Department 107
- health index 107
- health information 107
- health inventory 107
- hygiene consultation service 107
- illness 107
- retardation 111
- retardation protein, fragile 75
- retardation, alpha-thalassemia 24
- retardation, fragile 75
- state, geriatric 80
- status 111
- status examination 112
mental retardation
- alpha-thalassemia 24
mentoanterior
- left 100
mentoposterior
- left 101
mentotransverse
- left 101
mercaptopurine
- anti cancer drug 110
Mercurascan 112
mercury 85
- hydroxypropane hemiplegic migraine 107
- millimeters 109
mesangial
- cells 112
mesangium
- cell, glomerular 112
mesencephalon 112
mesenchymal
- stem cells 112
mesenteric
- arterial conductance, superior 154
- artery blood flow, superior 154
- artery embolism, superior 154
- artery occlusion, superior 155
- artery syndrome, superior 155

- artery, dog 60
- artery, superior 154
- superior 154
- vein, dog 61
mesioincisodistal 108
mesodermal
- tumor, malignant mixed 109
mesopic
- visual acuity 114
mesothelial
- cells 112
mesothelioma
- epithelial malignant 69
- malignant 109
- mixed malignant 109
- poorly differentiated malignant 129
mesoxalic acid 110
messenger RNA 111
metabolic
- acidosis, chronic 48
- display, differential 60
- heat load stimulator 107
- rate, basal 33
- rate, resting 144
metabolism
- basal 33
metacarpal
- phalangeal (also MCP) 110
metacarpophalangeal 113
- joint 105
metal 103
- halide 106
- oxide 110
- transporter 1, divalent 61
metalloproteinase
- matrix 109
- tissue inhibitor 162
metaplasia
- agnogenic myeloid 19
- duodenal gastric 59
- myelofibrosis 106
- myeloid 106, 109
- with myelofibrosis, agnogenic myeloid 19
metastases 106
- absent 103
- present 103
- unknown 114
metastasis
- cannot be, or has not been, assessed 114
- distant 103
- regional lymph node 114
metastatic
- carcinoma 104
metastatic melanoma 109
metatarsal
- phalangeal 113
- phalangeal joint 110
- veins, dorsal 61
meter 103
- kilogram, second 108
- oxygen saturation 126
metered-dose inhaler 105
methacrylate
- butyl 33
methadone
- maintenance 109
methamphetamine 106
methanococcus
- vannielii 114
methemoglobin 107
methicillin resistant staphylococcus aureus 111
methimazole 109
methionine 103, 106
- codon 25
- peptide histidine 132
method
- of adjustment 110
methotrexate 113
- cytoxan 48
methotrexate, vinblastine, doxorubicin, cisplatin 114
methoxy
- hydrophenylglycol 107
- propyl cyanoacrylate 110
- psoralen 110
methoxyacrylate 110
methoxypsoralen 110
methyl
- alcohol level, serum 155
- benzyloxycarbonyl 33
- ethyl ketone 105
- malonic acid 109
- methacrylate 109
- methanethiosulfonate 109
- mevinolinic acid 109
- phenidate treatment 111
- selenocysteine 112
- sulfonylmethane 61
- sulfonylmethane or dimethylsulfone 113
- trioxorhenium 113
- umbellyferyl-*-D-glucuronide 113
methylated
- domain.differentially 60
methylation-specific polymerase chain reaction 113
methylene
- blue, carbolic 48
- edianiline 105
- hydroxydiphosphonate 107
methylmalonyl 109
metropolitan
- Health Group 107
- Health Plan 107
mevalonic
- acid 114
- aciduria 114
mevinolinic
- acid 114
mezlocillin 114
MI
- subendocardial 151
mice
- transgenic line 19
micellar
- concentration, critical 48
Michaelis-Gutmann body 106
micro 181
microampere 181
microangiopathic
- hemolytic anemia 103, 107
microangiopathy
- thrombotic 163
microarray
- infostructure, tissue 163
microbar 181
microcytic 108
microembolic
- signals 106
microglobulin
- beta2 181

microgram 104, 181
microhemagglutination 107
- Treponema pallidum 107
microhodotermes viator corpus cardiacum peptide 108
microliter 181
micrometer 181
microparticle
- enzyme immunoassay 105
microphonic
- cochlear 48
microphtalmia
- gene 107
- transcription factor 108
microphysiometer
- silicon 154
micropouch gastric bypass 106
microscope
- atomic force 15
- electron 69
- scanning laser acoustic 153
- surgical 154
microscopic 108
microscopic polyangiitis 110
microscopy
- confocal laser scanning 47
- fluorescence digital imaging 73
- polarized light 133
microsecond 181
microsomal
- heme oxygenase 107
- membranes, dog pancreas 62
microtubule
- organizing centers 113
microvascular
- abnormalities, intraretinal 94
- anastomosis 114
- angina 114
- architecture 114
- cells 114
- endothelial cells, bone marrow 33
microvessel
- count 114
microvillar
- cells 114
microvilli
- long slender 102
microvillous
- atrophy 114
microvolt 181
microwatt 181
microwave
- assisted extraction 103
- thermotherapy, transurethral 167
mid
- expiratory flow rate, maximum 109
- stream specimen urine 113
- systolic click 112
- systolic click-late systolic murmur syndrome 112
midclavicular line 105
middle
- axillary line 104
- cerebral artery occlusion 104
- ear 105
- ear effusion 105
- finger 106
- meningeal artery 109
- subcutaneous adipose tissue 112
midexpiratory
- flow rate, maximal 109
- flow, maximal 109
midforceps delivery 106
midline 108
- deviation, left 100
- episiotomy 108
midnight 105, 110
midpalatal
- suture cartilage 112
midparental height 111
midsternal line 112
midstream
- clean catch (urine) 42
- specimen of urine 113
- urine 113
- urine, clean catch 42
midwives' board
- central 48
migraine
- basilar artery 28
- common 48
- menstrually related 109
- mercury-hydroxypropane 107
- ophthalmoplegic 124
- with aura 114
- without aura 110
migrating
- spike complexes 112
migratory
- contraction, giant 79
- motor complex, interdigestive 92
mild
- hypoxia 106
- traumatic brain injury 113
military
- antishock trousers 104
- medical exercise 105
milk
- of magnesia 110
- somatic cell 112
millicurie 105
milliequivalent 106
milliequivalents per liter 106
milligram 106
milliliter 108
millimeter 109
- of Mercury 109
- of mercury 107
millimolar 109
millimole 109
milliosmole 110
milliseconds 111
millivolt 113
Miltenberger class V-like molecule 108
min
- of visual angle 113
mineral
- base, standard 155
- content bone 33
- content, whole body bone 175
- oil adjuvant 110
mini stress test 113
miniature
- squamous cells 112
- synaptic currents 112
minimal 108
- concentration 47

- DiGeorge critical region 105
- head injury 107
- incision surgery 108
- inhibitory concentration 108
- inhibitory volumes 108
- medium 109
- sporocidal concentrations 112

minimally
- invasive directed coronary bypass 108
- invasive spinal surgery 108
- invasive surgery 108
- invasive surgery, computer assisted 38

mini-mental
- state examination 109

Mini-Mental State 109
minimum 103, 108
- alveolar concentration 103
- audible angle 103
- bactericidal concentration 104
- detectable concentration 105
- effective dose 105
- fatal dose 106
- hemolytic dilution 107
- hemolytic dose 107
- immobilizing viscosity 108
- infective dose 108
- inhibitory dose 108
- irradiation dose 108
- lethal concentration 108
- lethal dose 108
- lumen diameter 108
- significant change 112
- spirocheticidal concentration 112
- visible angle 114

minipig
- kidney cell line 111

Minnesota
- multiphasic personality inventory 109

minor 108
- breakpoint cluster region 104
- groove binder 106
- morphologic aberration 109
- surgery 111

minus 180
minute 108, 180
- counts per 50
- virus of canines 114

minutes
- double 61

mismatched 109
missing in action 107
mitochondrial
- diazepam binding inhibitor receptor 105
- glutamic-oxaloacetic transaminase 81

mitotane 123
mitotic index of proliferating cell population 134
mitoxantrone, etoposide and Ara-C regimen 105
mitral
- commissurotomy, percutaneous transvenous 139
- insufficiency 107, 108
- opening snap 110
- orifice area 110
- regurgitation 111
- stenosis 111
- valve 108, 113
- valve area 114
- valve defects 114
- valve prolaps 114
- valve replacement 114

mivacurium 108
mivazerol 108
mixed
- cellularity 104
- cellularity classical Hodgkin lymphoma 105
- connective tissue disease 105
- effect model, nonlinear 118
- gastric and intestinal type 113
- gonadal dysgenesis 106
- lymphocyte reaction 109
- lympohocyte culture 108
- malignant mesothelioma 109
- mesodermal tumor, malignant 109
- oligoastrocytomas 110

- venous hemoglobin saturation 159
- venous oxygen tension 140

mobile intensive care unit 108
mobility
- group, high 86

mobilization
- soft tissue 158

modality
- combined 48
- therapy, combined 49

model
- risk screening 146

moderate 110
- osteoarthritic 110

moderately advanced 103
modification
- clinical 48

modified
- barium swallow test 104
- derivative, glycopeptide moiety 80
- Hank balanced salt solution 107
- Health Assessment Questionnaire 107
- physiotherapy 111
- radical mastectomy 111
- sampling connections 112
- semi-circular 112
- synaptonemal complexes region 112
- vaccinia virus Ankara 114

modifier
- biological response 34

modifying
- drug, disease 61

modulation
- gap detection 106

Mohs micrographic surgery 109
Mohshardness
- Number 107

moiety
- modified derivative, glycopeptide 80

molar 103
molecular
- beacons 104
- dynamics, discontinuous 60

- shape comparison 112
- volume, gram 80
- weight 110, 114
- weight, gram 80
molecule
- T cell-activating 161
Moloney
- sarcoma cell 112
molt-inhibiting hormone 108
molybdopterin guanine dinucleotide 106
moment
- nulling, gradient 80
monitor
- blood temperature 35
- controller, oxygen ratio 125
- oxygen ratio 125
monitored
- stroke unit 113
monitoring
- blood 33
- trends in cardiovascular diseases study, Danish 56
monkey
- cell, grivet 79
- kidney, primary 134
monoamine
- oxidase 104
- oxidase inhibitor 104
- sulfating form of sulfotransferases 111
monoclonal
- antibodies 104, 110
- antibody immobilization of granulocyte antigens 104
- gammopathy of undetermined significance 106
- gammopathy, benign 33
- immunoglobulin deposition disease, renal 108
monocyte 103, 110
- chemoattractant protein 105
- chemotactic factor 104
- circulating 47
- synergistic cytotoxicity 112
monodigitoxoside
- digitoxigenin 60
monogalactosyl
- diacylglycerol 106
monoglucuronosyl
- bilirubin 106
monoiodotyrosine 108
monolayer
- growth defect 106
monomeric carboxylesterases 104
monomethyl
- adenosine 109
- aminoantipyrine 109
mononuclear
- cells, peripheral blood 128
- lymphocytes 110
- phagocyte system 111
monosodium
- glutamate 112
- urate 113
monosymptomatic
- hypochondriacal psychosis 107
monosynaptic
- connection 112
month(s) 110
Montserrat
- volcanic ash 114
mood
- States, profile of 134
morbidity 109
morbidity and mortality 109
morbus
- hemolyticus neonatorum 107
- Hodgkin 106
more
- or less 110, 180
- severe than 180
- than 113, 179
morning 19
morphine
- and cocaine 48
- sulfate 111, 113
- sulfate tablets 113
- sulphate Contin 112
morphogenetic
- protein, bone 33
- protein, recombinant human bone 143
morphologic
- aberration, minor 109
- index, red blood cell 142
- rubric of ICD-O 90
morrow
- assessment of nausea and emesis 104
mortality 103, 109
- and morbidity 109
- rate, relative standard 146
mosaic
- analysis with a repressible cell marker 104
- variegated aneuploidy 114
- virus 19
mosquito iridescent virus 108
moth
- codling 48
mother 103
- and father 106
motile
- sperm count 112
motion
- active 13
- aftereffect 103
- cervical range 51
- defined 105
- hand 86
- imaging, power 134
- machine, continuous passive 50
- normal range 119
- onset asynchrony 110
- rephasing, gradient 80
- systolic 154
motor
- activity, gross 79
- activity, spontaneous 154
- and sensory neuropathies, hereditary 86
- area, supplementary 154
- axonal neuropathy, acute 19
- complex, interdigestive migratory 92
- conduction studies 105
- evoked potentials 106
- gross 79
- layers superior colliculus 111
- neuron (signs), upper 171

- neuron, lower 101
- nucleus, dorsal 61
- sensory axonal neuropathy 19
- sensory cortex 112
- unit action potentials 113
- vehicle accident 114
- vehicle collision/crash 114

Motor Age Score 110
motor, sensory, pulse 113
mouse
- diaphragm assay 105
- double minute protein 105
- genome database 106
- potency level 111
- ribosome receptor protein 111
- Schwann cell line 112
- spinal cord 112
- splenocytes 112
- urinary protein 113

mouse apo A-I 110
mouth 125
- floor 75

mouth or other opening 125
movement 114
- bowel 33
- extraocular 70
- finger 75
- full passive 76
- limitation 101
- loss 101
- orthodontic tooth 126

movements
- periodic leg/limb 133
- rapid alternating 142

moves all extremities 103
moving
- Picture Experts Group 110

MRI 151
- enhancement, superparamagnetic iron oxide 156

mRNA
- early EBV 67

MS
- Contin tablets 112

mucin
- gastric-foveolar 113
- goblet cell 113
- human gastric 85
- ovine submaxillary 126
- pyloric-gland 113

mucinous
- antigen, small intestinal 152
- tumor of low malignant potential 109

mucocutaneous
- candidiasis, chronic 48

mucoepidermoid
- tumor of the jaws, central 48

mucopurulent
- cervicitis 110

mucosa
- associated lymphoid tissue 104
- gastric 79
- or mucus, cervical 47

mucosal
- barrier, gastric 79
- biopsy, selected 155
- starter culture 112

mucous
- membrane 109

mucus membranes moist 109
Mueller
- Hinton 106
- Hinton agar medium 107
- Hinton Base 107

Mulberry
- heart disease 107

Mullerian
- inhibiting hormone 108

multi angle
- polarised scatter separation 104

multi drug resistant 105
multichannel
- autoanalyzer, sequential 154
- autoanalyzer, simultaneous 154

multidimensional
- health locus of control 107

multidrug
- resistance protein 111

multifocal
- atrial tachycardia 104

multigated
- acquisition 113

multiglandular
- disease 106

multiheaded 106
multi-infarct
- dementia 108

multi-institutional
- arrangements 107

multilevel upper airways reconstruction 113
multimedia
- Super Corridor 112

multinodular
- goiter, toxic 163

multiorgan dysfunction syndrome 110
multiparity
- grand 79

multiple
- analysis, sequential 154
- angle reconstruction technique, simultaneous 155
- chemical sensitivity 105
- correspondence analysis 104
- daily insulin injections 105
- dose vial 105
- endocrine adenomatosis 105
- endocrine neoplasia 105
- fragment wounds 106
- ion detection 108
- module access 109
- myeloma 109
- organ failure 110
- organ system failure 110
- sclerosis 111
- sclerosis, chronic progressive 50
- sclerosis, clinically definite 43
- sclerosis, functional assessment 73
- sclerosis, primary progressive 136
- sclerosis, relapsing remitting 145
- sleep latency test 111
- soft tissue injuries 113
- synchronous cancer 112
- tumors 103

- vessel angioplasty 114
- vitamin injection 114
- wake latency test 114
multiplicative
- scatter correction 112
multiplicity
- of attachment 110
multiplied
- by times 176
multiply
- handicapped 106
multipotential
- subserosal cells 112
multipurpose
- phantoms 111
- phantoms, water MPP 176
- silastic catheters 112
multi-slice CT (scan) 112
multi-syringe time-based injection 113
multivalent
- influenza vaccine 108
multivariate
- analysis 114
- analysis of variance 104
multivesicular
- aggregates 114
multivessel
- coronary disease 104
municipal
- hospital 106
- solid waste 113
murex
- hybrid capture CMV DNA assay 84
murine
- aortic endothelial cells 103
- leukemia virus 109
murmur 103, 109
- cardiac 47
- continuous 48
- diastolic 60
- heart 86
- holosystolic 87
- rubs or gallops 111
- syndrome, mid-systolic click-late systolic 112
- systolic 154
murmurs 106, 111
muscimol 111
muscle 113
- activity 103
- autoantibody, antiheart 16
- balance 104
- band, creatine kinase 45
- cardiac 47
- circular 47
- function test 106
- group 106
- mass 109
- psoas minor 134
- rectus 143
- right superior oblique 146
- right superior rectus 147
- satellite cells 112
- score 112
- soleus 156
- stimulation, electrical 69
- strength 109
- superior rectus 157
- test 113
- test, manual 109
- testing, quantitative 141
muscles 109
- and tendons 113
- extraocular 70
- plantar 133
muscular
- atrophy, neurogenic 118
- atrophy, progressive 134
- atrophy, spinal 154
- dystrophies, Becker 33
- dystrophies, Duchenne and Becker 56
- dystrophy 105
- dystrophy, childhood 48
- dystrophy, congenital 48
- dystrophy, Duchenne 61
muscularis mucosae 109
musculo-aponeurotic
- system, superficial 155
musculoskeletal 112
mushroom bodies 104
mussel
- defensin, mediterranean 106
mutant
- dominant negative 61
- pertussis toxin 111
mutation
- point, repeat-induced 144
- rate 181
- restriction site 146
mutiple
- hamartoma 107
mutual 111
- legal assistance treaty 108
- recognition 111
myasthenia gravis 106
mycobacteria
- nontuberculous 121
mycobacterial
- disease, disseminated 61
mycobacterium avium complex 103
mycoplasma removal agent 111
myelin
- basic protein 104
- forming Schwann cells 112
- protein 22, peripheral 134
myelin-associated glycoprotein 103
myelinolysis
- central pontine 50
myeloblastic
- leukemia, acute 19
myelodysplastic
- myelproliferative syndromes 105
- syndrome 105
- syndrome, secondary 155
myelofibrosis 106
- chronic idiopathic 45
- metaplasia 106
- secondary 155
myelogenous
- leukemia, acute 19
- leukemia, chronic 48
myeloid
- leukemia, atypical chronic 11
- metaplasia 106, 109
- metaplasia with myelofibrosis, agnogenic 19
- metaplasia, agnogenic 19
- suppressor cells 112
myeloma
- multiple 109
myeloma, multiple 109

myelomeningocele 109
myelomonocytic
- leukemia, chronic 48
myeloperoxidase 111
- activity, neutrophil 111
myeloproliferative
- disease, chronic 48
- disorder 110
- disorder, transient 163
- disorders 110
- syndromes 111
myelovertebral
- abnormalities 114
myocardial
- dysfunction, diastolic 60
- infarction 107
- infarction, acute 19
- infarction, anterior lateral 18
- infarction, inferior 92
- infarction, non-Q-wave 119
- infarction, painless 134
- infarction, perioperative 134
- infarction, previous 134
- infarction, Q-wave 141
- infarction, right ventricle 149
- infarction, rule-out 144
- infarction, transmural perioperative 163
- infarctions, posterior 134
- injury, subendocardial perioperative 157
- revascularization, direct 61
myocardiopathy
- congestive 48
- of unknown origin 113
myoclonic
- absence epilepsy 103
- astatic epilepsy 103
- epilepsy, severe 155
myoclonus
- cherry red spot 51
myoepithelial sialoadenitis 106
myofibroma(tosis)
- of the skin, solitary 155
myoglobin 106
- serum 155
myohemoglobin 107
myointimal
- hyperplasia 108
myoneural
- junction (disease) 110
myopia 114
myosin
- anticardiac 11
- binding subunit 104
myotonic
- dystrophy gene 60
- dystrophy gene 2 60
mytilus
- galloprovincialis defensin 1 106
myxedema
- pretibial 139
myxofibrous
- tumor, liposclerosing 102
myxothiazol 110

N

N
- (2-chloroethyl)-N'-cyclo-hexyl-N-nitrosourea 42
- 4-acetylsulfisoxazole 121
Na
- channels 115
N-acetyl
- aminoantipyrine 10
- L-cysteine 115
- neuraminic, acid 115
- neuraminic, acid storage disorders 120
naftopidil
- phenyl-hydroxy 132
nagase analbuminemic rats 115
nail
- bed 115
Nairobi
- sheep disease 120
NANA 120
nanogram 117
naples low-excitability 117
naples random-bred rats 119
Naples-High Excitability rats 117
narcolepsy
- disorder of excessive somnolence 61
narcotic 115
- synthetic 111
narrow
- diameter endosseous screw implant 48
narrowing
- joint space 96
nasal
- airflow resistance 119
- airflow resistance in the basal state 119
- cannula 116
- discharge, anterior 19
- root breadth 119
- septal deformity 120
nascent polypeptide associated complex 115
nasogastric 117
- tube 117
nasopharyngeal 119
- carcinoma 119
nasopharynx 118, 119
nasotracheal
- tube 121
Nasu-Hakola syndrome 133
national
- Breast Screening Study, Canadian 115
- Health Interview Survey 117
- Health Service 117
- marrow donor program 118
natriuretic
- peptide, atrial 20
- peptide, brain 33
- peptide, porcine brain 128
natural
- head position 117
- health 117
- killer cells 117
- killer cells, subset 117
- latex gloves 117
- rubber latex 119
nausea
- and vomiting 20, 121
- and vomiting, postchemotherapy 135
- and vomiting, postinfusion 135

- and vomiting, postoperative 135
- vomiting 121
- vomiting, diarrhea 121
- vomiting/diarrhea/ constipation 121
navel 171
- orangeworm 119
navicular
- cast, long arm 98
N-benzoyl
- L-tyrosyl-p-aminobenzoic acid 35
N-bromosuccinimide 115
n-desmethyl-clobazam 116
near
- infrared 117
- infrared spectroscopy 117
nearly
- equal 180
nebulizer
- ultrasonic 172
neck
- asymmetrical tonic reflex 24
- of femur 118
- posterior 28
- vein pressure 135
necrobiotic
- xanthogranuloma 121
necrosis
- avascular 27
- bilateral acute retinal 29
- bone marrow 33
- massive hepatic 107
- renal tubular 148
necrotizing
- enterocolitis 116
- mediastinitis, descending 61
- pulmonary aspergillosis, chronic 49
needle
- ablation (prostatic), transurethral 167
- biopsy, aspiration 8
- biopsy, CT-guided 54
negative 116, 180, 181
- electron 65
- inspiratory force 117
- mutant, dominant 61
- predictive value 119
neocarzinostatin 116
neomycin sulfate
- and vancomycin hydrochloride 135
neonatal 118
- intensive care 117
- intensive care unit 117
- nurse practitioners 118
neonatally splenectomized (animals) 121
neoplasia
- cervical intraepithelial 45
- mammary intraepithelial 108
- multiple endocrine 105
- vaginal intraepithelial 172
neoplasm
- malignant 110
- papillary Hurthle cell 132
neostigmine 116
neovascularization
- iris 121
nephritis
- acute bacterial 9
- lupus 101
- passive Heymann 132
nephrogenic
- diabetes insipidus 116
nephrolithiasis
- X-linked recessive 176
nephropathy
- ablation 9
- acute vasomotor 27
- endemic balkan 67
nephrotic
- syndrome 119
nerv 114
nerve 114
- activity, sympathetic 155
- cervical 40
- conduction studies 116
- conduction velocities 116, 117
- cranial 37
- ending 116
- injury, peripheral 134
- irritation, acute 20
- net pulses 118
- pharyngeal branch of the vagus 132
- phrenic 132
- posterior interosseous 133
- root 119
- root involvement or irritation 119
- root irritation 20
- root, dorsal 61
- sheath tumor, granular cell 78
- stimulation, transient electric 161
- treatment 121
nerves 118, 119
- and muscles 118
nervi
- corpori cardiaci interni 116
nervous
- system 120
- system, autonomic 20
- system, central 49
- system, peripheral 134
- system, sympathetic 155
network
- digital x-ray prototype 65
neural tube defect 121
neuralgia
- post-herpetic 132
neuritic
- plaques 119
neuritis
- acute brachial 9
- demyelinating optic 61
- experimental allergic (autoimmune) 67
- optic 123
neuro
- Behçet 115
neuroblastoma 115, 119
- staging system, international 92
neuroblasts 115
neuroectodermal
- tumor, primitive 134
neuroendocrine
- carcinoma, large cell 99
neurofibrillary 116
neurofibrillary tangles 117

neurofibromatosis
- type 1 gene 116
- type 2 gene 116
neurofibromin 116
neurofilament 117
- protein 116
neurogenic
- muscular atrophy 118
neurography
- magnetic resonance 111
neurointensive
- care unit 117
neurokinin I receptor 117
neuroleptic
- malignant syndrome 118
neurologic
- deficit, prolonged reversible ischemic 138
- deficit, reversible ischemic 144
- examination 116
- history 117
- syndrome, high pressure 87
- test, alert, verbal, painful, unresponsive 27
neurological 116
neurology 116
neurometric
- battery 115
neuromuscular 118
- blocking agent 118
- facilitation, proprioceptive 134
- junction 118
neuron
- medial septum cholinergic 112
- specific enolase 120
- thalamic projection 163
neuronal
- intranuclear inclusion 117
neuropathology 119
neuropathy
- acute brachial 9
- acute motor axonal 19
- acute motor sensory axonal 19
- anterior ischemic optic 18
- diabetic autonomic 56
- hereditary motor and sensory 86
- optic nerve, amiodarone 20
- organophosphorus-induced delayed 123
- ulnar 171
- with liability to pressure palsies, hereditary 86
neurophysin
- bovine 33
neuropil threads 121
neuropsychiatric 119
- hospital 117
- inventory/nursing home 119
neuropsychiatry 119
neurosecretory
- cell, magnocellular 112
- cells 120
- dysfunction 120
- material 120
neurosensory
- deficit 120
neurosurgery 120
neurotensin
- like immunoreactivity 121
neurotrophic
- factor, ciliary 49
neurotropic
- melanoma, desmoplastic 61
neurovascular 121
neutral
- detergent fiber 116
- endopeptidase 116
- protamine Hagedorn - an intermediate acting insulin 119
- red bioassay 119
- to basic cytokeratin 45
neutrophil
- count, absolute 19
- myeloperoxidase activity 111
- polymorphonuclear 151
neutrophilic
- leukemia, chronic 49
never gave birth 121
new drug application 116
New York Heart Association 121
newborn 115
- hemolytic disease 84
- nursery 115
- persistent pulmonary hypertension 136
next of kin 118
N-formyl
- aminoantipyrine 72
niacin
- bound 33
nicotinamide
- adenine dinucleotide 115
- adenine dinucleotide phosphate 115
nicotine
- replacement therapy 119
nictitans lacrimal gland 117
night 118
- shift dose 120
nigrostriatal
- degeneration 120
Nijmegen breakage syndrome 115
nil per os 119
nitrate-reducing bacteria 119
nitric
- oxide 118
- oxide synthase 118
- oxide, inhaled 92
nitrofurazone
- soluble dressing 120
nitrogen 114
- antibody 9
- assimilation control protein 115
- dioxide 118
- nonprotein 119
nitroglycerine 121
nitroprusside infusion 121
nitrous
- oxide-barbiturate 115
N-methyl
- 1-deoxynojirimycin 118
- D-aspartate 118
- D-glucamine dithiocarbamate/ferrous sulfate mixture 106
- N-isopropyl) amiloride 93
N-nitroso
- 2-nitrophenacetin 118
- piperidine 118

Ix

- propranolol 118
- pyrrolidine 118
no 180
- abnormalities 114
- action required 115
- active disease 115
- acute disease 115
- acute distress 115
- acute infection 115
- added salt 115
- apparent abnormalities 114
- apparent distress 115
- apparent respiratory distress 115
- bone injury 115
- carbon required paper 116
- cardiac resuscitation 116
- change 116, 156, 179
- complaint 116
- complaints offered 116
- complications, no sequelae 116
- contraction 181
- effort detected 116
- evidence of disease 116
- evidence of recurrence 116
- evidence of recurrent disease 116
- infection present 117
- inflammation present 117
- insurance 117
- known allergies 117
- known disease 117
- known drug allergies 117
- light perception 118
- observable adverse effect level 118
- observable effect level 118
- ocular pain 118
- organisms seen 118
- pathologic diagnosis 119
- previous complaint 119
- previous history 119
- regular medications 119
- response 181
- return necessary 119
- sequelae, no complications 116
- show 120
- sign of infection, inflammation 120
- sign of significant disease 120
- significant abnormalities 120
- significant change 120
- significant defect 120
- significant differences 120
- significant findings 120
- sleep deprivation 120
- test 121

nocte 118
nocturnal
- dyspnea, paroxysmal 134
- hemoglobinuria, paroxysmal 134

nodal
- marginal zone b-cell lymphoma 118

node
- atrioventricular 27
- sentinel lymph 153

nodular
- hyperplasia, focal 75
- lymphocyte predominant Hodgkin lymphoma 118
- melanoma 118
- poorly differentiated lymphocytes 119
- poorly-differentiated lymphocytic lymphomas 129
- sclerosing Hodgkin's disease 120
- sclerosis 120
- sclerosis classical Hodgkin lymphoma 120

noise
- artificial background 10
- broad band 30
- ratio, vessel-to-tissue 174

nominal
- absorbed radiation dose 115
- ocular hazard area 118
- standard dose 120

non
- accidental injury 115
- alcoholic steatohepatitis 115
- aligned proximal tooth surfaces, number 118
- amyloid component 115
- cardiac cerebral ischemia 116
- cholera vibrios 116
- contributory 116
- disabling 116
- dissociative, carpal instability 45
- distended 116
- esterified fatty acids 116
- gonococcal urethritis 117
- histone nuclear proteins 118
- Hodgkin's lymphoma 117
- Ig superfamily 118
- insulin-dependent diabetes mellitus, type II 117
- invasive blood pressure 115, 117
- invasive ventilation 117
- ketotic coma, hyperosmolar 86
- ketotic hyperglycinaemia 117
- ketotic hyperosmolar syndrome 117
- lactating 118
- lactating, non-pregnant 118
- linear mixed effect model 118
- mast cell lineage disorder, associated clonal hematopoietic 16
- matching-to-sample, delayed 61
- melanoma skin cancer 118
- myelinating Schwann cells 118
- neoplastic pneumopathy 118
- neoplastic polyps 118
- neuropathic, diabetic 118
- obese diabetic 118
- preferring (alcohol) 119
- pregnant normotensive women 118
- pregnant, normal 118
- protein nitrogen 119
- protein-bound estradiol 119
- Q-wave myocardial infarction 119
- rebreather mask 119
- rebreather oxygen mask 119
- rejoining break 119
- segmental defect 120

- serrated cells 120
- significant result 120
- small cell lung cancer 120
- soap detergent 120
- specific 120
- specific damage 120
- specific defense 120
- specific dermatitis 120
- specific duodenitis 120
- specific esterase 120
- steroidal anti-inflammatory drugs 120
- stress test 121
- structural protein 5A 120
- sudden death 120
- suicidal depressed 120
- surgical doctors 120
- susceptibility to DNV 120
- syndromic prelingual deafness 120
- thrombocytopenic preterm 121
- thrombocytopenic term 121
- tuberculous mycobacteria 121
- walking cast, short leg 153
- weight bearing 121
- weight bearing cast, short-leg 153

none 121, 180
noon
- before 19

noradrenaline
- reuptake inhibitor with 5-HT3 receptor blocking action, new selective 105

norbromide 119
noreleagnine 117
norepinephrine 116
norethisterone
- acetate 116

normal 72, 114, 117, 179
- and well 121
- breath sounds 115
- brooding temperature 119
- controls 49
- coordinate structural decomposition 120
- delivery, full term 77
- light perception 118
- limits 117
- non-pregnant 118
- plantar reflex 179
- plasma, pooled 134
- pressure and temperature 119
- pressure hydrocephalus 119
- range 121
- range of motion 119
- saline 120
- saline (solution) 120
- saline solution 121
- salt diet 120
- sinus rhythm 120
- size and shape 121
- sodium dialysate 120
- spontaneous delivery 120
- spontaneous vaginal delivery 121
- temperature 121
- temperature and pressure 121
- tissue complication probability 121
- value, practical 135

normalized
- protein nitrogen appearance rates 119
- relative backscatter 119
- slope descriptors 120
- spin density 120
- standard deviation 120

normoactive bowel sounds 115
normoblast 115
normocephalic 116
- atraumatic 116

normotensive
- sedentary 120
- women, non-pregnant 118

norpramin 61
Norway
- electrical inspection agency 130

nose 118
- and throat 121

not
- admitted 114
- applicable 114
- available 114
- considered disabling 116
- detected 116
- diagnosed 116
- done 116
- equal to 180
- for resuscitation 116
- known 117
- less than 180
- lower than 118
- measured 118
- mentioned 118
- more than 118
- necessary to return 118
- otherwise provided for 118
- otherwise specified 118
- palpable 119
- recommended 119
- remarkable 119
- specific 120
- tender 121
- tested 121, 180
- verified 180
- yet diagnosed 121

nota bene 115
note well 115
nothing 117
- abnormal detected 115
- by mouth 115, 119
- by mouth after midnight 119
- to do 121

novel nuclear protein 118
N-tosyl-L-lysine chloromethyl ketone 162
nuclear
- antigen, Epstein-Barr 67
- antigen, proliferating cell 129
- bodies 115
- coefficient of variance 116
- cytoplasmic (ratio) 116
- FMRP-interacting protein 121
- localization signal 118
- magnetic resonance (scan) 118
- protein, novel 118
- proteins, non-histone 118
- RNA-binding protein 119

nucleated red blood cells 119

lx

nucleic
- acid amplification testing 115
nucleocytoplasmic
- area ratio 116
nucleoside
- analogue reverse transcriptase inhibitors 119
- diphosphates 116
- yttrium, tyrosine, pyrimidine 177
nucleotide 121
- guanine 80
- releasing bacterial Lumac 119
- releasing somatic Lumac 119
- sugar 120
- triphosphates 121
nucleotide-binding site 115
nucleus
- abducens 9
- accumbens 115
- dorsal vagal 64
- paraventricular hypothalamic 132
- perihypoglossal 132
- pulposus, herniated 86
- tractus solitarius 121
- tractus solitarius, caudal region 49
null
- type 121
nulling
- gradient moment 80
number 118, 180
- needed to treat 118
- of non-aligned proximal tooth surfaces 118
- of pregnancies 128
- of step-down 120
- wave 181
numbers
- Roman 183
numbness and tingling 121
nurse
- anesthetist, certified registered 51
- army head 16
- clinician, geriatric 80
- notes 118
- operating room 125
- ophthalmic 124
- orthopedic 125
- practical 134
- practitioner 22, 119
- practitioner, family 75
- practitioner, geriatric 80
- practitioner, gerontologic 80
- practitioners, advanced 20
- practitioners, neonatal 118
- private duty 129
- public health 132
- registrated 144
- service, visiting 174
- visiting 174
- vocational practice 174
nursery
- intensive care 90
- newborn 115
nursing 120
- arched-back 10
- assistance, general 80
- care, general 80
- coronary care 42
- critical care 42
- facility, skilled 155
- home 117
nutrient
- broth 115
- pH 132
nutrition
- associated cholestasis, total parenteral 163
- parenteral 131
- peripheral parenteral 136
nystagmus
- gaze 80

O

oak ridge analytical system 124
object 122
- relations technique 125
- sorting test 126
- unidentified bright 169
objective 121, 122
- structured clinical examination 126
- test 126
oblique 122
- left anterior 98
- superior 155
- talus 126
obliterans-organizing
- pneumonia, bronchiolitis 34
obliteration
- prediction index 123
obliterative
- pulmonary hypertension 123
observable
- cholinomimetic effects 122
observation 122
- and examination 122
- unit, intensive therapy 93
observe for 180
observed 180
observer 122
obsessive
- compulsive 122
- compulsive disorder 122
obstetric prediabetic 123
obstetrics 122
- and gynecology 122
obstruction
- bladder neck 33
- bladder outlet 34
- congenital duodenal 43
- intestinal 93
- small bowel 150
obstructive
- airways disease, chronic 49
- cardiomyopathy, hypertrophic 86
- jaundice 123
- lung disease, chronic 49
- pulmonary disease, chronic 50
- pulmonary emphysema, chronic 50
- sleep apnea 125
- sleep apnea syndrome 125
obturator internus bursa 122
obtuse marginal artery 123
occasionally 122
occipital 122
- acoustic window 121
- posterior, left 101

occipital-frontal
- circumference 122
occipitoanterior
- left 101
occipitolateral
- left 101
occipitosacral 125
occiput 122
- anterior 121
- anterior, right 144
- posterior 121, 123
- posterior, right 144
- transverse, right 144
occluded
- pressure, pulmonary artery 127
occluder
- Amplatzer septal 23
occludin-related gene 125
occlusal
- conditions social acceptability scale 149
occlusion
- (in coronary artery stenting), side branch 150
- acute coronary 12
- centric relation 48
- middle cerebral artery 104
- portal triad 139
- time 126
occlusions
- recurrent aortic 142
occlusive
- disease, arteriosclerotic 20
- disease, arteriosclerotic peripheral vascular 22
- pressure, pulmonary artery 128
occult
- blood 122
- primary malignancy 124
occupation 122
occupational
- disease 122
- history 122
- medicine 123
- noise-induced hearing loss 123
- safety 125
- therapist 126
- therapy 126
- therapy assistant 126
oct motif 44
octamethylcyclotetrasiloxane 123
oct-containing
- composite elements 122
octopamine-IR 60
ocular
- pain, no 118
- plethysmodynamography 123
- pneumoplethysmography 123
- tension 126
oculocephalic reflex 122
oculopalatocerebral (syndrome) 123
oculoparalytic
- illusion 123
oculopneumoplethysmography 124
oculus
- dexter 122
- sinister 125
- uterque 127
odd-carbon fatty acid enriched 122
odds ratio 124
odontectomy and alveolectomy 121
odontoblast layer, lingual 101
odor
- anodal closure 12
oestrogen
- receptor 124
- receptor, human 86
of 180
- each 5
- soil vapor extraction 158
office
- audit, medical 110
- call 122
- clinical trials 54
- general accounting 77
- surgery 125
- therapy 126
- visit 127
officer of the day 122
ofloxacin 122
oil
- adjuvant, mineral 110
- red 0 125
- retention 124
- retention enema 124
- seed rape 126
ointment 123, 171
old
- english sheepdog 122
- term (in anatomy) 126
- tuberculin 126
olfactory
- reference syndrome 125
- threshold 126
oligoastrocytomas 121
- malignant 110
- mixed 110
oligodeoxynucleotide 122
oligomenorrheic
- polycystic ovary syndrome 123
oligomeric
- carboxylesterases 122
oligonucleotides
- antisense 24
olivopontocerebellar
- atrophy 123
- degeneration 123
Omenn syndrome 125
omental 123
omnibus
- personality inventory 123
on
- call 122
- day of admission 122
- examination 122
once 181
- a day 141
- daily 122
oncogene
- cellular 49
- cellular erythroblastosis 43
- proto-, feline sarcoma 74
- proto, simian sarcoma 152
- viral 174
- viral avian erythroblastosis 173
- viral feline sarcoma 173

lx

oncology 123
one
- half 157
- hour 181
- liter per minute 100
- to-one 181
- type of breast reconstruction 164
online
- medical control 123
- survey, certification and reporting system 126
open
- canalicular system (about platelets) 122
- fracture 122
- heart surgery 122
- label 123
- reading frame 124
- reduction 124
- reduction and fixation 124
- reduction jaw fracture 125
- reduction, external fixation 124
- reduction, internal fixation 125
- systems interconnection 126
opening 123, 125
- aortic valve 27
- atrioventricular 27
- pressure 123
- snap 125
- snap, mitral 110
operating
- curve analysis, receiver 144
- room 124
- room nurse 125
- room personnel 125
- room technician 125
- room, general 81
- system 125
- system, prime 138
operation 123
operations 124
- and training 126
operative dentistry 123
Oph ophthalmology 123
ophthalmia 123
- neonatorum, gonococcal 81
ophthalmic
- nurse 124
ophthalmociliary artery
- distal segment 61
- middle segment of 110
ophthalmology 123
- doctor 123
ophthalmopathy
- thyroid associated 159
ophthalmoplegic
- migraine 124
ophthalmoscope 123
ophthalmoscopy 123
opiate
- receptor agonist 124
- receptor delta 124
- receptor kappa 124
- withdrawal 124
opiates 123
opponens pollicis 123
opportunistic
- infection in AIDS 18
- infections 122
opposite 124
optic
- density 122
- nerve damage, glaucomatous 81
- nerve, amiodarone neuropathy 20
- neuritis 123
- neuritis, demyelinating 61
- neuropathy, anterior ischemic 18
- radiation 124
- tract 126
optical
- immunoassay 122
- path difference 123
- position sensor 124
- rotation 181
- rotatory dispersion 124
- scanning 124
optician 124
optics 124
optimal AVD 121
optimal hemodialysis 124
optimus 124
optokinetic 123
oral 121
- antibiotics 124
- attenuated poliovirus with types 1, 2, and 3 163
- cholecystogram 122
- conjugated estrogens 122
- contraceptive 122
- contraceptive pills 122
- contraceptive therapy 122
- glucose tolerance test 122
- osmotic 125
- polio vaccine 124
- poliovirus vaccine 124
- radiation death 124
- rehydration 124
- rehydration solution 125
- rehydration therapy 125
- squamous cell carcinoma 126
- surgeon 125
- surgery 125
orally 135
orange juice 123, 125
orangeworm
- navel 119
orbis sigma valves type I 126
orbital
- medial 110
orbitale 124
orchitis 124
order
- verbal 174
- voice 174
ordered subset expectation maximization 126
organ
- at risk 121
- failure, multiple 110
- specific 125
- system failure 126
organic 125
- brain syndrome 122
- carbon, total 163
- heart disease 122
- mental syndrome 123
organisms
- pleuropneumonia-like 136
organizing
- centers, microtubule 113

organophosphate utilization 124
organophosphorus
- induced delayed neuropathy 123
orientation
- test 126
oriented 6, 12, 124
orifice 125
- aortic valve 27
original sampling connections 126
original tuberculin 126
ornithine 125
- decarboxylase 122
- transaminase 126
- transcarbamylase 126
oropharynx 123
orosomucoid 124, 125
orotate
- phosphoribosyltransferase 124
orotracheal 126
orphan
- virus, enteric cytopathogenic bovine 67
orthodontic tooth movement 126
orthodontist
- judgment 123
orthogonal projection approach 123
ortho-iodobenzoate 122
orthopaedic
- surgery 125
orthopantomograin 123
orthopedic 124, 125
- examination 122
- nurse 125
- research 124
- special assessment examination 125
- surgeon 125
- surgery 125
- treatment 126
- web links 127
orthopedics 125
orthophosphate, inorganic 132
orthorhythmic
- pacemaker 125
orthoses
- ankle-foot 15
orthosis
- hip-knee-ankle-foot 85
- reciprocating gait 143
- thoracolumbosacral 163
orthostatic
- tachycardia syndrome, postural 135
orthotoluidine
- arsenite 126
orthotopic liver transplantations 123
oryzacystatin 122
os 125
- tibiale mediale 126
oscillation 126
- systemic arterial pressure 149
oscillatory
- ventilation, high-frequency 85
oscilloscope
- cathode ray 51
Osler-Rendu-Weber (syndrome) 125
osm TRPC 127
osmiophilic inclusion bodies 122
osmium 125
osmolality 126
osmole 126
osmoles
- per kilogram 126
- per liter 126
osmosis 126
osmotic 126
- oral 125
- pressure 181
- pressure of plasma 124
osseointegrated implant bridge 122
osseous 126
ossification
- heterotopic 86
- periarticular 127
osteoarthritic
- moderate 110
osteoarthritis 121, 126
- generalized 81
- post-traumatic 139
osteoarthropathy 121
- hypertrophic 86
osteoblastic
- proliferation index 123
osteocartilaginous
- exostoses 122
osteochondral
- autograft transfer system 121
osteochrondritis
- dissecans 122
- dissecans, juvenile 96
osteoclast
- activating factor 121
- resorption stimulating activity 125
- stimulating factor 126
osteodysplastica
- geroderma 80
- hereditaria, gemderma 81
osteodystrophy
- Albright, hereditary 16
osteogenesis imperfecta 122
osteogenic
- sarcoma 125
osteogenic sarcoma 125
osteoid
- osteoma 123
osteoma
- osteoid 123
osteomyelitis 126
- skull base 150
osteomyelosclerosis 123
osteonecrosis
- of the femoral head 123
osteopathic
- manipulation 123
osteopathy 126
- doctor 61
osteopontin 124
osteoporosis
- pseudolipoma syndrome 124
osteoprotegerin 123
osteosarcoma 125
osteosclerosis 125
osteotomy
- closing wedge, high tibial 55
- vertical ramus 174

- vertical sagittal split 174
Oswestry
- disability score 122
other
- party liability 123
- regulated material 125
otitis
- externa 122
- externa, bilateral 33
- media 123
- media effusion, persistent 135
- media with effusion, acute 123
- media, acute 20, 33
- media, bilateral 33
- media, left 101
- media, right 144
otolaryngology 126
otology 126
otopalatodigital (syndrome) 123
otorhinolaryngology 125
otospondylometaphyseal
- dysplasia 126
Ottawa Ankle Rules 121
oubain
- sensitivity 125
ounce(s) 127
out
- of bed 123
- of hospital 123
- of plaster 123
- patient 123
outcome
- score, Glasgow 81
outer
- diameter 122
- domain, inverted repeat 96
- membrane protein, H. pylori 86
- plexiform layer 123
- quadrant, left 101
- quadrant, left upper 102
- spiral fiber 126
- subcutaneous 126
outflow
- dorsal 61
- dorsolateral 60
- rate 124
- resistance, total 163
- ventrolateral 174
outlet
- obstruction, bladder 34
- relaxed vaginal 149
outpatient 124
- clinic 123
- department 123
- dispensary 123
- service 124
- surgery 124
- treatment 124
output
- basal acid 28
- brachial artery 28
- cardiac 49
- fecal 75
- maximal acid 104
- total cardiac 141
- urine 171
ova
- and parasite 123
- blood and parasites 122
ovarian
- papillary serous adenocarcinoma 124
- sectional area 125
ovaries
- polycystic 129, 136
over the counter 126
overall survival 125, 158
overbite
- and horizontal overjet (OJ) ratio 122
overdose 122
overgrowth
- stimulating factor 126
overjet
- type of maloclusion 123
overloading
- test, cervical compression 42
overproduction
- inhibition 123
over-the-shoulder strap 126
overwhelming
- postsplenectomy infection 124
ovine
- placental lactogen 123
- submaxillary mucin 126
ox red blood cell 124
oxidase
- lysyl 101
oxidation-
- reduction 124
- reduction potential 125
oxide
- barbiturate, nitrous 115
oxidized glutathione 82
oxidoreductase 124
- human 86
- hydroxysteroid 86
oximetry
- pulse 135
oxygen 121
- alveolar 127
- arteriovenous 27
- capacity 121
- content, peripheral arterial 127
- difference, arteriovenous 26
- in arterial blood, partial pressure 127
- mask, non-rebreather 119
- partial pressure 124, 135
- pressure 135
- radical scavengers 125
- ratio monitor 125
- ratio monitor controller 125
- ratio, arteriovenous 27
- saturation 121, 125
- saturation (%), systemic arterial 149
- saturation by pulse oximeter 157
- saturation difference basal, arteriovenous 26
- saturation difference, arteriovenous 26
- saturation meter 126
- saturation, regional 146
- saturation, room-air 142
- tension difference, alveolo-arterial 7
- tension, alveolo-arterial 6
- tension, mixed venous 140
oxygenase
- microsomal heme 107

oxygenation
- extracorporeal membrane 67
oxypolygelatin 123
oxytocin 126, 127
oxytryptamine 126
ozone safe 125

P

PACAP
- receptor I 137
paced
- cycle length 47
pacemaker
- atrial triggered 7
- orthorhythmic 125
pacemakers
- rate responsive 145
- respiratory-dependent 143
- ventricular single-chamber synchronous 175
pachyman
- polysaccharides 136
pacing
- atrial 21
- rate responsive 145
- right atrial appendage 142
- transcutaneous 160
pack
- hot wet 88
- years (of cigarettes) 140
package
- zigzag In-line 177
Packard
- Radioimmunoassay System 137
packed
- cell volume 84
- cell volume (hematocrit) 129
- red blood cells 137
packs
- hot moist 86
- per day 136
Paget's disease 129
pain 134
- back 33
- biliary tract 35
- chest 50
- killer 133
- lumbo-dorsal 99
- management index 134
- management inventory 134
- on palpation 135
- rating index 137
- rating intensity score 137, 138
- sympathetic maintained 155
- syndrom, patellofemoral 131
- syndrome, complex regional 51
- syndrome, pelvic 136
- threshold, mechanical 111
- zoster associated 177
painless
- myocardial infarction 134
pair model
- reversible radical 145
paired 136
- stimulation, potentiating 136
palate
- cleft 46
pallido
- ponto-nigral degeneration 136
palmar
- adductors 127
- crease, distal 62
- skin temperature 139
palpable 127
palpate 127
palpated 127
palpation
- and auscultation 21
- percussion and auscultation 135
palsy
- cerebral 50
pamidronate 21
pancreas
- microsomal membranes, dog 62
pancreatectomy
- total 163
pancreatic
- ductal adenocarcinoma, infiltrating 93
- extract 130
pancreatico
- cholangiography 129
pancreatitis
- acute 21
- acute hemorrhagic 16
- chronic relapsing 51
panencephalitis
- subacute sclerosing 157
panoramic
- mandibular index 134
Papanicolaou
- smear 128
paper
- electrophoresis 130
- no carbon required 116
- radioimmunosorbent test 138
papillary
- carcinoma of the thyroid, warthin-like 176
- carcinomas 129
- conjunctivitis, giant 82
- Hurthle cell neoplasms 132
- serous adenocarcinoma, ovarian 124
- thyroid carcinomas, diffuse sclerosing variant 63
papilloma virus
- bovine alimentary 29
- human 87
papillomatosis
- recurrent respiratory 145
papular
- xanthoma 140
papulosis
- lymphomatoid 103
para 127
- iodobenzoate 132
paracervical
- ganglion 129
paracetamol 21
paraganglioma
- gangliocytic 81
parallel 180
- bars 180
- conductance 81
paralysis
- acute atrophic spinal 7
- acute flaccid 15

- bilateral abductor vocal cord 29
- bilateral facial 32
- general 81
- progressive general 132
paramedic 133
parameter
- ventricular inotropic 173
paraparesis
- tropical spastic 165
paraplegic 128
parasegment 138
paraspinous 138
parathyroid
- hormone 139
- hormone, C-terminal 139
- hormone-related peptide 139
paraventricular
- hypothalamic nucleus 132
- nuclei 140
paraventriculospinal
- tract 140
paravertebral 140
- block 140
parenchyma
- acinar 21
- dense 65
parent 127
- adolescent relationship questionnaire 128
parental
- acceptance/rejection questionnaire 128
parenteral
- nutrition 131
- nutrition, peripheral 136
- nutrition, total 163
- nutrition-associated cholestasis, total 163
paresis
- general 81
paresthesias 128
parietal
- cell, gastric 82
Parkinson
- disease 129
- disease questionnaire 129
Parkinson's disease
- late 101
paroxysmal
- atrial fibrillation 127
- atrial tachycardia 128
- cold hemoglobinuria 129
- nocturnal dyspnea 134
- nocturnal hemoglobinuria 134
- positional vertigo, benign 34
- supraventricular tachycardia 139, 140
- tachycardia 139
- ventricular tachycardia 140
part
- equal 5
part per trillion 136
partial
- disability, permanent 136
- epilepsy 130
- pressure in arterial blood, carbon dioxyde 127
- pressure of carbon dioxide 129
- pressure of carbon dioxide in arterial blood 127
- pressure of oxygen 135
- pressure of oxygen in arterial blood 127
- pressure, oxygen 124
- remission 136
- remission, good 82
- response 136
- thromboplastin time 139
- thromboplastin time, automated 22
- weight bearing 140
particle
- alpha 181
- beta 181
- signal recognition 157
particles
- immuno magnetic 92
particulate
- air/adsorption, high-efficiency 84
- total suspended 165
partner
- abuse, intimate 93
parts per million 136
parturition
- after 21
- to conception interval 129
party
- liability, other 123
parvovirus
- 2 50
- B19 140
pasiniazid 93
passage
- extrahepatic biliary 69
- time, arteriovenous 27
passed urine 139
passive
- cutaneous anaphylaxis inhibition 128
- Heymann nephritis 132
- movements, full 76
- range of motion 138
- sampling devices 138
past
- history 132
- medical history 134
- medical illness 134
- pertinent history 136
- surgical history 139
Pasteurella
- haemolytica 106
patellar
- tendon bearing 139
- tendon reflex 139
patellofemoral
- joint 131
- pain syndrom 131
patent
- ductus arteriosus 129
- foramen ovale 131
paternal
- grandfather 131
- grandmother 132
- HLA antigens, inherited 93
- meiosis I 134
- meiosis II 134
path
- difference, optical 123
pathologic
- stage 138
pathological 127
pathology 128

- clinical 47
pathway
- accessory 21
- atrioventricular 21
- Embden-Meyerhof 69
- intermediate tectobulbar 160
patient 127, 139
- care, direct 62
- controlled analgesia 128
- in office 135
- out 123
- refused test 138
- review instrument 137
- survey, initial 93
pattern
- analysis, interference 93
paucity of lymph node T cell mutation 133
payment
- error prevention program 131
- system, prospective 62, 136
PBS 127
PCO2 difference
- arterial-end tidal 127
peak
- electron volts 131
- expiratory flow 131
- expiratory flow rate 131
- expiratory velocity 131
- scatter factor 138
- systolic velocity 139
- velocity prosthetic flow, diastolic 64
pediatric 130
- advanced life support 127
- intensive care unit 133
- life support 22
- Risk Index 137
pediatrics 130
pelvic
- examination 130
- examination under anesthesia 130
- hematoma necessitans 132
- inflammatory disease 133
- lymph node dissection 133
- pain syndrome 136
- vascular injury 140
pemphigoid
- bullous 34
pemphigus vulgaris 140
penetrating coronary artery injury 128
penicillase-resistant penicillin 138
penicillin 129, 131
- binding protein 128
- penicillase-resistant 138
- relatively resistant 145
penile
- erection 130
penis
- dorsal vein 64
pennyweight 65
pentamidine
- aerosol 21
pentosan polysulfate 136
pentylenetetrazol 139
peplomycin 133
- emulsion in saline 156
peplomycin emulsion in hydroxypropylcellulosum 87
pepsin
- active 21
- extract of type-24 M protein 131
peptic
- ulcer 139
- ulcer disease 140
peptidase
- A isozyme 131
- B isozyme 131
- C isozyme 131
- D isozyme 131
- D-alanyl-D-alanine 58
- S isozyme 131
peptide
- atrial natriuretic 20
- elongation factor 68
- gastric inhibitory 79
- glucose-dependent insulinotropic 79
- histidine isoleucine 132
- histidine methionine 132
- ion transport 95
- microhodotermes viator corpus cardiacum 108
- parathyroid hormone-related 139
- porcine brain natriuretic 128
- RNA III-inhibiting 144
- vasoactive intestinal 173
- vasoinhibitory 173
per 180
- capita annual income 128
- day 55
- diem 129
- minute, counts 50
- os 135
- protocol 135
- rectum 136
- rectum (L) 137
- vagina bleed 140
perceived stress scale 139
perception
- fuzzy logical model of 75
percussion and auscultation 21, 127
percussion and postural drainage 136
percutaneous
- catheter drainage 129
- coronary intervention 129
- endoscopic gastrostomy 131
- ethanol injection 131
- transhepatic cholangiography 139
- transluminal angioplasty 139
- transluminal coronary angioplasty 139
- transmyocardial revascularization 139
- transvenous mitral commissurotomy 139
perforating dermatosis
- acquired 21
perforator
- compression, septal 156
performance
- incentive award 132
- rating instrument 137
- test, physical 136
- visual impact 173
perfused
- rat kidney, isolated 93

perfusion
- chemotherapy, intraperitoneal hyperthermic 93
- isolated limb 91
periarteriolar
- lymphocyte sheath 127
- lymphocyte sheath (about spleen) 127
periarthropatia homero scapularis 132
periarticular
- ossification 127
pericardial
- effusion 130
peridinin
- chlorophyll A protein 131
perihypoglossal
- nucleus 132
perinatal
- death 129
- respiratory insufficiency 137
perineal 20, 131
perineoscrotal
- hypopospadias, pseudovaginal 136
perinuclear
- antineutrophil cytoplasmic antibodies 127
period
- absolute refractory 23
- effective refractory 70
- last normal menstrual 101
- menstrual 110
- relative rest 145
- retrograde refractory 145
periodic
- leg/limb movements 133
periodic safety update report 139
periodontal
- ligament 129
perioperative
- myocardial infarction 134
- myocardial infarction, transmural 163
- myocardial injury, subendocardial 157
periparturient relaxation of immunity 136
peripheral
- arterial disease 127
- arterial occlusive disease 127
- arterial oxygen content 127
- arteriosclerotic disease 127
- blood 128
- blood mononuclear cells 128
- blood progenitor cells 128
- blood stem cell 128
- intravenous (line) 133
- intravenous line 133
- lymph nodes 133
- myelin protein 22 134
- nerve injury 134
- nervous system 134
- parenteral nutrition 136
- pulmonary stenosis 136
- pulses present 136
- renin activity 137
- resistance, total 163
- stem cell rescue 138
- stem cell transplant 138
- vascular 140
- vascular disease 140
- vascular disease, arteriosclerotic 24
- vascular occlusive disease 22
- vascular resistance 140
peripherally
- inserted catheter 132
periprostatic
- vein thrombosis 140
perirenal
- adipose tissue 136
peristalsis
- antral 21
peristomal
- pyoderma gangrenosum 136
peritoneal
- cancer, disseminated 62
- dialysis, acute 21
- dialysis, automated 21
- dialysis, chronic 50
- dialysis, continuous ambulatory 38
- dialysis, continuous cycling 42
- exudate 130
- exudate cells 130
- lavage, diagnostic 62
peritonitis
- gonorrheal, invasive 79
peri-urethral
- diathermy 140
periventricularis
- hypothalami 132
permanent
- and stationary 138
- and total 139
- partial disability 136
- total disability 139
permanently
- implantable 132
permeability
- factor, vascular 174
- increasing protein, bactericidal 34
permeation liquid membrane 133
permissible
- concentration, maximum 110
- dose, maximum 110
- exposure limit 131
permit
- access 21
pernicious anemia 127
peroxidase antiperoxidase 128
peroxisome proliferator activated receptor-alpha 136
peroxisome proliferator activated receptor-gamma 136
persistent
- bioaccumulative and toxic 128
- fetal circulation 131
- generalized lymphadenopathy 132
- otitis media effusion 135
- pigmented purpuric eruption 136
- pulmonary hypertension of the newborn 136
personal
- computer 128
- edition 130

- injury 132
- preference scale 136
- protective equipment 136
- Reaction Inventory 137
personality
- disorder, borderline 34
- Five-Factor Model 74
personnel
- Expertise and Resource Listing 130
- operating room 125
pertussis
- toxin, mutant 111
pervasive
- developmental delay 129
petit mal 133
petri
- enteropathogen count (plate) 130
Peyer's patches 135, 136
P-glycoprotein 132
pH
- change 181
- nutrient 132
- values 132
phagocyte
- system, mononuclear 111
phagocytic activity 127
phantoms
- multipurpose 111
pharmaceutical
- Education Advisory Committee 130
- Manufacturers Association 134
pharmacy 132
- practices, good 82
pharyngeal
- branch of the vagus nerve 132
- Retention Index 137
pharyngoesophageal 130
phase
- 1 studies, maximum tolerated dose 113
- acute 20
- difference method 156
- encoded 130
- encoded artifact reduction 130
phasic
- contractions, spontaneous 156
phenacetin 132
phenanthrene 132
phenazinium 132
phencyclidine 129
phenobarbital 128
phenol
- red impurity 137
phenoxymethylpenicillin 135
phentolamine 132
phenyl 181
- alanine 72, 132
- dimorpholinomethyl-hydroxy)-benzoyl-indole 88
- ephrine 130, 132
- ethanolamine-N-methyl-transferase 134
- ethyl alcohol 130
- ethylamine 130
- hydroxy-naftopidil 132
- isothiocyanate 132
- ketonuria 133
- nitrene 132
- N-tert-butyl nitrone 128
- sulfonphthalein test 139
- sulphonylbenzenesulphonamide 120
- thiohydantoin 139
- valerate 132
phenytoin
- equivalent 130
- hypersensitivity syndrome 132
pheochromocytoma 128
Philadelphia
- chromosome 132
phone
- call 128
phoneutria nigriventer spider venom 135
phonocardiogram 129
phosphat
- raw rock 145
phosphatase
- acid 12, 21
- alkaline 18, 21
- prostate-specific acid 12
phosphate
- acid 11
- and tensin homolog 139
- buffered saline 128
- choline 50
- diisopropyl 60
- reabsorption index 137
- saline, bovine albumin 28
- specific transporter 139
- yeast glucose 131
phosphatidyl
- choline anthrylvinyl-labeled 22
- choline egg 70
- choline soybean 156
- choline, desaturated 62
- ethanolamine 130, 131
- inositol glycan-class A 133
- inositol-4,5-biphosphate 133
- inositolglycan A 133
phosphodiesterase 129
phosphoenol
- pyruvate 131
- pyruvate synthase gene 136
phosphogluconate
- dehydrogenase 131
phosphoinositide 94
pholemman 133
phospholipases 133
phospholipomannan 133
phosphomannose
- isomerase 134
phosphoprotein
- phosphatase 135
- phosphatases 136
phosphoribose
- isomerase 137
phosphorous-31 nuclear magnetic resonance spectroscopy 118
phosphorus 127
phosphorylated product of Rb gene 137
phosphotransferase
- system 139
phosphotungstic
- acid 139

- acid hematoxylin 139
phosrestin 137
photo differential scanning calorimeter 132
photobioreactors
- tubular undulating row 167
photochemical
- reflectance index 137
photodynamic therapy 130
photographic
- effect 130
photometric
- method, direct 62
photon 181
photoreceptors 132
phrenic 132
- artery, inferior 93
- nerve 132
phthalate
- dibutyl 56
phycoerythrin 130
physic
- general 81
physical 132
- activity index 127
- activity readiness questionnaire 128
- activity recall questionnaire 128
- education 130
- engineering 130
- examination 130, 140
- examination, complete 50
- exercise 130
- medicine and rehabilitation 134
- performance test 136
- status 138
- therapy 139
- therapy, chest 50
- therapy, register 145
physician
- assistant 127
- assistant house 16
- attending 24
- data query (CancerNet) 129
- desk reference 129
- emergency 70
- extender 130
- modalities, rehabilitation, injections, cross training, evaluation, salicylates 137
- patient and society 136
- practice management companies 136
- private 135
physiological
- ecology 130
physiology 132
physiotherapy
- modified 111
physostigmine 132
phytane
- isoprenoid 132
phytohemagglutinin 132
Pick
- body dementia 128
- disease 133
picogram 131
pig enteropathogenic E.coli 131
pigeons
- show racer 157
- white carneau 175
piggyback
- infusion, intravenous 95
pigment
- dispersing hormone 129
pigmented
- epithelium 130
- purpuric eruption, persistent 136
- villonodular synovitis 140
pills
- birth control 31
pilocarpine
- epinephrine 130
pinealectomy 140
pink, warm and dry 140
pint 139
pipe-associated
- irrigation 93
piperacillin 133
Pitocin 133
pituitary
- adenylate-cyclase-activating polypeptide 127
- anterior 21
- growth hormone 132
- hormone, anterior 22
pityriasis rubra pilaris 138
placebo 128
- controlled food challenge, double-blind 56
placenta 133
placental
- alkaline phosphatase 133
- extract 130
- lactogen, human 87
- membrane inflammation 134
- ribonuclease inhibitor 137
- RNase inhibitor 137
- site, trophoblastic tumor 139
plan 127
plankton
- reactivity in the marine environment 138
plans
- assessment and 21
plant
- engineering 130
plantar
- muscles 133
- reflex, normal 179
- response 179
planus-like
- keratosis, lichen 101
plaque
- atherosclerotic 21
plaques
- neuritic 119
plasma
- antihuman thymocyte 17
- cell apoptotic index 128
- cell labeling index, bone marrow 129
- cell membrane receptor 43
- cells 128
- coagulation, argon 21
- exchange 130
- flow, contralateral renal 51
- flow, renal 145
- fresh frozen 74
- glucose, post prandial 136
- membrane integrity 134
- osmotic pressure 124
- pooled normal 134
- pregnancy test 136

- protein 181
- reagin, rapid 145
- renin activity 137
- volume 140
- zoster immune 177

plasmactytic
- hyperplasia 132

plasmacytoma
- variant translocation-1 gene 140

plasmepsin 133
plasmids
- root-inducing 137

plasminogen
- activator, tissue 163
- activators in plasma, functional activity 72
- activators in urine, functional activity 72
- plasmin system 136

plasmodium
- falciparum, chloroquine-resistant 51

plaster of Paris 135
plastic surgery 138
plate
- blood-agar 28

platelet 133
- activating factor 127
- activation, indices 93
- derived growth factor 129
- endothelial cell adhesion molecule (CD-31) 130
- factor 4 131
- reactivity index 137

platelets 133
platform
- system, biomechanical ankle 28

plating
- efficiencies 130

platinum
- cis-diamminedichloro- 45
- diamminedichloro 58
- etoposide 130
- total 163

play
- the-winner 139

pleckstrin
- homology 132

plethysmodynamography
- ocular 123

plethysmography
- respiratory inductance 144
- venous impedance 173

pleural
- effusion 130

pleuropneumonia
- contagious, bovine 39
- like organisms 136

plexiform
- layer, outer 123

pluripotential
- hematopoietic stem cell 132

plus 180
- or minus 180

pneumatic
- anti-shock garment 128
- foot compression, intermittent 93

pneumatosis
- gastric 81

pneumo 134
pneumococcal
- polysaccharide, polyvalent 136

pneumoconiosis
- coal worker 55

pneumocystis
- carinii pneumonia 129

pneumoencephalogram 131
Pneumonia 134
pneumonia 134
- acute 21
- acute interstitial 18
- aspiration 21
- bronchiolitis obliterans-organizing 34
- giant cell interstitial 79
- pneumocystis carinii 129
- usual interstitial 171

pneumonitis
- desquamative interstitial 60
- lymphoid interstitial 100

pneumopathy
- non-neoplastic 118

pneumoplethysmography
- ocular 123

pneumothorax 135, 139
- artificial 21

p-nitrophenoxycarbonyl
- methyl disulfide 119

PO 135
Poa pratensis group IX allergen 135
podiatric
- medicine, doctor 62

point
- attachment 20
- average, grade 81
- Bolton 29
- of entry 130
- of exit 135
- of maximum impact 134
- of-care 135
- replication initiation 144
- respiratory inversion 137

polar
- cataract, anterior 21

polarised
- scatter separation, multi angle 104

polarized
- light microscopy 133

Police Department 129
policy coordination unit 129
polio
- vaccine, oral 124

poliovirus
- types 1, 2, and 3, oral attenuated 163
- vaccine, inactivated 94
- vaccine, oral 124

pollen mitosis one 134
pollicis
- brevis, flexor 75
- longus, flexor 75

poly (ADP-ribose) polymerase 128
poly D, L-lactic acid 129
polyacrylamide gel electrophoresis 127
polyactive 127
polyangiitis
- microscopic 110

polyarteritis nodosa 127
polybrominated
- biphenyls 128
polychlorinated
- biphenyls 128
polycyclic
- aromatic hydrocarbon 127
polycystic
- kidney disease 129, 133
- ovarian disease 129
- ovaries 129, 136
- ovary syndrome, oligomenorrheic 123
polycythemia vera 140
polydimethylsiloxane 129
polydioxanone 129
- suture 130
polyetheretherketone 130
polyethylene 130
- high-density 84
- ultra-high molecular weight 171
polyglycolic acid 131
polyhydroxynonanoate 132
polylactic acid 133
polymerase
- chain reaction 129
- chain reaction, differential-display 58
- chain reaction, methylation-specific 113
- chain reaction, reverse transcriptase 148
polymethylmethacrylate 134
polymorphic
- ventricular tachycardia 140
polymorphism
- restriction-fragment length 143
- single nucleotide 155
polymorphonuclear
- cells 135
- leukocyte 134
- leukocytes 135
- neutrophil 151
polymyalgia rheumatica 134
polymyositis 133
polymyxin B sulfate 135
polyneuropathy
- chronic inflammatory demyelinating 45
poly-p-dioxanone suture 130
polypeptide
- associated complex, nascent 115
- factors of thymus, low-molecular 76
- pituitary adenylate-cyclase-activating 127
polyphosphate 135
- kinase 136
polyposis
- adenomatous 21
- familial adenomatous 73
polyposis coli
- adenomatous 21
polyps
- nonneoplastic 118
polyradiculoneuropathy
- acute inflammatory demyelinating 18
polysaccharide
- egg antigen 130
- pachyman 136
- polyvalent pneumococcal 136
- vaccine, hemophillus influenzae type B 83
polysomnography 138
polysubstance abuse 138
polytetrafluoroethylene 131, 139
polyunsaturated
- fatty acids 140
polyurethane 140
- segmented 156
polyvalent
- pneumococcal polysaccharide 136
polyvinyl
- alcohol fixative 140
pontine
- myelinolysis, central 50
pool
- readiliy releasable 145
pooled
- normal plasma 134
poor
- progesterone surge 136
poorly
- differentiated lymphocytes, nodular 119
- differentiated lymphocytic lymphomas, diffuse 129
- differentiated lymphocytic lymphomas, nodular 129
- differentiated malignant mesothelioma 129
- nourished 134
popliteal 135
- pterygium syndrome 136
- vein transplant 140
popliteus tendon 135
porcine
- brain natriuretic peptide 128
- somatotropin 139
porous
- alumni 18
- alumni (ceramic), hydroxyapatite coated 83
- apatite ceramics 127
portal
- hypertension 132
- triad occlusion 139
- vein 140
- vein thrombosis 140
- vein, diameter 62
Porta-Neb Sidestream jet nebulizers 135
portosystemic
- pressure gradient 136
- shunt, transjugular intrahepatic 162
- stent shunts, transjugular intrahepatic 162
position
- natural head 117
positional
- vertigo, benign paroxysmal 34
positive 135, 180
- airway pressure, continuous 50
- end airway pressure 130
- end-expiratory pressure 25, 131

- indices 132
- mental attitude 134
- or negative 180
- predicitive value 136
- pressure 135
- pressure breathing 50
- pressure breathing, intermittent 93
- pressure respiration, intermittent 93
- pressure ventilation device 136
- pressure ventilation, intermittent 93
- pressure, inflation with oxygen, intermittent 93

positron 65
- emission tomography 131

possible 135, 180

possibly
- significant 180

post 127
- anesthesia care unit 127
- anesthesia recovery unit 128
- cenam 128
- chemotherapy nausea and vomiting 135
- coital bleeding 128
- exponential growth 130
- exposure prophylaxis 131
- herpetic neuralgia 132
- infusion nausea and vomiting 135
- liver transplantation 133
- menopausal 133
- menopausal bleeding 134
- meridian 133
- mitotic cells 133
- mortem 133
- mortem interval 134
- nasal 133
- natal day 134
- necrotic liver cirrhosis 134
- operative 135
- operative care 135
- operative day 135
- operative nausea and vomiting 135
- operative(ly) 135
- ovulatory 135
- ovulatory day 135
- oxygen consumption, excess 70
- partum 135
- partum hemorrhage 136
- partum psychiatric syndromes 136
- partum resumption interval 137
- partum sterilization 136
- partum thyroiditis 136
- partum tubal ligation 136
- perfusion syndrome 136
- pericardiotomy syndrome 136
- polio syndrome 136
- prandial 135
- prandial blood sugar 136
- prandial bood sugar 128
- prandial plasma glucose 136
- pump syndrome 136
- radiosurgical imaging 137
- recurrence induction 137
- remission intensification 137
- sophomore fellow 138
- splenectomy infection, overwhelming 124
- stimulus time histograms 139
- streptococcal glomerulonephritis 138
- surgical, prosthetics, immediate 93
- synaptic potential, excitatory 70
- synaptic potential, inhibitory 94
- synaptic potentials, depolarizing inhibitory 60
- transfusion hepatitis C 139
- transplant lymphoproliferative disorder 139
- traumatic osteoarthritis 139
- traumatic stress disorder 139
- void residual 140

posterior 135
- axillary line 127
- cerebral artery infarction 128
- cervical 128
- cervical fusion 129
- chamber intraocular lens 129
- cruciate ligament 129
- descending artery 129
- fascicular block, left 101
- hemiblock, left 101
- interosseous artery 132
- interosseous nerve 133
- longitudinal ligament, ossification 124
- lumbar fusion 133
- myocardial infarctions 134
- occiput 121, 123
- right occiput 144
- spinal fusion 138
- spinous process 139
- superior iliac spine 139
- tibial artery pulse 139

postero
- anterior 127
- anterior (x-ray) 127
- inferior cerebellar artery 133
- lateral 133
- lateral interbody fusion 133

postural orthostatic tachycardia syndrome 135

posture
- relaxed resting 145

potassium 97
- chloride 97
- hydroxide 97
- iodide 97
- iodine, saturated solution 157

potency
- level, mouse 111

potential
- acuity meter 127
- antidromic 21
- corneal-retinal 51
- cortical somatosensory evoked 53
- difference (in volts) 168
- energy 130
- excitatory postsynaptic 70
- inhibitory postsynaptic 94
- life lost, years 177
- oxidation-reduction 125
- rivalry-related 145

- short latent evoked 153
- sphenoidal evoked 156
potentials
- brain stem auditory evoked 34
- depolarizing inhibitory postsynaptic 60
- motor evoked 106
- motor unit action 113
- reaction related 145
- somatosensory cerebral evoked 157
- spinal somatosensory evoked 156
- visually evoked 173
potentiating
- paired stimulation 136
potentiation
- long-term 102
potentiel évoqué visuel (french) 131
pouch
- conduit, aorto-pericardial 22
pound 98
pound(s) 99
pounds 180
- per square inch 139
powder 129, 140
powdered
- extract 130
power
- motion imaging 134
- ratio index 137
- respiratory-related 145
p-phetiylenediamine 123
practical
- incidence estimators 133
- normal value 135
- nurse 134
- nurse, licensed 101
practice
- cost index, geographic 82
- general 81
- good clinical research 78
- good laboratory 79
- management companies, physician 136
- nurse, vocational 174
- standards, professional 136
practices
- good pharmacy 82
practitioner
- general 81
- nurse 119
practitioners
- advanced nurse 20
- neonatal nurse 118
Prader-Willi syndrome 140
prealbumin
- tryptophan-rich 164
preamplification
- primer-extension 131
precipitate 179
precipitated
- alum 21
precursor
- protein, Alzheimer amyloid 22
- protein, beta amyloid 28
- uptake 22
prediabetes
- genetic 81
prediabetic
- obstetric 123
prediction
- index, obliteration 123
predictive
- value, negative 119, 135
- value, positive 136
prednisone
- methotrexate, doxorubicin, cetoposideyclophosphamide, cytarabine, bleomycin, vincristine, methotrexate 138
preeclampsia 130
preejection
- to ejection time 131
preexcitation 130
preferred
- Health Network 132
prefix 181
- for multiple 135
prefrontal cortex 131
pregastricin 131
pregnancy 82
- acute fatty liver 15
- ectopic 70
- first 138
- induced hypertension 133
- intrauterine 95
- intrauterine term 95
- prevention program 136
- rapid repeat 145
- risk assessment monitoring system 137
- risk category 137
- specific beta-1-glycoprotein 156
- term 163
- term intrauterine 162
- test, plasma 136
- test, urinary 171
- urine 140
- voluntary interruption 173
prehospital
- trauma life support 132
preinoculation 137
preinstallation
- maintenance 133
preleukemic
- syndrome, primary acquired 136
preliminary
- anatomic diagnosis 127
prelingual
- deafness, nonsyndromic 120
premarital
- residential independence 137
premature
- adrenarche, idiopathic 93
- atrial contraction 127
- beat, atrial 21
- contraction, atrial 21
- contraction, junctional 96
- contractions, ventricular 174
- junctional contraction 133
- rupture of membranes 138
- ventricular beat 140
- ventricular contraction 140
prematurity
- retinopathy 144
premenstrual
- dysphoric disorder 134
- experiences, calendar of 50
- syndrome 134
- tension syndrome 134

prenatal
- care 134
- environmental stress 131
- psychological stress 136
- vitamins 135
preoperative 137
preoperative(ly) 137
preoptic
- area, anterior hypothalamic 16
- area, medial 111
preparation 137
prepare as 137
prepare for 137
preprotachykinin B 136
preputial
- separation 136
prereduced
- anaerobically sterilized 137
preresponse
- interval 137
prescription 140
- (L. recipe) 149
presenile
- dementia (Alzheimer) 129
- dementia of Alzheimer type 129
- vascular dementia 140
present 180
- complaint 128
- evaluation 130
- illness 132
- illness, history 87
- symptoms 138
presentation
- breech 34
- vertex 175
presenting
- problem 135
preservation
- reperfusion injury 137
pressure 127
- airway, biphasic intermittent positive 32
- and temperature, normal 119
- aortic 21
- arterial 21
- arterial blood 10
- atmosphere, chemical ionization 21
- brachial artery 28
- brachial artery, mean 28
- center of 49
- cerebrospinal fluid 54
- change 181
- colon anastomosis bursting 39
- diastolic 62
- diastolic ventricular 64
- distal airway 56
- equalization 130
- equalization tube 131
- intracranial 90
- intraocular 93
- jugular venous 97
- left atrial 98
- management indicator 134
- neck vein 135
- of oxygen 135
- on expiration 130
- opening 123
- osmotic 181
- positive 135
- positive end airway 130
- positive end-expiratory 131
- positive, breathing 50
- product, rate 145
- pulmonary artery 128
- pulmonary artery diastolic 127
- pulmonary artery end-diastolic 127
- pulmonary artery occluded 127
- pulmonary artery occlusive 128
- pulmonary artery systolic 128
- pulmonary artery wedge 128
- pulmonary capillary wedge 129
- pulmonary wedge 140
- reduced renal perfusion 145
- relief index 137
- resting venous 149
- right ventricular 149
- saturated 24
- self-administered positive expiratory 156
- self-controlled positive end-expiratory 25
- systolic 156
- venous 174
- ventilation device, positive 136
- ventilation, intermittent positive 93
- zero end-expiratory 177
pre-study site visit 139
presumed 180
presumptive
- eligibility 130
preterm
- nonthrombocytopenic 121
preterm labor 139
pretibial myxedema 139
prevention
- marketing initiative 134
preventive
- care group 129
previous
- menstrual period 134
- myocardial infarction 134
pricing
- system, prospective 136
primary 137, 181
- acquired preleukemic syndrome 136
- biliary cirrhosis 128
- brain lymphoma 128
- care evaluation of mental disorders 138
- care extender 138
- care physician 129
- cell culture 128
- cell cultures, liver 101
- central nervous system lymphoma 129
- cerebral lymphoma 129
- chronic adrenal insufficiency 128
- closure, delayed 62
- cutaneous lymphoma 129
- effusion lymphoma 131
- hyperparathyroidism 132

lx

- lymphoplasmacytic lymphoma 133
- malignancy, occult 124
- mediastinal B-cell lymphoma 134
- monkey kidney 134
- progressive aphasia 135
- progressive multiple sclerosis 136
- pulmonary hypertension 136
- sclerosing cholangitis 138
- tumor, extent 159
primase 138
primate
- chorionic gonadotropin 129
primates 137
prime
- operating system 138
primed
- lymphocyte tests 133
primer
- extension preamplification 131
primidone 137
primipara 138
primiparity 138
primitive
- neuroectodermal tumor 134
primordial germ cell 131
primosome
- assembly site 128
prinedil 137
printed
- circuit board assembled 128
prion protein 138
prior
- births 128
- to admission 139
- to admission medication 139
- to arrival 139
- to exposure 130
prism
- down, base 31
pristane
- isoprenoid 137
Pristinamycin 137
private
- duty nurse 129
- medical doctor 134
- physician 135
privately owned vehicle 135
pro re nata 138
probable
- error 130
problem-
- based learning 128
- intervention-evaluation (system) 133
- oriented medical record 135
- solving therapy 139
procalcitonin 129
procedure
- comprehensive renal scintillation 51
- debridement and drilling 57
process
- analytic hierarchy 16
processing
- rapid information 144
- regulated ubiquitin/ proteasome-dependent 148
proctology 137
produced by 179
produces 179
product 127
- fross 81
- of conception 135
- of Rb gene 137
- rate pressure 145
product of Rb gene
- phosphorylated 137
production
- cell bank 128
- index, reticulocyte 145
productive 138
products
- fibrin degradation 74
- fibrin(ogen) degradation 75
- of incomplete combustion 133
professional
- engineer 130
- practice standards 136
- shortage area, health 87
- team physicians 139
ProFile
- Ni-Ti rotary instruments 137
profile
- behavior activity 28
- hematology 84
- length, functional 75
- of Mood States 134
- velocity/time 174
progenitor
- cell, granular 82
- cells, hematopoietic 87
- cells, peripheral blood 128
progesterone 70
- receptor 132
prognosis 138, 140
prognostic
- index, international 93
prognostically high-risk sites for malignant melanoma 28
program
- evaluation 130
- pregnancy-prevention 136
- psychosocially enhanced treatment 131
programmed cell death 129
programs
- designated driver 58
progress record 137
progressing 179
progression
- free survival 131
- geometric 81
progressive
- aphasia, primary 135
- Deterioration Scale 130
- disease 129
- general paralysis 132
- multiple sclerosis, chronic 50
- multiple sclerosis, primary 136
- muscular atrophy 134
- renal insufficiency 137
- resistance exercises 137
- retinal atrophy, x-linked 176
- spinal muscular atrophy 139
- subcortical gliosis 138
- systemic sclerosis 139
progressively
- transformed germinal centers 139

projection
- filtered back 73
- maximum intensity 108
- neuron, thalamic 163
projects
- in controlled environments 138
prolactin 138
- release inhibiting hormone 138
prolaps
- mitral valve 114
prolapse
- recurrent rectal 145
prolapsed
- intervertebral disc 133
proliferating cell nuclear antigen 129
proliferation
- index 97
- index, osteoblastic 123
- rate index 137
proliferative
- acute 21
- glomerulonephritis, diffuse 62
- index 156
- unit, epidermal 70
proliferator
- activated receptor-alpha, peroxisome 136
- activated receptor-gamma, peroxisome 136
- peroxisome 136
proline 127, 138
- codon 40, 41, 42
prolonged
- mechanical inspiration 134
- reversible ischemic neurologic deficit 138
prolymphocytic leukemia 133
promoter
- membrane ovalbumin under the control of the rat insulin 144
- rat insulin 144
- region, proximal 137
promyelocytic
- leukemia 134
- leukemia protein 134
pronation 138
pronator 138
prophylaxis 138
- postexposure 131
proportional
- error 130
- to 181
proportionate to 180
proprioceptive neuromuscular facilitation 134
propylthiourcil
- antithyroid drug 139
prospective
- payment system 62, 136
- pricing system 136
prostacyclin 132
Prostaglandin 131
prostaglandin 131
- E 131
- E1 131
prostate 138
- benign hypertrophic 32
- malignancy index 134
- message, testosterone-repressed 164
- specific acid phosphatase 12
- specific antigen 138
- symptom score, Danish 56
prostatectomy
- radical retropubic 145
- transurethral 167
- transurethral ultrasound-guided, laser induced 167
prostatic 138
- acid phosphatase 128
- acid phosphatase, total serum 165
- hypertrophy, benign 34
prosthesis 138
- blood vessel 37
- threaded titanium acetabular 166
prosthetic
- flow, diastolic peak velocity 64
- immediate postsurgical 93
protamine
- Hagedorn, neutral 119
- zinc insulin 140
protease
- inhibitor 132
- inhibitor, barley alkaline 28
- inhibitor, secretory leukocyte 153
- inhibitors 137
protection
- factor, assigned 22
- relative rest, ice, compression, elevation 137
- relative rest, ice, compression, elevation, modalities, medication 137
- rest, ice, compression, elevation, support 137
protective
- device, electrosensitive 71
- dose 50 % 129
- equipment, personal 136
- services, children's 50
protein 138
- A, surfactant 156
- alpha-transducing, guanine nucleotide-binding 80
- bactericidal permeability, increasing 34
- Bence Jones 33
- beta amyloid precursor 28
- binding, competitive 50
- bound iodine 128
- C, activated 21
- capsid 50
- cartilage matrix 51
- cell wall 55
- chymotrypsin-like 47
- coat 50
- complex, dystrophin-associated 56
- C-reactive 50, 51
- cross-reacting 51
- cyclic AMP receptor 51
- derivative (of tuberculin), purified 136
- dystrophin associated 56
- energy malnutrition 131
- enhanced green fluorescent 69

- equivalent of total nitrogen appearance 134
- glial fibrillary acidic 78
- green fluorescent 78
- guanine nucleotide-binding 80
- intake 137
- invasion plasmid antigens 93
- kinase, death-associated 56
- monocyte chemoattractant 105
- mouse double minute 105
- mouse ribosome receptor 111
- mouse urinary 113
- multidrug resistance 111
- neurofilament 116
- nitrogen appearance rates, normalized 119
- nuclear FMRP-interacting 121
- nuclear RNA-binding 119
- nutritional value 135
- plasma 181
- plasma fractional 136
- plasma substitute 136
- prion 138
- promyelocytic leukemia 134
- receptor related 145
- receptor-interacting 144
- regA-regulated 145
- response, unfolded 171
- retinol-binding 142
- rhomboid-related 145
- ribosome receptor 145
- ribosome-inactivating 144
- transition 163
- tyrosine kinases 139

proteinaceous
- infectious particle 138

proteinase 3 137

proteins
- GTPase-activating 77

proteinuria
- Bence Jones 33

proteoglycan 131

proteolysis
- regulated intramembrane 144

proteolytic
- activity, thrombo 163

protestant 138

prothrombin time 138, 139

protocol 138
- resident assessment 142

protonic
- magnetic resonance (analysis) 134

protoporphyrin
- free erythrocyte 74

prototype
- digital x-ray 65

proximal 179
- convoluted tubule 129
- femoral focal deficiency 131
- interpalangeal 133
- interphalangeal joint 133
- promoter region 137, 138
- radioulnar joint 138
- radioulnar ligament 138
- row carpectomy 137
- straight tubule 139
- straight tubules 139

pruritic
- urticarial papules and plaques of pregnancy 140

pseudo 181

pseudoexfoliation 130

pseudogene
- glutamate dehydrogenase 79

pseudogout 131

pseudomembranous
- colitis, antibiotic-associated 6

Pseudomonas
- exotoxin 130

pseudostratified
- ciliated columnar epithelium 128

pseudovaginal
- perineoscrotal hypopospadias 136

pseudoxanthoma
- elasticum 140

psittacosis
- lymphogranuloma-trachoma group viruses 133

psoas
- minor muscle 134

psoriatic diatheses 129

psych scale
- inpatient multidimensional 92

psychiatric 181
- rating, brief 34
- syndromes, postpartum 136

psychiatry 139
- adolescent 21

psychiatry and neurology 134

psychogenic nonepileptic seizures 134

psychokinesis
- recurrent spontaneus 147

psychological
- stress, prenatal 136

psychomotor retardation 134

psychopathy
- Resemblance Index 137

psychophilic
- marine bacterium 9

psychosis
- monosymptomatic hypochondriacal 107

psychosocially
- enhanced treatment program 131

psychotic 138

psychrophilic
- marine bacterium 173

pterygium
- syndrome, popliteal 136

public
- health nurses 132
- Health Nursing 132
- Health Nutrition 132
- Responsibility in Medicine & Research 138

pubococcygeus 129

pulmonary
- arteries, intralobar 93
- artery 127
- artery (systolic) pressure 128
- artery diastolic pressure 127
- artery end-diastolic pressure 127
- artery occluded pressure 127
- artery occlusive pressure 128
- artery pressure 128

- artery systolic pressure 128
- artery wedge pressure 128
- artery, left 101
- aspergillosis, chronic necrotizing 49
- aspergillosis, invasive 93
- capillary wedge 129
- capillary wedge pressure 129
- disease 129, 140
- disease, chronic obstructive 50
- disease, chronic restrictive 51
- disease, diffuse 62
- edema 130
- embolism 130
- embolus 130
- emphysema, chronic 50
- emphysema, chronic obstructive 50
- function tests 131
- HTN 132
- hypertension 132
- hypertension, obliterative 123
- hypertension, primary 136
- infiltration with eosinophilia 133
- intensive care unit 133
- stenosis 138
- stenosis, peripheral 136
- thromboembolism 139
- vascular resistance 140
- venous congestion 140
- wedge pressure 140

pulmonic
- heart sound, second 127
- insufficiency 132

pulsation
- ascending aorta, synchronized 7

pulse 127
- amperometry, integrated 93
- apical 21
- blood volume 37
- deep 62
- dorsalis pedis 62
- jugular venous 97
- markedly impaired 181
- moderately impaired 181
- normal 181
- oximeter, oxygen saturation 157
- oximetry 135
- per second 136
- rate 137
- separation time 139
- slightly impaired 181
- volume recorder 140

pulseless
- electrical activity 130

pulses
- distal 62
- nerve net 118

pulsus paradoxus 135

pulvinar 140
- medial 140
- posterior-lateral complex 140

puncture
- lumbar 101

pupillary
- defect, relative afferent 142
- distance 129
- light reflex 133

pupils
- equal and reactive to light 130
- equal, reactive to light + accommodation 131
- equally round and reactive to light 131
- equally round and reactive to light and accommodation 131
- round, regular and equal 138

pure
- red cell aplasia 137
- red cell aplasia caused by parvovirus B19 34

purified
- protein derivative 136

Purkinje fibers 131

purpura
- autoimmune thrombocytopenic 24
- Henoch-Schönlein 87

purpuric
- eruption, persistent pigmented 136

push
- fluids 131
- intravenous 95

pyelogram
- intravenous 95
- retrograde 144, 145

pyelography
- rapid-sequence intravenous 146

pyloric-gland mucin 113

pyoderma
- gangrenosum, peristomal 136

pyrexia of unknown origin 140

pyridoxal
- isonicotinoyl hydrazone 133

pyrogenic
- exotoxin 130

pyrogens
- endogenous 70

pyropoikilocytosis
- hereditary 87

pyrrolidine
- dithiocarbamate 130

Q

QT syndrome
- long 101

quadrant
- abdomen, left 100
- abdomen, right upper 148
- left inner 100
- left lower 179
- left outer 101
- left upper 179
- left upper, outer 102
- lower 101
- lower right 101
- right lower 179
- right upper 179
- upper left 171
- upper right 172

quadrants
- both lower 33
- both upper 36

quadriplegic 141

quality
- adjusted life year 140

- assurance 140
- control 140
- control, instrument 94
- improvement, continuous 50
- level, acceptance 22
- of life 141
- of life, health-related 87

quantitative 141
- autoradiography 140
- autoradiography, in vitro 95
- computed tomography 140
- coronary angiography 140
- muscle testing 141

quantity 141
- not sufficient 141
- sufficient 141

quantum
- libet 141
- vis 141

quaque 140
- in die 141
- quarta hora 141

quart 141
question
- of 180

questionable 180
questionnaire
- behavior style 35
- Parkinson's disease 129

questions
- frequently asked 73

quiet 141
quotient
- brain-age 29
- glucose oxidation 81
- respiratory 145

Q-wave
- myocardial infarction 141

R

rabbit
- kidney 144
- limbal epithelial 144
- liver esterase 144
- serum albumin 146

rabies
- immunoglobin, human 87

radial 142
radiating to 179
radiation
- absorbed dose 142
- death, oral 124
- dose, absorbed 56
- dose, indicative 60
- dose, nominal absorbed 115
- optic 124
- related pericardial effusion 145
- safety officer 146
- therapy 142, 176
- therapy, cranial 51
- therapy, external 70, 176
- treatment planning 148

radical retropubic prostatectomy 145
radioactive
- iodine metaidobenzoguanidine 107
- iodine uptake 142

radioactive iodine 88
radiocarpal joint 142
radiofrequency ablation 143
radiogram
- chest 50

radiography
- cervical spine 51, 54

radioimmunoassay 143
- coated tube 54
- double-antibody 56

radioimmunoimaging 144
radioimmunoprecipitation 144
radioimmunosorbent
- test,paper 138

radiologic
- technologist 147

radiological
- sciences unit 147

radiology
- diagnostic 62
- interventional 95
- interventional vascular 95

radionuclide ventriculography 144, 149
radioscaphoid 145
radioscapholunate
- ligament 146

radiosensitivity test 147
radiotelemetry 147
radiotherapy 142, 147, 176
- cranial 51
- dedicated computed tomography 148
- hyperfractionated 85
- intensity-modulated 92
- intraoperative 93
- thoracic 164

radioulnar
- joint, distal 63
- joint, proximal 138
- ligament, proximal 138
- ligaments, distal 63

radium 142
radium therapy 147
radon
- transform, diffraction 62

rainbow
- trout gonadal tissue cells 148

raised 179
raising
- test, straight leg 153

Rancho Los Amigo Scale 144
random
- control trial 147
- response technique 145
- sample 145

randomized
- controlled trial 142

randomly
- bred White Carneau pigeons 142

range
- normal 121
- of motion (of joint) 144
- of motion, active 23
- of motion, active assertive 7
- of motion, active assisted 7
- of motion, full 76
- of motion, full free 74
- of motion, full joint 75
- of motion, normal 119
- of motion, resistive 145
- of movement, full 76

rape
- oilseed 126
- treatment center 147

rapid
- alternating movements 142
- atrial fibrillation 142
- eye movement 143
- fluorescent focus inhibition test 143
- information processing 144
- plasma reagin 145
- repeat pregnancy 145
- sequence induction 146
- sequence intravenous pyelography 146
- sequence intubation 146
- shallow breathing index 146
- spin-echo 146
- tranquilization 147
- urease test 148
rapidly progressive glomerulonephritis 145
rare earth elements 143
rat
- biobreeding 29
- biobreeding/Worcester 30
- insulin promoter 144
- kidney, isolated perfused 93
- liver epithelial cells 144
- lung epithelial cells 144
- spleen cell 146
- stomach strip 147
rate
- age-adjusted incidence 5
- contraceptive prevalence 50
- inspiratory flow 91
- mutation 181
- of outflow 124
- peak expiratory flow 131
- pressure product 145
- responsive pacing/ pacemakers 145
- single chamber 5
rating
- brief psychiatric 34
- instrument, performance 137
- of medication influences scale (psychiatry) 144
- scale, behaviorally anchored 29
- scale, brief Carroll depression 30
- scale, Burks' behavior 30
- schedule 145
ratio 180
- albumin/globulin 15
- basal acid output to maximal acid output 28
- benefit/cost 30
- blood urea nitrogen/creatine 36
- contrast-to-noise 49
- glucose/nitrogen 79
- index, power 137
- lecithin/shingomyelin 102
- nucleocytoplasmic area 116
- odds 124
- of fat area 143
- ventilation-perfusion 174
- vessel-to-tissue noise 174
rats
- Dahl salt-resistant 63
- inbred strains 20
- nagase analbuminemic 115
- naples random-bred 119
- Naples-High Excitability 117
rauwolfia
- serpentina 145
raw rock phosphat 145
ray tracing algorithm 147
Raynaud
- syndrome 145
reabsorption
- index, phosphate 137
react to light and accommodation 148
reaction 149
- acid 180
- active avoidance 7
- adverse drug 14
- alkaline 180
- antigen-antiglobulin 7
- antihyaluronidase 16
- cerebrospinal fluid-Wassermann 54
- chain, ligase 99
- graft vs. host 83
- related potentials 145
- reversible 179
- time 147
- time, choice 51
- time, complex 51
- time, discriminative 62
- time, disjunctive 62
- times 148
- to degeneration 142
reactive
- airway disease 142
- amyloidosis 5
- lysis, membrane inhibitor 108
- oxygen species 144
reactivity
- digital vascular 64
- index, platelet 137
readily releasable pool 145
readiness
- test, device 62
reading
- frame, open 124
- test 147
reagin
- rapid plasma 145
- screen test 147
real time scan 148
recalcification
- time, blood-activated 29
recall
- delayed word 65
receiver operating curve analysis 144
receptor
- (o)estrogen 124
- agonist, opiate 124
- alpha-peroxisome proliferator activated 136
- alpha-retinoic acid 142
- beta-adrenergic 29
- colony-stimulating factor 54
- gamma-peroxisome proliferator activated 136
- glutamate 79
- gonadotropin-releasing hormone 80
- homing 86
- human oestrogen 86
- intracellular 94
- mitochondrial diazepam binding inhibitor 105
- PACAP I 137

- peripheral, benzodiazepine 37
- plasma cell membrane 43
- potential channel proteins, transient 164
- potential, transient 164
- progesterone 132
- related protein 145
- retinoid 149
- signal sequence 157
- steroid and xenobiotic 159
- tyrosine kinase 148
receptor-interacting protein 144
recessive
- nephrolithiasis, X-linked 176
recipe 149
recipient's serum 145
reciprocating
- gait orthosis 143
- tachycardia 147
- tachycardia, atrioventricular 27
reclassification sensitivity 145
recognition
- mutual 111
recombinant
- human bone morphogenetic protein 143
- ribosomal P 145
- tissue plasminogen activator 148
- tumor necrosis factor 148
recombinase-activating gene 1/2 142
recombination
- meiotic sister-chromatid 111
- sister-chromatid 150
recommended
- daily intake 142
- dietary allowance 142
reconditioning exercise 143
reconstruction
- anterior capsulolabral 11
- images, three dimensional (surface) CAT scan 57
- latissimus dorsi flap 99
- technique, simultaneous multiple angle 155
record
- electronic medical 69
- emergency drug identification 68
- hospital 87
- problem orientet medical 135
recorder
- pulse volume 140
recovery
- in vivo 95
- room 145
- time, corrected sinus 54
recreational
- therapist 148
- therapy 147
rectal 141, 143, 148
- examination, digital 62
- pressure, resting 145
- prolapse, recurrent 145
- sinus 145
- suction biopsy 146
- suppository 145
- temperature 142, 147
rectosigmoid 145
rectosigmoidoscopy 147
rectum 143
- abdominal perineal resection 21
rectus
- lateral 101
- medial 111
rectus muscle 143
recurrence
- induction, post 137
recurrent
- aortic occlusions 142
- depression, unipolar 171
- disease, no evidence 116
- rectal prolapse 145
- respiratory papillomatosis 145
- sinus barotrauma 146
- spontaneous psychokinesis 147
recursive partitioning analysis 145
red
- blood cell 142
- blood cell, morphologic index 142
- blood cell, ox 124
- blood cell, turnover rate 148
- blood cells, nucleated 119
- blood cells, packed 137
- blood cells/count 142
- blood count 142
- blood per rectum, bright 34
- blood, bright 34
- cell aplasia caused by parvovirus B19, pure 34
- cell distribution width 143
- cells, volume packed 174
- pulp 144
redistribution
- intramolecular vibrational energy 95
- pattern, reverse 145
redox potential 66
reduced
- glutathione 82
- renal perfusion pressure 145
- vascular response 149
reducing substance 145
reduction
- and cast, closed 50
- and fixation, open 124
- and percutaneous fixation, closed 51
- closed 50
- external fixation, open 124
- open 124
- program, restraint 145
- test, copper 51
- time 147
Reed-Sternberg cell variants 100
Reed-Sternberg cells 145
reentrant
- atrioventricular junctional 27
- tachycardia, atrioventricular 27
reentry
- atrioventricular nodal 27
- intraventricular 96
- tachycardia, atrioventricular node 27
refer to 43

reference lumen diameter 144
refill
- time, capillary 51
reflectance
- index, photochemical 137
reflex
- asymmetrical tonic neck 24
- Bezold-type 35
- biceps tendon 36
- conditioned 50
- inhibiting pattern 144
- light 101
- normal plantar 179
- oculocephalic 122
- sympathetic dystrophy 146
- sympathetic dystrophy syndrome 146
- triceps 162
reflexes
- average 181
- brisk 181
- low normal 181
- very brisk 181
reflux
- disease, gastroesophageal 78
- duodenogastric 59
- gastroesophageal 81
- hepatojugular 85
- index, venous 174
refractory
- anemia 142
- anemia with excess blasts 142
- cytopenia with multilineage dysplasia 142
- period, absolute 23
- period, atrioventricular 27
- period, atrioventricular node functional 27
- period, effective 70
- period, relative 145
refuse/s medical assistance 144
regarding 143
regA-regulated protein 145
regimen
- intravenous 96
region
- complementarity-determining 43
- gene, immunoglobulin variable 91
- I, variable 174
- left iliac 100
- modified synaptonemal complexes 112
- of interest 144
- proximal promoter 137, 138
regional
- anesthesia, intravenous 96
- cerebral blood flow 142
- lymph node metastasis 114
- oxygen saturation 146
- thresholding, dynamic 62
- trauma center 147
- wall motion 149
regions
- scaffold/matrix attachment region 155
register
- physical therapy 145
registered 148
- dietician 142
- health information administrator 143
- health information technician 143
- nurse 144
- nurse practitioner 22
- trademark 148
registrar 143
regression
- syndrome, caudal 51
regular 143
- rate and rhythm 145
- rate and rhythm, heart 87
- sinus rhythm 147
- spiking activity 146
- uterine contraction 148
regular(ly) 143
regulated intramembrane proteolysis 144
regulated ubiquitin/proteasome-dependent processing 148
regulation
- isovolumetric 96
regulator
- antiviral 27
- antiviral repressor 27
- cell matrix adhesion 48
regulators
- response 145
regulatory volume decrease 149
regurgitation
- mitral 111
rehabilitation 143
- index, vocational 174
- program, coronary 51
- registered nurse, certified 51
rehydrated
- hemoccult 86
rehydration
- oral 124
- solution, oral 125
- therapy, oral 125
reinforcement
- brain stimulation 35
reinforcing
- stimulus 146
Reiter
- syndrome 146
relapse free survival 143
relapsing
- pancreatitis, chronic 51
- remitting multiple sclerosis 145
related to 147
relation
- occlusion, centric 48
relations
- technique, object 125
relationship
- structure-activity 149
relative
- afferent pupillary defect 142
- biological effects 142
- fluorescence index 143
- humidity 143
- refractory period 145
- rest period 145
- retention time 145
- risk 145
- slow sinus rate 147
- specific activity 146
- standard accuracy 146
- standard deviation (Srel) 146
- standard mortality rate 146

- stimulus 146
- survival rate 147
relatively resistant to penicillin 145
relaxation
- isovolumic 96
- of immunity, periparturient 136
- time 181
- times 148
relaxed
- resting posture 145
- skin tension lines 147
- vaginal outlet 149
relaxing
- factor, endothelium-derived 68
release 143
- carpal tunnel 54
- endoscopic carpal tunnel 68
- sustained 157
- test, chromium 51
released
- in vitro 95
releasing
- factor, growth hormone 79
- incisions, mandibular lingual vertical 109
relief
- nurse, disaster 62
REM behavioral disorders 142
remaining lifetime fracture probability 144
remission
- complete 50
- continuous complete 42
- good partial 82
- partial 136
remitting
- multiple sclerosis, relapsing 145
- seronegative symmetrical synovitis with pitting edema 147
removable silicone plug 146
removal
- agent, mycoplasma 111
- of drain 144
- of sutures 144
renal
- blood flow 142
- disease, atheroembolic 22
- disease, end stage 71
- failure 143
- failure index, UNa/(UCr/PCr) 143
- failure, acute 22
- failure, chronic 51
- failure, dosage adjustment 56
- failure, end stage 71
- function, residual 145
- hypertensive disease 143
- insufficiency, chronic 51
- insufficiency, progressive 137
- monoclonal immunoglobulin deposition disease 108
- perfusion pressure, reduced 145
- phosphorus threshold, theoretical 164
- plasma flow 145
- plasma flow, contralateral 51
- scintillation procedure, comprehensive 51
- specialist 146
- tomography, computerized 51
- transplant, cadaveric 51
- transplantation 147
- transplantation patient 148
- tubular acidification defect 147
- tubular acidosis 147
- tubular cell 147
- tubular defect 148
- tubular necrosis 148
- vein thrombosis 149
renin
- activity, peripheral 137
- activity, plasma 137
renin-angiotensin system 142
repair 143
- of sublethal damage 146
repeat 143
- higher-order 86
- once if urgent 156
repeat-induced point mutation 144
repeats
- inverted 96
- long terminal 102
repetition
- strain injury 146
- time/echo time 164
repetitions 143
repetitive
- transcranial magnetic stimulation 148
rephasing
- gradient motion 80
replacement
- aortic valve 27
- double valve 64
- mitral valve 114
- therapy, dopamine 62
- therapy, enzyme 70
- therapy, estrogen 70
- therapy, hormone 87
- therapy, nicotine 119
- therapy, testosterone 164
- tricuspid valve 167
replication error 143
replication initiation point 144
report
- incident 94
repressor
- regulator, antiviral 27
reproductive
- health 143
reprojection
- intermediate view 95
required 143
requisition
- clinical materials 49
re-replacements 145
rescue
- peripheral stem cell 138
research
- health outcomes 86
- orthopedic 124
- practice, good clinical 78
resection
- bilateral carotid body 30
- gastric 82
- of bladder tumor, transurethral 167
- of bladder, transurethral 167

- of the prostate, transurethral 167
- of the rectum 21
- submucous 155
- transurethral 167

residence times 148

resident
- assessment protocol 142
- legal advisor 144
- surgical officer 146

residential
- treatment center 147

residual
- capacity, functional 76
- limits, maximum 111
- post-void 140
- renal function 145
- tumor after treatment 141
- volume of lung 148

resin
- T3 uptake 148
- uptake 148

resistance 141
- active 22
- basal skin 35
- exercises, progressive 137
- high outlet 86
- index, vascular 174
- laryngeal 144
- low outlet 101
- nasal airflow 119
- respiratory 145
- systemic 145
- total 147
- transfer 147
- transfer factor 148
- unit, respiratory 145

resistant
- multi drug 105
- to penicillin, relatively 145

resistive
- index 143
- range of motion 145

resonance
- electron spin 71

resorption
- stimulating activity, osteoclast 125

resource utilization groups 148

respiration 141, 143
- artificial 22
- assisted 22
- frequency 76
- intermittent positive pressure 93

respiratory 143
- bronchiolotis interstitial lung disease 142
- care unit 142
- compliance, static 37
- control index 142
- control ratio 142
- dependent pacemakers 143
- disease 142
- disease, acute 22
- disease, bovine 34
- disease, chronic 51
- disease, upper 171
- distress 142
- distress syndrome 143
- distress syndrome, acute 22
- distress syndrome, adult 22
- distress syndrome, infant 94
- distress, no apparent 115
- disturbance index 142
- failure, acute 22
- failure, acute hypoxemic 16
- inductance plethysmography 144
- infection, acute viral 27
- infection, viral 174
- insufficiency, perinatal 137
- inversion, point 137
- quotient 145
- rate 145
- rate, tidal volume ratio 149
- related power 145
- resistance 145
- resistance unit 145
- resistance, total 164
- syncytial (virus) 146
- syncytial virus 147
- system, compliance 51
- therapist 147
- therapists 148
- therapy 147
- therapy technician, certified 52
- tract fluid 148
- tract infection 148
- tract infection, lower 102
- tract secretions 148
- tract, lower 102

responder
- medical first 106

response
- audiometry, auditory brainstem 10
- audiometry, evoked 70
- brain stem auditory evoked 28
- complete 50
- cortical somatosensory evoked 53
- double ventricular 64
- eyes, motor, verbal 70
- frequency following 74
- long-latency 100
- no 181
- partial 136
- regulators 145
- regulators, genes encoding 145
- stimulus 157
- task, discriminative 62
- task, empathy 70
- technique, random 145
- time 147
- time, diffusional 62
- to stimulus 146
- unconditioned 169
- visual evoked 173

rest
- ice, compression, and elevation 144
- in peace 144
- tremor 147

rested state contraction 146

restenosis
- target site 165
- target vessel 167

restin 146

resting
- metabolic rate 144
- rectal pressure 145
- subject 146
- venous pressure 149

restless legs
- periodic leg movements during sleep 144
- syndrome 144
restraint reduction program 145
restricted 179
restriction
- enzyme from bacillus amyloliquefaciens H 28
- enzyme from Escherichia coli 68
- enzyme from haemophilus aegyptius 83
- enzyme from haemophilus influenzae Rd 85
- enzyme from Nocardia otitidis-cavarium 118
- enzyme from Staphylococcus aureus 3A 149
- enzyme from streptomyces stanford 158
- factor, homologous 87
- fragment length polymorphism 143
- site mutation 146
restrictive
- pulmonary disease, chronic 51
result
- checked 45
- non significant 120
resulting from 179
results in 179
resumption
- interval, postpartum 137
resuscitation
- bystander cardiac pulmonary 37
- cardiopulmonary 50
- no cardiac 116
retardation
- alpha-thalassemia-mental 24
- mental 111
- psychomotor 134
retarded 148
retention
- Index, pharyngeal 137
- time 23
- time ratio 148
- time, corrected 51
reteplase 145
reticular
- nucleus, dorsal 62
reticulated siderocyte 146
reticulo
- cyte, production index 145
- cyte, standard buffer 146
- endothelial system 143
- endotheliosis virus 143
- histiocytosis, congenital self-healing 54
reticulum
- cell sarcoma 142, 146
- cells, fibroblastic 76
retinal
- necrosis, bilateral acute 29
- pigment epithelium 145
- schiff base 146
- vein occlusion, central 52
- vein, central 52
retinoblastoma gene 142
retinoic
- acid receptor-alpha 142
- acid.all-trans 24
retinoid
- receptors 149
retinol-binding protein 142
retinopathy
- diabetic 62
- of prematurity 144
retinoschisis 146
retransformation 147
retrieval
- heat induced epitope 85
- sonication-induced epitope 152
retrograde
- cholangiopancreatography, endoscopic 70
- pyelogram 144, 145
- refractory period 145
- urethogram 148
retrolental fibroplasia 144
retroperitoneal gasless
- balloon-assisted, endoscopic 32
retroperitoneal hematoma 145
retropharyngeal
- soft tissue space 147
Rett syndrome 146, 148
return
- to clinic 147
- to office 148
revascularization
- direct myocardial 61
- percutaneous transmyocardial 139
- target lesion 163
- target vessel 167
- transmyocardial 163
reverse
- redistribution pattern 145
- transcriptase 147
- transcriptase assay 147
- transcriptase inhibition 148
- transcriptase inhibitors, nucleoside analogue 119
- transcriptase polymerase chain reaction 148
- transcriptase, polymerase chain reaction 148
- transcriptase-producing (agent) 148
- transcriptases 148
- transcription 147
- triiodothyronine, rT3 147
reversible
- chemical reaction 179
- ischemic neurologic deficit 144
- radical pair model 145
- reaction 179
- sickle-cell 146
review
- board, institutional 94
- of symptoms 144, 146
- of systems 144
revised
- trauma score 148
- trauma scores 148
Reye syndrome 146
rhabdoid
- tumor of the kidney 148
rhesus
- (monkey) factor 143
- factor, negative 143

- factor, positive 143
- rotavirus vaccine-tetravalent 145
rheumatic
- factor 143
- fever 22, 143
- heart disease 143
rheumatism
- aute articular 7
rheumatoid
- arthritis 142
- arthritis, joint space 96
- factor 143
rhomboid-related protein 145
rhyme
- task, dichotic 62
rhythm
- accelerated ventricular 27
- atrioventricular junction 27
- idioventricular 95
rhythmic
- theta (waves), diffuse 62
riboflavin 143
ribonuclease
- inhibitor, placental 137
ribonucleic acid 144
ribonucleotide
- aminoimidazole carboxamide 17
ribose 143
ribose-5-phosphatase 146
riboside
- uric acid 169
ribosomal P, recombinant 145
ribosome receptor protein 145
ribosome-inactivating protein 144
ribothymidine 147
Richter's
- syndrome 146
ricinus
- communis agglutinin 142
rickets
- sex-linked hypophospbatemic 153
ridging
- intervascular 95
right 141, 147
- anterior oblique 142
- arm sitting 142
- atrial appendage pacing 142
- atrial enlargement 142
- atrial pressure 142
- atrium 142
- axis deviation 142
- bundle branch block 142
- bundle-branch block 94
- circumflex 142
- coronary artery 142
- costal margin 142
- ear 13
- ear-bone conduction threshold 180
- eye 122, 143
- eye, vision 174
- frontoanterior 143
- frontoposterior 143
- frontotransverse 143
- heart failure 143
- hepatic artery 143
- hypertrophia 143
- inguinal hernia 144
- lateral 144
- lateral (L) 147
- leg 144
- lower extremity 144
- lower lobe (lung) 144
- lower quadrant 179
- lower quadrant (abdomen) 144
- lung 144
- mediolateral 144
- mentoanterior 144
- mentoposterior 144
- mentotransverse 144
- middle lobe (lung) 144
- occiput anterior 144
- occiput posterior 144
- occiput transverse 144
- otitis media 144
- quadrant, lower 101
- sacroanterior (fetal position) 146
- sacrolateral (fetal position) 146
- sacroposterior (fetal position) 146
- sacrotransverse (fetal position) 147
- sacrum 146
- salpingo-oophorectomy 146
- scapuloanterior (fetal position) 146
- scapuloposterior (fetal position) 146
- septum 146
- side 146
- somatosensory evoked potential 146
- stellate (ganglion) 146
- sternal border 146
- subclavian 146
- subclavian artery 146
- subclavian vein 147
- substantia nigra 146
- superior oblique (muscle) 146
- superior rectus (muscle) 147
- superior vena cava 147
- thigh 147
- toe off 148
- toestrike 148
- upper lobe (lung) 148
- upper quadrant 179
- upper quadrant (abdomen) 148
- ventricle 148
- ventricle diastolic collapse 149
- ventricle myocardial infarction 149
- ventricular assist system 149
- ventricular dysplasia, arrythmogenic 23
- ventricular failure 149
- ventricular failure, congestive 52
- ventricular hypertrophy 149
- ventricular pressure 149
- ventricular volume, total 164
rigidity 15
ring
- biofragmentable anastomosis 29
- intravaginal 96
Ringer
- lactate 144

- solution 146
rising 179
risk
- category, pregnancy 137
- factor 143
- ratio 145
- relative 145
- screening model 146
risks
- against all 7
risperidone 144
rivalry-related potential 145
RNA
- dependent RNA polymerases 145
- III-inhibiting peptide 144
- messenger 111
- polymerases, RNA-dependent 145
RNase
- inhibitor, placental 137
road traffic accident 147
roasted soybeans 146
Roberts syndrome 146
Rocky Mountain spotted fever 144
rod
- gram-negative 80
- intramedullary 92
roentgen 141
- ographic stereogrammetric analysis 146
- per second 145
Roman
- numbers 183
room
- air 142
- air oxygen saturation 142
- temperature 147
root
- breadth, nasal 119
- dorsal 62
- ganglion, dorsal 62
- inducing plasmids 137
- mean square 144
Rorschach Mutuality 110
Rosenberg
- Self-Esteem Scale 146
rostral ventrolateral medulla 149
rotation
- and extension, external 72
- external 70
- in extension, external 70
- in extension, internal 94
- in flexion, external 70
- in flexion, internal 94
- internal 94
- lower trunk 102
- optical 181
- phase-cycled, B1-independent 32
rotatory
- dispersion, optical 124
- instability, antero-lateral 19
Rothmund-Thomson syndrome 148
round
- regular, and equal 145
round the clock 147
RoundupReady* oilseed rape 145
Rous
- sarcoma 146
- sarcoma virus 147
routine
- admission chemistry 154
- maintenance 144
- test dilution 148
- urinalysis 148
Roux-Y choledocho-jejunostomy 149
row
- carpectomy, proximal 137
rT3 reverse triiodothyronine 147
rub 141
rubber
- ethylene propylene diene 70
- latex, natural 119
- styrene butadiene 150
rubella
- syndrome, congenital 51
Rubinstein
- Taybi (syndrome) 147
- Taybi syndrome 148
rubrospinal tract 147
rubs 106
rubs, gallops, murmurs 143
rule
- of thumb 144
- out 144
rule-out myocardial infarction 144
rumination
- time, daily 62
rupture
- of membrane, spontaneus 157
- of membranes 144
- of membranes, artificial 23
- of membranes, premature 138
Russell-Silver syndrome 147
Russian
- spring-sununer encephalitis 147

S

sacralization 98
sacroanterior
- (fetal position), right 146
sacroiliac joint 151
sacrolaeva
- anterior 152
- posterior 153
- transversa 154
sacrolateral
- (fetal position), right 146
sacroposterior
- (fetal position), right 146
sacrotransverse
- (fetal position), right 147
- left 154
sacrum
- anterior, lateral 102
- anterior, left 102
- posterior, left 102
- right 146
- transverse, left 102
sad, hostile, anxious, frustrating, tenacious syndrome 151
sadomasochism 154

safe
- medical devices act (of 1990) 155
- ozone 125

safety
- occupational 125
- officer, radiation 146

saiboku-to
- a herbal preparation 162

saiko-keishi-to
- herbal medicine 162

salicylic acid 149

saline 149
- normal 120
- solution, normal 121
- volume expansion 158

salivary
- gland carcinoma 151

salivation
- lacrimation, urination, defecation 154
- lacrimation, urination, defecation, gastrointestinal upset, emesis 154

salmonella-shigella agar 157

salpingo-oophorectomy
- bilateral 35
- left 102
- right 146

salt
- diet, normal 120
- resistant rats, Dahl 63
- sensitive, Dahl 63
- solution, balanced 35
- solution, buffered 35

samarium 154

sambucus nigra agglutinin 155

same as 179

sampling
- chorionic villous 55
- connections, modified 112
- devices, passive 138

saphenofemoral bypass 151

saphenous
- vein graft 159
- vein, aortocoronary 13
- vein, aortocoronary bypass graft 13
- vein, dog 63

sarcolemma 152

sarcoma
- cell, Moloney 112
- endometrial stromal 71
- Kaposi's 18
- Karposi 97
- mast cell 105
- oncogene, viral simian 174
- osteogenic 125
- reticulum cell 146

satellite
- cells, muscle 112

saturated
- fatty acids 151
- solution of potassium iodine 157

saturating
- dose, single 157

saturation
- oxygen 121, 125
- room-air oxygen 142
- transferrin 164

Sauve
- Kapandji (procedure) 152

scaffold/matrix attachment regions 155

scalded skin syndrome 157

scale
- hospital anxiety and depression 83
- Progressive Deterioration 130
- Rancho Los Amigo 144

scalp 28
- current densities 150

scan
- hepatobiliary 85
- ventilation/perfusion 174

scanning
- automatic computerized transverse axial 13
- calorimeter, photo differential 132
- calorimetry, differential 63
- electron microscopy 151
- electron microscopy, low-voltage 103
- laser acoustic microscope 153
- liquid ionization chamber 153
- optical 124

scapho
- capitate 150
- lunate 152
- lunate advanced collapse (wrist) 153
- lunate interosseous ligament 153
- trapezial 158
- trapezo-trapezoidal 158

scapulo
- anterior (fetal position), right 146
- posterior (fetal position), right 146

scar
- skin viroid, apple 24

scatter
- correction, multiplicative 112
- separation, multi angle polarised 104

scavengers
- oxygen radical 125

schedule
- for affective disorders and schizophrenia 97

scheduling
- clinic 52

scheme
- youth exchange 177

schiff
- base, retinal 146

schizophrenia 150, 159
- chronic 52

Schwann
- cell line, mouse 112
- cells, myelin-forming 112
- cells, nonmyelinating 118

science
- clinical behavioral 39

scientific
- manpower commission 155

scientist
- clinical laboratory 52

scintigraphy
- cerebral 52

sclerosing
- cholangitis, primary 138
- leukoencephalopathy 152

lx

- panencephalitis, subacute 157
sclerosis
- amyotrophic lateral 19
- anterolateral 19
- nodular 120
- progressive systemic 139
- systemic 157
- transverse spinal 165
- tuberous 164, 165
sclerotherapy
- endoscopic 70
scoliosis
- adolescent idiopathic 18
score
- French Society of Arthroscopy 151
- Glasgow outcome 81
- manual function 106
- motor age 110
- muscle 112
- pain rating intensity 137, 138
scrape
- endocervical 68
- endometrial 69
screen
- film angiography 151
- test, reagin 147
screening
- detected breast cancer 149
- high throughput 87
- test, bacteriuria 35
- test, thromboplastin 166
screw
- placement, variable 174
seasonal
- schizo-affective DO 149
second 44, 151, 180
- compartment volume 172
- degree 181
- pulmonic heart sound 127
- sound, aortic 5
secondary 181
- leukemia 152
- lymphoid organ chemokine 153
- myelodysplastic syndrome 155
- myelofibrosis 155
- thyroid carcinoma 158
- to 179
secretion
- bronchial 34
- conjunctival 52
- respiratory tract 148
secretory
- component, membrane 111
- leukocyte protease inhibitor 153
section
- breast tumor frozen 35
- frozen 76
- transverse 164, 165
sectional
- area, ovarian 125
sedation
- conscious 52
sedentary
- normotensive 120
sedimentation
- rate 151, 157
- rate, blood 35
- rate, erythrocyte 71
- rate, zeta 177
segment
- length 152
- length, anterior 152
- length, inferior 152
- length, lateral 153
- length, septal 152
- long-spacing 153
segmental
- limb systolic pressure 153
segmented polyurethane 156
seizure 159
seizures
- psychogenic nonepileptic 134
selected mucosal biopsy 155
selective
- bronchial brushing, transtracheal 165
- lymphoid irradiation 153
- noradrenaline reuptake inhibitor with 5-HT3 receptor blocking action, new 105
- serotonin reuptake inhibitor 157
self
- administered positive expiratory pressure 156
- controlled positive end-expiratory pressure 25
- evaluation (questionnaire), clinical-symptom 53
- examination, breast 34
- examination, testicular 165
- healing reticulohistiocytosis, congenital 54
- monitored blood glucose 155
- monitoring 154
semi
- circular, modified 112
seminal
- vesicles 151
seminal vesicle epithelium 158
sendai virus envelopes 158
Sendai viruses 151
senile
- dementia of Alzheimer's type 150
- macular choroidal degeneration 155
- macular degeneration 155
senior house officer 151
sensation 149, 151
sensation level 152
sensitive 149
sensitivity
- colchicine 46
- contact 52
- diagnostic 63
- function 53
- index, international 94
- multiple chemical 105
- oubain 125
- reclassification 145
sensor
- optical position 124
sensory 151
- aphasia, transcortical 165
- cortex, motor 112
- deficit, functional 76
- latency 152
- latency, terminal 165
- perception, decreased 63
sensu lato 152

sentinel
- lymph node 153
- lymph node biopsy 153
separation
- immunomagnetic 92
- multi angle polarised scatter 104
- preputial 136
- time, pulse 139
sepsis
- catheter-related 51
septal
- defect, atrial 23
- defect, atrioventricular 27
- defect, interventricular 96
- defect, ventricular 174
- deformity, nasal 120
- hypertrophy, asymmetrical 23
- leaflet 152
- occluder, Amplatzer 23
- perforator compression 156
- velocity, diastolic 63
septic
- abortion 151
- complications, major 112
septostomy
- balloon atrial 29
septum
- cholinergic, medial 112
- complex, medial 112
- right 146
sequence
- cryptidin-related 51
- differential upstream 64
- tag, expressed 71
sequencing
- auditory vocal 27
sequential
- compression device 150
- multichannel autoanalyzer 154
- multiple analysis 154
- multiple analysis in-six different serum tests 154
- multiple analyzer 154
- multiple analyzer computer 154
- ventriculo-atrial pacing 158
serial line interface protocol 153
series
- acute abdominal 7
- gallbladder 77
- upper gastrointestinal 171
serin
- protease inhibitors 151
serine 149, 151
- codon 10, 15
serious
- adenocarcinoma, ovarian papillary 124
- adverse event 149
serological
- test 151
- test for syphilis 158
serology 151
séroneutralization 155
serotonin
- reuptake inhibitor, selective 157
serratia marcescens 154
serum 149
- a -fetoprotein, maternal 111
- albumin, bovine 34
- albumine, human 87
- antihuman lymphocyte 16
- antihuman thymus 17
- antirat thymocyte 25
- antitetanus 25
- antithymocyte 25
- bilirubin, total 165
- chemistry value, critical 53
- cholesterol 44
- corticosterone 42
- creatinine 150
- fetal calf 73
- gamma- glutamyl transpeptidase 151
- globulin, immune 94
- glutamic-oxalacetic transaminase 151
- glutamic-pyruvic transaminase 151
- guinea pig anti-insulin 81
- hepatitis 151
- inhibition factors 152
- iron 151
- lactate dehydrogenase 153
- leucine aniinopeptidase 153
- lipophosphoprotein 153
- methyl alcohol level 155
- myoglobin 155
- protein electrophoresis 156
- protein, total 165
- radioallergosorbent test 142
- vitamin E 158
service
- blood transfusion 36
- emergency medical 69
- outpatient 124
- social 157
services
- children's protective 50
severe
- aphasia, boston assessment 29
- combined immunodeficiency disease 150
- myoclonic epilepsy 155
- torso injury 158
severity
- of burns 180
- of wounds 180
sewage sludge ashes 157
sex
- chromosome, female 176
- chromosome, male 176
- hormone binding globulin 151
- limited protein 153
- linked hypophospbatemic rickets 153
sexual
- intercourse, unprotected 171
- maturity ratings 155
- size dimorphism 157
sexuality 84
sexually
- transmitted disease 158
seychelles child development study 150
SGOT 24
shaded-surface display 157
shape
- comparison, molecular 112
shear
- vertical 174

sheath
- carotid 52
- periarteriolar lymphocyte 127
sheep
- erythrocyte antibody 153
- Nairobi, disease 120
sheffield child development study 150
shell
- vial assay 158
- vial assay-indirect immunofluorescent assay 158
Shieh-Qing-Wan 157
shift
- dose, night 120
- value, diethylamine 63
shock
- cardiogenic 52
- index 151
- syndrome, dengue 63
- therapy, insulin 95
- wave lithotripsy, extracorporeal 71
short
- bowel, congenital 53
- latent evoked potential 153
- leg (brace) 152
- leg brace 153
- leg cast 153
- leg cylinder cast 153
- leg nonwalking cast 153
- leg non-weight bearing cast 153
- leg splint 153
- leg walking cast 154
- luteal phase 153
- michigan alcoholism screening test 155
- TRPC 158
- wave diathermy 159
shortage
- area, health professional 87
shortening
- fraction, left ventricular 103
shortness
- of breath 156
- of breath on exertion 149
sho-saiko-to
- a herbal medicine 162
- go-keishi-ka- shakuyakuto 162
shoulder
- arthroplasty, total 165
- disarticulation 150
show racer pigeons 157
shows 179
shunt
- arteriovenous 27
- bidirectional Glenn 32
- distal splenorenal 63
- fraction 141
Shwachman-Diamond syndrome 150
Shwartzman local reaction 153
Shy-Drager syndrome 150
sialadenitis
- focal lymphocitic 76
sialoadenitis
- myoepithelial 106
Sibley-Lehninger (unit) 152
sibling 152
sick
- euthyroid syndrome 151
- sinus syndrome 157
sickle
- cell 150
- cell crisis 150
- cell disease 150
- cell diseases 150
- cell, reversible 146
sickness
- decompression 57
side
- branch occlusion (in coronary artery stenting) 150
- scatter (flow cytometry term) 157
- -to-side duodenoplasty 157
siderocyte
- reticulated 146
sides
- both 32
sievert 158
sight
- loss 101
sigmoid 181
signal
- detectability, theory 165
- detection 150
- level 152
- microembolic 106
- nuclear localization 118
- recognition particle 157
- regulatory proteins 152
- sequence receptor 157
- transducers and activators of transcription 158
- transduction, tyrosine kinase 177
significant 180
- change, minimum 112
- other 155
- possibly 180
- villous edema 159
signs
- and symptoms 149, 157, 158, 159
- and symptoms (also SAS) 157
- vital 174
silastic
- catheters, multipurpose 112
silica glass powder 151
silicone
- microphysiometer 154
- plug, removable 146
- prosthesis, intraocular 94
- rubber, low viscosity 103
silver
- stain, gomori methenamine 80
simian
- sarcoma proto-oncogene 152
- vacuolating virus no. 40 158
- virus 158
similar 180
simple mastectomy 154
simultaneous
- laryngoscopy and abdominal thrusts 153
- multichannel autoanalyzer 154
- multiple angle reconstruction technique 155
- stimulation, double 63
sin nombre virus 155

since 180
Sinding Larsen (syndrome) 152
sine 149
single
- cell liquid cytotoxic assay 153
- lens reflex 153
- limb support 153
- lung transplantation 154
- nucleotide polymorphism 155
- photon emission computed tomography 156
- photon emission tomography 156
- saturating dose 157
- strand damage (DNA) 157
- substrate, buffered 35
- supernumerary teeth 157
- twitch response (EMG) 158
- twitch stimulation (EMG) 158
- use diagnostic system 158
- vision, binocular 35
sinoatrial 149
- node 149
sinus
- barotrauma, recurrent 146
- carcinoma, maxillary 112
- carotid 52
- coronary 52
- flow, coronary 53
- of valsalva aneurysms 158
- rate, relative slow 147
- recovery time, corrected 54
- rectal 145
- rhythm, normal 120
- rhythm, regular 147
- superior sagittal 158
- tachycardia 158
- transverse 164
sister
- chromatid exchange 150
- chromatid recombination 111, 150
site
- nucleotide-binding 115
- primosome assembly 128
- support center, investigative 95
sitogluside 35
sitting
- right arm 142
size
- and shape, normal 121
- dimorphism, sexual 157
- of tumor in staging cancers 159
Sjogren-Larsson
- (syndrome) 152
- syndrome 153
skeletal 152
skilled nursing facility 155
skim milk 154
skin
- cancer, non melanoma 118
- fold thickness, tricipital 166
- fold triceps 165
- graft, full thickness 77
- graft, split thickness 158
- prick test 157
- response, sympathetic 157
- signs, warm, pink, dry 176
- temperature 164
- temperature, palmar 139
- tension lines, relaxed 147
- test antigen, toxoplasmin 166
- test dose 158
- test, tumor 166
- viroid,apple scar 24
- wound breaking strength 175
SK-SD streptokinase-streptodomase 152
skull
- base osteomyelitis 150
- pin head holder, Mayfield 106
SLDH 153
sleep
- apnea syndrome, obstructive 125
- apnea, obstructive 125
- attacks 149
- deprivation 150
- deprivation, no 120
- light fragment 100
- related breathing disorders 157
- related hallucinations 157
- time, total 166
- transitional 164
sleepiness
- excessive daytime 68
slide
- latex agglutination 153
slip
- of the upper femoral epiphysis (radiograph) 158
slipped
- capital femoral epiphysis 150
slips made out 155
slit
- lamp 152
- lamp examination 153
slope
- descriptors, normalized 120
slow
- sinus rate, relative 147
- twitch red (skeletal muscle) 158
- wave activity 159
small 154
- animal 154
- bowel follow through series 150
- bowel follow-through 155
- bowel obstruction 150
- bowel syndrome, contaminated 53
- bowel, contaminated 53
- cell lung cancer 150
- cleaved cell lymphomas, follicular 76
- for-gestational age 151
- intestinal disease, immunoproliferative 94
- intestinal mucinous antigen 152
- intestinal submucosa (hernia repair) 152
- intestine allotransplantation, total 165
- lymphocyte 152
- lymphocytic lymphoma 47, 153
- volume expansion 159
smart
- card, medical 112
Sm-C 155
smear 154

- Papanicolaou 128
Smith
- (antigen) 154
- Lemli-Opitz syndrome 153
- Magenis chromosome region 155
smoke
- environmental tobacco 71
- evacuator, disposable 63
- less tobacco 154
smoker
- cigarette 52
- current 52
smooth
- muscle 154
- muscle activating factor 154
- muscle antibody 154
- muscle cell 155
- muscle contracting agent 155
- muscle myosin heavy chain (gene 16p13) 114
snap
- opening 125
soap suds enema 157
social
- acceptability scale of occlusal conditions 149
- history 151
- security disability 157
- service 157
- services, department of 63
- worker 159
- worker, children 54
- worker, licensed clinical 99
socioeconomic status 151
sodium 114, 156
- bicarbonate 115
- chloride 115
- dialysate, normal 120
- dodecyl sulfate-polyacrylamide gel electrophoresis 151
- fractional excretion 74
- hornan 115
- lactate 152
- nitroprusside 118, 155
- N-methyl dithiocarbamate 155
- tetrathionate 115
soft
- tissue infections 158
- tissue injuries, multiple 113
- tissue lateral neck 158
- tissue mobilization 158
- tissue space, retropharyngeal 147
software 159
- for statistical analysis of correlated data 158
soleus muscle 156
solid
- logic technology 154
- waste, municipal 113
solidified liquid 152
solitary
- myofibroma(tosis) of the skin 155
soluble
- liver antigen 153
- membrane attack complex 154
solution 156
- boric acid 29
- glucose-saline 82
- modified Hank balanced salt 107
- oral rehydration 125
somatic
- cell, milk 112
somatogravic illusion 151
somatomammotropin
- A, chorionic 53
- chorionic 52
somatomedin
- (insulin-like growth factors) 154
- A 154
- C 155
- C/insulin-like growth factor 155
somatomedin C 155
somatosensory
- cerebral evoked potentials 157
- evoked potential, cortical 53
- evoked potential, right 146
- evoked potentials 157
- evoked response 157
- evoked response, cortical 53
somatostatin 157
- like immunoreactivity 153
somatostatin-
- like immunoreactivity 153
somatotropin 158
- porcine 139
- release-inhibiting factor (somatostatin) 157
sonic
- accelerated fracture healing system 149
sonication-induced epitope retrieval 152
sonogram 156
sonography
- duplex doppler 58
- emergent abdominal 67
sonohysterography 151
soon 23
sorbitol
- deshydrogenase 150
- MacConkey agar 154
sorting
- test, object 126
sound
- aortic first 5
- level 152
- level meter 153
sounds
- bowel 34
- breath 34
source
- data verification 151
- delivery unit 151
- skin distance 157
- surface distance 157
south african territories 149
soybean
- inhibitor, Bowman-Birk 30
- meal 150
- oil 150
- phosphatidylcholine 156
soybeans
- roasted 146
space
- gas chromatography, head 87
- medicine 154

spastic
- paraparesis, tropical 165
spatial disorientation 150
special
- assessment examination, orthopaedic 125
- care unit 150
- supplemental food program for women, infants, and children 175
specialist
- (physician) 149
species
- reactive oxygen 144
specific
- absorption rate (MRI) 149
- activity, relative 146
- gravity 151, 156
- immunotherapy 23
- macrophage arming factor 154
- not 120
- pathogen-free 156
specimen
- (urine), clean voided 47
- lipemic, unable to perform 102
spectral
- analysis, computerized 53
- assay, compressed 53
spectrometric
- method, enzymatic 70
spectrometry
- mass 78, 111
spectrophotometry
- atomic absorption 7
spectroscopy
- near infrared 117
- phosphorous-31 nuclear magnetic resonance 118
- surface enhanced laser desorption/ionization mass 151
speech
- sound discrimination 157
speech and hearing 156
sperm
- count, motile 112
- injection, intracytoplasmic 90
S-phase fraction 156
sphenoidal evoked potential 156
spherocytosis
- hereditary 87
sphincter
- anal 23
- lower esophageal 99
- upper esophageal 170
sphingomyelin 154
sphingosylphosphorylcholine 156
spike
- complexes, migrating 112
- frequency adaptation 151
spiking
- activity, regular 146
spin
- density, normalized 120
- echo (MRI) 151
spinal 156
- chord stimulation 150
- cord 156
- cord injury 150
- cord injury without radiologic abnormality 150
- cord intensive care unit 150
- cord, mouse 112
- fluid 156
- fusion, anterior 23
- fusion, posterior 138
- muscular atrophy 154
- muscular atrophy, progressive 139
- nucleus, lateral 102
- paralysis, acute atrophic 7
- sclerosis, transverse 165
- somatosensory evoked potentials 156
- stenosis, lumbar 102
- surgery, minimally invasive 108
spindle
- epithelial tumor with thymus-like differentiation 151
- frequency activity 151
- shaped cells, malignant 112
spine 156
- anterior superior 24
- anterior superior, iliac 23
- cervical 52, 54
- dorsal 63
- lumbar 102
- posterior superior, iliac 139
- radiography, cervical 54
- thoracic 63
spin-echo
- conventional 53
- rapid 146
spinocerebellar
- degenerations 150
spinous
- process, posterior 139
spiral
- fiber, outer 126
spirocheticidal
- concentration, minimum 112
spleen
- cells 156
- colony-forming units 44
splenectomized
- neonatally 121
splenic
- localization index 153
- macrophage 154
- vein, diameter 63
splenocytes
- mouse 112
splenomegaly
- syndrome, tropical 166
splenorenal
- shunt, distal 63
splint
- long leg 100
- short leg 153
split
- osteotomy, vertical sagittal 174
- thickness skin graft 158
Spodoptera frugiperda cells 151
spondylitis
- ankylosing 23
spondylometaphyseal
- dysplasia 155
spondylometaphyseal dysplasia 155
sponge 156

spongiform
- encephalopathy, bovine 34
- encephalopathy, zoological 177
spongiotic
- dermatitis, autosensitization 23
spontaneous 157
- abortion 149
- echo contrast 151
- lymphocyte-mediated cytotoxicity 153
- motor activity 154
- phasic contractions 156
- psychokinesis, recurrent 147
- rupture of membrane 157
- vaginal delivery 158
- vaginal delivery, normal 121
spontaneously
- hypertensive rats 151
sporocidal
- concentrations, minimal 112
sports
- medicine 154
- vision evaluations 159
spotted fever group 151
spreading
- melanoma, superficial 157
sprue
- celiac 52
- tropical 164
squamocolumnar
- junction 150
squamous 157
- cell carcinoma 150
- cell carcinoma antigen 150
- cell carcinoma, cutaneous 53
- cell carcinoma, oral 126
- cells, atypical 23
- cells, miniature 112
- intraepithelial lesion, high-grade 85
- intraepithelial lesion, low grade 102
- intraepithelial lesions 152
square
- centimeter 47
- deviations, sum 157
- root mean 144
squats with rebound 143
squats without rebound 119
St. Jude Medical 152
St.Louis
- encephalitis 153
- encephalitis virus 153
stability
- factor, cold 53
stabilization
- test, compost 50
stabilized
- liposomes 152
stable 179
- disease 150
- vital signs 174
stachybotrys
- microspora triprenyl phenol 155
staff 118
stage
- clinical 52
- of disease 158
staging
- cancers, size of tumors 159
stagnant
- loop syndrome 153
stain
- hematoxylin and eosin 84
- May-Grünwald-Giemsa 106
staining regions
- homogeneous 87
standard 158
- accuary, reletive 146
- buffer, reticulocyte 146
- clearance 37
- clinical criteria 150
- deviation 150, 181
- deviation units 151
- deviation, normalized 120
- deviation, relative 146
- dose, nominal 120
- electrode potential 66
- error of the mean 151
- method agar 154
- mineral base 155
- mortality rate, relative 146
- operating protocol 156
- test method, american 24
- unit, british 35
- valves, cordis 54
standardized
- incidence ratio 152
standards
- for medical device communication 155
standing
- foot angle 151
- order 155
standing vertical jump and reach 152
staphilococcus
- aureus 149
staphylococcal
- enterotoxin B 151
- enterotoxins 151
- scalded-skin syndrome 158
staphylococcus 158
- aureus 3A, restriction enzyme 149
- aureus, methicillin resistant 111
- aureus, methicillin-sensitive 113
- epidermis, methicillin-resistant 111
starch
- methylenedianiline 155
starter
- culture, meat 112
state
- children's health insurance program 150
static
- respiratory compliance 37
statistical
- analysis system 149
- mean 181
status
- cardiovascular 55
- clinical 52
- Karnofsky performance 97
- physical 138
- post 156
steady 72, 179
steatohepatitis
- nonalcoholic 115
steel (mouse) 151

Stein-Leventhal
- syndrome 152, 153
stellate
- right 146
stem
- cell factor 150
- cell rescue, peripheral 138
- cell transplant, peripheral 138
- cell transplantation 18
- cell, peripheral blood 128
- cell, pluripotential hematopoietic 132
- cells, mesenchymal 112
- temporal 164
stemline 152
stenosis
- aortic 23
- aortic valve 27
- idiopathic hypertrophic subaortic 91
- lumbar spinal 102
- mitral 111
- peripheral pulmonary 136
- pulmonary 138
- tricuspid 164
stents
- endoluminal colonic wall 68
step
- down latency 150
- down, number of 120
stepping
- digital subtraction angiography 150
stereotactic
- interstitial brachytherapy, computer-assisted frameless 38
sterile
- dressing, dry 63
- gauze, dry 63
- vaginal examination 159
sterilization
- postpartum 136
sterilized (media)
- prereduced anaerobically 137
sternal
- border, left 102
steroid
- and xenobiotic receptor 159
- contraceptive drugs 150
- injection, epidural 71
steroidogenic acute regulatory 158
stiatopallidonigral 157
stick
- finger 76
stillborn 149
stimulated cultures
- long-time 102
stimulating
- factor, granulocyte and macrophage colony 79
- factor, overgrowth 126
- hormone, corpus luteum 47
stimulation
- beta-adrenergic 29
- cervical 52
- double simultaneous 63
- electrical 70
- electrical muscle 69
- potentiating paired 136
- spinal cord 150
- transcranial electrical 161
- transcranial magnetic 163
- vibroacoustic 172
stimulator
- metabolic heat load 107
stimulus
- conditioned 52
- duration, critical 53
- reinforcing 146
- relative 146
- response 157
- therapy, brief 35
- unconditioned 170
stock
- master cell 105
stomach 158
- volume, total 166
stomatitis
- acute herpetic gingival 16
stone
- cholesterol 52
- kidney 97
storage
- cells, mantle 112
- container, cryogenic 53
strabismus
- divergent unilateral 64
straight
- leg raising (Lasègue) 153
- leg raising test 153
- tubule, distal 63
- tubule, proximal 139
- tubules, proximal 139
strain
- injury, repetition 146
strains
- of rats, imbred 20
strap
- chest 52
- over-the-shoulder 126
stratum corneum 150
streak
- virus, digitaria 63
strength
- concentrated 52
- current 52
streptococcus 158
- beta hemolytic 32
streptokinase 152
streptolysin 152
- O 153
streptomyces
- stanford, restriction enzyme 158
streptomycin 154
- dependent, conditionally 53
streptozotocin 158
stress 181
- ful vital events 159
- prenatal environmental 131
- prenatal psychological 136
- syndrome, medial tibial 113
- test, treadmill 166
stria
- terminalis, bed nucleus 33
striatonigral degeneration 155
stroke 55
- complete 52
- index 151
- unit, monitored 113
- volume 158
- volume echocardiography 158

- volume index 159
- volume, aortic valve 27

stromal
- cells, marrow 112
- hyperplasia, cortical 54
- sarcoma, endometrial 71

structural
- adjustment facility, enhanced 70
- or karyotypic anomalies, extra-cardiac 67
- unit, basic 35

structure-activity relationship 149

Strumpell-Marie
- (syndrome) 154

studies
- motor conduction 105
- nerve conduction 116

styrene butadiene rubber 150

sub cutis 158

subacute
- bacterial endocarditis 150
- sclerosing panencephalitis 157

subaortic
- stenosis, idiopathic hypertrophic 91

subarachnoid
- hemorrhage 149
- venous pressure, cerebral 53

subclavian 150
- artery, right 146
- right 146
- vein, right 147

subcortical
- gliosis, progressive 138
- ischemic vascular disease 152
- vascular encephalopathy 159

subcutaneous 150, 157, 158
- (sub cutis) 158
- adipose tissue, middle 112
- insulin infusion, continuous 54

subdural
- hematoma 150
- hematoma, chronic 54

subendocardial
- MI 151
- perioperative myocardial injury 157

suberate
- disuccinimidyl 63

subjective, objective assessment plan 156

subjects
- treated, all 24

sublentiform nucleus 153

sublethal
- damage 153
- damage repair 153
- damage, repair 146

sublingual 152, 158

subluxation
- of the patella 153

submandibular 154

submanubrial
- dullness 155

submaxillary 154
- mucin, ovine 126

submergence
- vehicle, deep 63

submucosa
- (hernia repair), small intestinal 152

submucous 154
- resection 155

submuscular
- aponeurotic system 155

subserosal
- cells, multipotential 112

substance
- abuse treatment, center 53
- body, isolation 34
- exophtalmos-producing 70
- P 156
- users 158
- vasoconstrictor 173

substances
- act, controlled 53

substantia
- nigra, right 146

substernal
- chest pain 157

substitute
- protein plasma 136

substraction
- angiography, digital 63

substrate
- buffered single 35

subtilisin
- inhibitor, barley alpha-amylase 29

subtract 180

subtraction
- angiography, stepping digital 150
- venacavography, digital 63
- venography, digital 63

subunit
- myosin-binding 104

succinate semialdehyde dehydrogenase 157

succinylmonocholine 155

suckling
- mouse 154
- mouse brain 155
- mouse, cataract agent 155

sucrose medium 154

suction
- biopsy, rectal 146
- method 154

sudan
- black 149
- black B 149

sudden
- cardiac death 150
- cardiac death syndrome 150
- death syndrome 157
- infant death syndrome 152

sufficient
- quantity 141

sufficient quantity 141

sugar
- blood, post prandial 136
- nucleotide 120

sugars
- total reducing 164

suggested 181

suggestive 180

suicide attempt 149

sulfamethoxazole 155

sulfate 156, 158

sulfisoxazole 159

sulfolobus solfataricus 157

sulfotransferases 158
- dehydroepiandrosterone 59

- monoamine-sulfating form 111
sulfur 181
- adenosylmethionine 149
sulphate
- Contin, morphine 112
sum
- of square deviations 157
sum of 181
summary 181
- dictated, discharge 63
- discharge 63
- of product characteristics 156
- of safety, integrated 95
sun protection factor 156
superficial
- femoral artery 151
- keratitis, chronic 54
- linear array 153
- musculo-aponeurotic system 155
- spreading melanoma 157
superior 158, 179
- cervical ganglionectomy 150
- labrum anterior posterior (lesion) 153
- laryngeal nerve 153
- limbic keratoconjunctivitis 153
- mesenteric 154
- mesenteric arterial conductance 154
- mesenteric artery 154
- mesenteric artery blood flow 154
- mesenteric artery embolism 154
- mesenteric artery occlusion 155
- mesenteric artery syndrome 155
- oblique 155
- rectus muscle 157
- sagittal sinus 158
- vena cava 158
- vena cava syndrome 158
superparamagnetic
- iron oxide MRI enhancement 156
supination 158
supplementary motor area 154
supply
- management, clinical 54
- room, central 54
support
- advanced life 19
- center, investigative site 95
- fixed arm 75
- for people with oral and head and neck cancer 157
- system, decision 63
supposed 180
suppository 158
- rectal 145
suppression
- test, dexamethasone 63
suppressor
- cells, myeloid 112
suprapubic 156
supraventricular 158
- arrhythmia 158
- ectopy 159
- extrasystole 159
- tachycardia 159
- tachycardia, paroxysmal 139, 140
surface
- antigen, hepatitis B 83
- area 149
- enhanced laser desorption/ionization mass spectroscopy 151
- immunoglobulins 152
- tension 181
surfactant
- extract, calf lung 47
- like activity 153
- protein A 156
surge (cycles)
- poor progesterone 136
surgeon
- oral 125
- orthopedic 125
surgery
- breast conservation 31
- cardiovascular 55
- colon and rectum 51
- computer assisted, minimally invasive 38
- conservative 52
- date 61
- minimal incision 108
- minimally invasive 108
- minimally invasive, spinal 108
- minor 111
- Mohs micrographic 109
- office 125
- open heart 122
- oral 125
- orthopaedic 125
- orthopedic 125
- outpatient 124
- plastic 138
- sinus, functional endoscopic 74
- thoracic 164
- trauma 164
- unit, ambulatory 24
- upper abdomen 169
surgical 158
- assistance, technical 165
- doctors, non 120
- intensive care unit 152
- microscope 154
- officer, resident 146
- wound infection 159
surrogate
- marker cost-efficacy 154
- mother 154
surveillance
- examinations 159
- scheme, suspected adverse reaction 149
- system, behavioral risk factor 34
survey
- national health interview 117
- youth risk behaviour 177
survival
- disease free 59
- event free 69
- failure-free 74
- overall 125
- progression free 131

lx

- rate, relative 147
- relapse free 143
- time, mean 113
- times, median 113

survivor
- long-term glioblastoma multiforme 102

susceptibility 149
- Coxsackie B3 virus 39
- does-dependent 150
- magnetic 181
- testing, antimicrobial 24

suspected
- adverse reaction 149
- adverse reaction surveillance scheme 149
- child abuse or neglect 150

suspended
- solids, total 166

suspension 158

sustained
- medication 154
- release 135, 157
- release, theophylline 166
- volume expansion 159

suture
- black silk 35
- cartilage, midpalatal 112
- removal 144

swallow
- barium 29

Swan-Ganz 151

swine
- fever 151
- fever, african 23
- fever, classical 53
- vesicular disease 158

switch
- valves, dual 63

Syh-Mo-Yin 155

Syh-Nih-San 155

symbol
- subtest, digit 63

sympathectomy
- bilateral upper, dorsal 36

sympathetic
- maintained pain 155
- nerve activity 155
- nervous system 155
- skin response 157

sympathomimetic
- activity, intrinsic 94

symptom 159
- complex, major 112

symptoms 154
- anticipatory nausea and vomiting 20
- B 28
- extrapyramidal 70
- no 5
- objective, assessment, and plan 156

synaptic
- currents, miniature 112
- membrane 154

synaptonemal
- complexes 150
- complexes region 112

synchronized
- pulsation, ascending aorta 7

synchronous
- cancer, multiple 112
- intermittent mandatory ventilation 152
- pacemaker 156

syncytial
- virus, respiratory 146

syncytiotrophoblast 158

syncytium
- inducing viral phenotype 152

syndrome
- acid aspiration 7
- acquired immunodeficiency 18
- acute coronary 13
- acute hemolytic uremic 17
- alveolar hypoventilation 16
- aseptic meningitis 19
- B27-arthritis-sacroiliitis-extra-articular features 29
- battered woman (or wife) 37
- blue diaper 31
- blue toe 36
- Brachmann-Cornelia de Lange 30
- bradycardia-tachycardia 36
- brown bowel 30
- cancer family 53
- carbohydrate-deficient glycoprotein 43
- carpal tunnel 54
- cervicobrachial 39
- cervico-dorsal 43
- chronic brain 39
- chronic fatigue and immune dysfunction 43
- contaminated small bowel 53
- culture-bound 39
- Dandy-Walker 65
- Dejerine-Sottas 63
- dengue shock 63
- fragile X 77
- frozen shoulder 76
- goodpasture 81
- hantavirus cardiopulmonary 84
- hemolysis, elevated liver enzymes, low platelets 84
- hemolytic uremic 87
- hereditary nonpolyposis colon cancer 86
- herniated disc 84
- high pressure neurologic 87
- infant respiratory distress 94
- infection-associated hemophagocytic 88
- intestinal obstruction from peritoneal bands 98
- irritable bowel 89
- mid-systolic click-late systolic murmur 112
- multiorgan dysfunction 110
- myelodysplastic/ myelproliferative 105
- myeloproliferative 111
- neuroleptic malignant 118
- Nijmegen breakage 115
- non-ketotic hyperosmolar 117
- obstructive sleep apnea 125
- oculo-reno-cerebellar 124
- of inappropriate antidiuretic hormone secretion 152
- of sudden death 157
- oligomenorrheic polycystic ovary 123
- organic mental 123

- osteoporosis-pseudolipoma 124
- photosensitivity, ichthyosis, brittle hair, impaired intelligence, decreased fertility 132
- polyneuropathy, organomegaly, endocrinopathy, monoclonal gammopathy, and skin lesions 135
- postural orthostatic tachycardia 135
- reflex sympathetic dystrophy 146
- restless legs 144
- Rubinstein-Taybi 147
- scalded skin 157
- Shwachman-Diamond 150
- Shy-Drager 150
- superior vena cava 158
- uveitis-glaucoma-hyphema 171
- uveitis-glaucoma-hyphema plus vitreous hemorrhage 171
- velocardiofacial 173
- virus-associated hemophagocytic 172
- Wilms' tumor, aniridia, genotourinary anomalies, and mental retardation 175
- Zollinger-Ellison 177

synergistic
- cytotoxicity, monocyte 112

synovial
- like interface membrane 153
- membrane 154

synovitis
- of the hip, transient 165
- pigmented villonodular 140
- with pitting edema, remitting seronegative symmetrical 147

synthetic
- amino acid 149
- glucose monomycolate 151
- latex gloves 153
- narcotic 111

syphilis 181
- (Latin lues) 98
- congenital 52
- serological test 158

system 159
- cardiovascular 55
- decision support 63
- disease, combined 53
- membrane anaerobic 104
- nervous 120
- phosphotransferase 139
- prime operating 138
- prospective-payment 62
- reticuloendothelial 143
- review 157
- sympathetic nervous 155

systemic
- arterial hypertension 149
- arterial oxygen saturation (%) 149
- arterial pressure oscillation 149
- arterial resistance 146
- blood pressure 150
- flow, total 165
- inflammatory response syndrome 152
- lupus erythematosus 153
- lupus erythematosus activity measure 153
- lupus erythematosus disease activity index 153
- mast cell disease 155
- mastocytosis 23, 154
- mastocytosis with associated clonal hematopoietic non-mast cell lineage disorder 155
- mastocytosis, indolent 94
- meningococcal disease 155
- resistance 145
- resistance, induced 95
- resistance, total 166
- sclerosis 157
- sclerosis, progressive 139
- to pulmonary collaterals 156
- vascular resistance 159

systems
- fixed-rate atrial single-chamber 5

systolic 159
- blood pressure 150, 179
- delay time index 151
- diameter, total end 161
- ejection murmur 151
- hypertension, isolated 94
- motion 154
- murmur 154
- pressure 156
- pressure, pulmonary artery 128
- pressure, segmental limb 153
- time intervals 158
- velocity, peak 139
- wall thickening 159
- wave, latent 152

T

T
- cell-activating molecule 161
- helper type 1 cell 161
- helper type 2 cell 161
- lymphocyte-associated antigen-4 (CD152), cytotoxic 54
- lymphocytes, cytotoxic 54
- suppressor (cell) 164

T helper cells
- functional subset 161

tablespoon 160

tablet 159
- triturate 166

tablets
- MS Contin 112

tachycardia 159
- artificial circus movement 11
- atrioventricular node reentry 27
- atrioventricular reciprocating 27
- atrioventricular reentrant 27
- automatic atrial 7
- multifocal atrial 104
- paroxysmal 139
- paroxysmal atrial 128
- paroxysmal supraventricular 139, 140

- paroxysmal ventricular 140
- polymorphic ventricular 140
- reciprocating 147
- sinus 158
- supraventricular 159
- syndrome, postural orthostatic 135
- ventricular 174

tachypnea
- transient 166, 167

tacrine hydrochloride 161
tactile
- tension 166
- threshold 166

tag
- expressed sequence 71

tail
- blood flow 160
- flick 161

Takayasu syndrome 164
talipes equinovarus
- congenital 54

tall-cell
- variant of papillary thyroid carcinomas 161

talus
- oblique 126

tamoxifen 159
tangential flow filtration 161
tangles
- neurofibrillary 117

tap water 167
tardive dyskinesia 161
target
- lesion revascularization 163
- organ damage 163
- site restenosis 165
- skin distance 165
- symptom evaluation scale 165
- value tailored apheresis 167
- vessel failure 167
- vessel restenosis 167
- vessel revascularization 167

tartrate
- resistant acid phosphatase 164

task
- discriminative response 62
- empathy response 70
- related unit 164

Tay-Sachs
- (disease) 164
- disease 165

T-cell
- attracting chemokine, cutaneous 54
- leukemia 24
- lymphoma, adult 24
- receptor 160
- receptor gene rearrangement (study) 160
- rich B-cell lymphoma 160
- translocation gene 166

TCR J beta 160
TdT-mediated-dUTP nick end labeling 167
team
- cardiac resuscitation 51

teaspoon 164, 165
technetium
- 99m 2-methoxyisobutylisonitrile 107
- sulfur colloid 165

technical
- assistance 159
- error measurement 161
- surgical assistance 165

technical components 160
technician
- automated defibrillator 14
- emergency medical 69
- operating room 125

technique
- coital alignment 38
- object relations 125

technologist
- radiologic 147

technology
- best available 29
- solid logic 154

tectobulbar
- pathway, intermediate 160

teeth
- single supernumerary 157

tegmental
- field, central 54

telangiectasia
- macularis eruptiva perstans 163

telemetry 161
telephone
- order 163

telethermography 166
tellurite
- taurocholate, and gelatin 166
- taurocholate, and gelatin agar 166

temperature 159, 161, 180, 181
- airway wall 160
- high brooding 85
- initial body 160
- interval 181
- mean peripheral 111
- normal 121
- normal brooding 119
- pulse, respirations 163
- rectal 142, 147
- skin 164
- wet bulb 167

temporal
- (beat-to-beat) variability of repolarization in amplitude 167
- (beat-to-beat) variability of repolarization in time 167
- acoustic window 160
- stem 164

temporalist
- mandibulae junctio 163

temporary
- duty 161
- total disability 166

temporomandibular joint 163
tender loving care 162
tenderness
- CVA 55
- low back 99

tendon
- Achilles 159
- bone bone-patellar 34
- interposition, ligament reconstruction 102
- popliteus 135
- reflex(es), deep 63
- reflex, patellar 139

- transfer 166
teniposide
- (anti cancer drug) 174
Tennessee
- self-concept scale 165
tensile
- strength 164
- strength, diametral 63
tension
- free vaginal tape 167
- ocular 126
- surface 181
- syndrome, premenstrual 134
- tactile 166
- time index 167
tentacle ball formation 160
terbinafine 160
term
- birth living child 160
- intrauterine pregnancy 162
- nonthrombocytopenic 121
- old 126
- pregnancy 163
terminal
- deoxynucleotide transferase 161
- dorsal root 62
- duct-lobular-units 161
- hepatic venule (central vein) 162
- interphalangeal 162
- sensory latency 165
- warm blood cardioplegia 167
termination
- of pregnancy 163
terminology
- current procedural 50
tertian
- malaria, benign 35
tertiary 181
test
- Ascheim-Zondek 28
- block design 31
- blood serologic 35
- brief vestibular disorientation 36
- Buschke selective reminding 35
- endurance run 70
- exercise tolerance 71
- galveston orientation and amnesia 81
- glucose oxidase 81
- high solids anaerobic digestion 87
- Mantel-Haenszel 106
- mini stress 113
- multiple sleep latency 111, 112
- multiple wake latency 114
- non-stress 121
- object sorting 126
- phenylsulfonphthalein 139
- serological 151
- serological, for Syphilis 158
- skin prick 157
- solution 164
- tube 166
testes
- descended 179
- undescended 179
testicular
- feminization syndrome 165
- regression syndrome 164
- self-examination 165
- torsion 166
testing
- cardiopulmonary exercise 50
- fecal occult blood 75
- nucleic acid amplification 115
testis
- specific protein 165
testosterone
- repressed prostate message 164
- total 167
tetanus
- antitoxin 160
- immune globulin 162
- toxin 166
- toxoid 166
- toxoid antibody 166
tetany
- duration 63
tetra
- hydrofurfuryldisulfide 166
- hydroindazolone carboxylic acid 85
- joule 162
- methylene glutaric acid 163
- methylrhodamine-iodoacetamide 88
- polar bioelectrical impedance 160
- sodium pyrophosphate 165
- thionate 166
- zol 166
tetralogy of Fallot 163
tetrodotoxin 167
Texas
- red 164
texture
- defined 161
thalamic
- projection neuron 163
thalassemia
- mental retardation 24
thalassemia-mental retardation 24
thanks in advance 162
the
- bethesda system 160
- dairy information system (UK) 56
- morrow assessment of nausea and emesis 104
thematic
- apperception test 160
theophylline
- sustained release 166
theoretical
- renal phosphorus threshold 164
theory
- delay-reduction 62
- of signal detectability 165
therapeutic 162
- absence, timed 166
- touch 166
- trial visit 167
therapist
- occupational 126
therapy 162, 168
- assistant, occupational 126
- autolymphocyte 19

- combined modality 49
- deep x-ray 65
- electroconvulsive 68
- electroshock 71
- external radiation 176
- growth hormone 79
- hormone replacement 87
- H-wave 88
- individual 95
- inhalation 95
- insulin coma 90
- intensive 95
- intradiscal electrothermal 90
- mechanical pressure 111
- occupational 126
- office 126
- oral rehydration 125
- photodynamic 130
- physical 139
- physical, chest 50
- radiation 176
- recreational 147
- testosterone replacement 164
- ultraviolet laser 172
therefore 180
thermal
- expansion, coefficient 54
- stability 164
- unit, british 35
- vascular test 167
thermogenesis
- digestion-related 62
thermokeratoplasty
- laser 102
thermoluminescent
- dosimeters 163
thesia
- electroanes 66
theta (waves)
- diffuse rhythmic 62
thiamin
- pyrophosphate 163
thiazolobenzimidazole 160
Thiers
- syndrome 25
thin
- film transistor 161
- layer chromatography 162
Thioguanine
- anti cancer drug 161
thioredoxin
- trx traction 164
thiosemicarbazide 165
thiosulfate
- sulfur-transferase 166
thiotepa 165
third
- compartment volume 172
- order dispersion 163
- trimester bleeding 166
- upper 168
- ventricle, anteroventral 27
thoracic 162
- diameter, transverse 166
- fluid content 161
- gas volume 161
- impedance 162
- outlet syndrom 163
- radiotherapy 164
- spine 63
- surgery 164
- surgery, video-assisted 173
- to be followed by number designating specific thoracic vertebra 159
- vertebrae 55, 159
thoracoabdominal
- wounds 160
thoracolumbosacral
- orthosis 163
thoracostomy
- tube 166
thorax 162
thorazine 50
threaded
- titanium acetabular prosthesis 166
three
- dimensional (surface) CAT scan reconstruction images 57
- dimensional magnetic resonance angiography 61
- dimensional visualization 64
- hours 181
- letter abbreviation/acronym (ha) 162
- times 181
- times a day 162
- times a day (L. ter in die) 162
- times a week 162
- times per week 162
threonine 159, 162
- codon 10, 11, 13
threshold
- limit values 163
- olfactory 126
- tactile 166
thresholding
- dynamic regional 62
thrombin
- clotting time 160
- sensitive protein 165
- time 166
thrombo proteolytic activity 163
thrombocythemia
- essential 71
- idiopathic 95
thrombocytopenia
- heparin induced 85
- heparin-assosiated 83
thrombocytopenic
- purpura, autoimmune 24
- purpura, idiopathic 95
thromboembolic
- complications 161
- deterrent stockings 161
thromboembolism
- pulmonary 139
- venous 174
thrombolysis
- in myocardial infarction 162
thrombolytic
- therapy 166
thromboplastin
- Bilbao 160
- index, total 167
- screening test 166
- time, automated partial 22
- time, partial 139
thrombopoiesis
- stimulating factor 165
thrombopoietin 163
thrombosis
- cerebral 54
- deep venous 64

- device-related 62
- hepatic artery 83
- periprostatic vein 140
- portal vein 140
- renal vein 149
thrombospondin 165
thrombotic
- brain infarction 160
- microangiopathy 163
- thrombocytopenic purpura 167
thromboxane
- A2 168
- B2 168
thrombus
- formation time 161
- tumor 166
through
- series, small bowel follow 150
throughput
- screening, high 87
thymectomy
- adult 25
thymidine
- labeling index 163
- tritiated 167
thymidylate synthetase 164
thymine 159
thymocyte
- cortisone resistant 51
- dexamethasone-resistant 62
- globulin, antihuman 17
- plasma, antihuman 17
- serum 25
thymol turbidity 166
thymopentin 163
thymus
- derived chemotactic agent 160
- extract, bovine 35
- like differentiation, carcinoma showing 38
- serum, antihuman 17
thyroglobulin
- low iodine 102
- lysosomal 102
thyroid 181
- associated ophthalmopathy 159
- binding globulin 160
- binding index 160
- blood flow 160
- function test 161
- hormone binding ratio 162
- stimulating antibody 165
- stimulating hormone 165
- stimulating hormone receptor 165
- stimulating hormone, alpha chain 165
- stimulating hormone, beta chain 165
- stimulating hormone, bovine 36
- stimulating hormone-releasing factor 165
- stimulating hormone-releasing hormone 165
- stimulating immunoglobulin 165
- stimulator, long-acting 99
- to serum ratio 166
- transcription factor 1 166
thyroiditis
- chronic lymphocytic 47
- postpartum 136
thyropharyngeus muscle 163
thyrotropic hormone 167
thyrotropin
- binding inhibition 160
- releasing hormone 164
thyroxine 159
- binding index 160
- free 76
- specific activity 165
- total 166
tibial
- torsion, internal 95
- tubercle 166
tibiale
- mediale, os 126
tibialis anterior 159
tic
- disorder, transient 166
tick-borne fever 160
tid 162
tidal volume 167, 174
tight
- filum terminale 161
- junctions 162
tilt table 166
time
- absolute retention 23
- acceleration 13
- activated clotting 13
- and temperature 166
- automated partial thromboplastin 22
- based injection 160
- bleeding 33
- central conduction 42
- clotting 47
- derivative of left ventricular pressure 62
- ejection 71
- histograms, poststimulus 139
- interval 181
- intervals, systolic 158
- of arrival, estimated 71
- of departure, estimated 71
- pulse separation 139
- relaxation 181
- required to complete the S phase of the cell cycle 164
- tension index 167
- thrombin clotting 160
timed
- exposure diffusive sampler 161
- therapeutic absence 166
timed vital capacity 167
timepto-intubation 167
times 176
- median survival 113
- relaxation 148
- three 181
tincture 164
tingling
- and numbness 121
- on percussion (Tinel's sign), distal 63
tissue
- antigen, tumor-specific 166
- Banks International 160
- blood flow 160
- cage fluid 160

lx

- culture infectious dose 50 % 160
- factor pathway inhibitor 161
- growth, lean 102
- inhibitor of metalloproteinase 162
- microarray infostructure 163
- middle subcutaneous (adipose 112
- perirenal adipose 136
- plasminogen activator 163
- plasminogen activator, recombinant 148
- space 164
- specific extinguisher 165
- tolerance dose 166

titanium
- dioxide 162
- interbody spacers 162

titer
- antihyaluronidase 17
- geometric mean 80

to 179, 180
- affected areas 163
- be determined 160
- be scheduled 160
- come in (hospital) 160
- keep open 162
- the left 179
- the right 179

tobacco
- EIN3-like 161
- mosaic virus 163
- rattle virus 164
- ringspot virus 164
- smoke, environmental 71
- smokeless 154

toe
- brachial index 160
- touch weight bearing 167

toestrike
- right 148

tolerance
- dose 161
- dose, tissue 166
- low zone 103
- test 166
- test, borderline glucose 32
- test, exercise 71
- test, glucose 82
- test, oral glucose 122
- weight bearing to 175

tolfenamic acid 159

toluene
- diamines 161
- diisocyanate 161
- sulfonic acid 165

tomographic
- helical computed 84

tomography
- computed body 39
- computerized 54
- electron-beam computed 67
- magnetic resonance 111
- positron emission 131
- quantitative computed 140
- single photon emission 156
- single photon emission computed 156

tonsillectomy
- and adenoidectomy 159

tonsils
- and adenoids 159

too
- numerous to count 163

tooth
- brushing instruction 160
- decay test 161
- movement, orthodontic 126
- surfaces, number of non-aligned proximal 118

topical(ly) 163

topographic rubric of ICD-O 90

topography
- deviation ratio 62

torque-time interval 167

torsion
- testicular 166

tosylate 164

total
- abdominal hysterectomy 159
- active motion 159
- anomalous pulmonary venous connection 159
- bilirubin 160
- binding index 160
- body clearance 47
- body fat 160
- body impedance 160
- body iron 160
- body irradiation 160
- body muscle mass 160
- body surface area 160
- body water 160
- bone index 160
- cardiac output 141
- diiodothyronine 166
- disability, permanent 139
- disability, temporary 166
- ear canal ablation 161
- end systolic diameter 161
- functional hemolytic complement 44
- hip arthroplasty 162
- hip prosthesis 162
- hip replacement 162
- hip revision 162
- hysterectomy with bilateral salpingo-oophorectomy 162
- iron-binding capacity 162
- joint arthroplasty 162
- Kjeldahl nitrogen (waste waters treatment) 162
- knee arthroplasty 162
- knee extension 162
- knee replacement/revision 162
- lung capacity 162
- lymphoid irradiation 163
- needed irradiation 163
- nodal irradiation 163
- organic carbon 163
- outflow resistance 163
- pancreatectomy 163
- parenteral nutrition 163
- parenteral nutrition-associated cholestasis 163
- peripheral resistance 163
- platinum 163
- reducing sugars 164
- resistance 147
- respiratory resistance 164
- right ventricular volume 164
- score, maximum mean 109
- serum bile acids 165
- serum bilirubin 165

- serum prostatic acid phosphatase 165
- serum protein 165
- severity assessment score 165
- shoulder arthroplasty 165
- skin electron beam 165
- skin examination 165
- small intestine allotransplantation 165
- solids (in urine) 164
- solute absorption 165
- stomach volume 166
- suspended particulate 165
- suspended solids 166
- systemic flow 165
- systemic resistance 166
- systemic vascular resistance 166
- testosterone 167
- thromboplastin index 167
- thyroxine 166
- time 166, 167
- toe arthroplasty 166
- triiodothyronine 166
- vaginal hysterectomy 167
- ventilation time 167
- viable cells 167
- viable count 167
- volume 167
- volume capacity 167
- weight gain 168
- worm burden 167

totally
- unexplained sudden infant death syndrome 165

touch
- and tone 166
- therapeutic 166

Tourette syndrome 164
toward 179
tower building 167
toxic 163
- multinodular goiter 163
- shock antigen 165
- shock syndrome 166
- shock syndrome exotoxin 166
- shock syndrome toxin 166
- shock syndrome toxin-1 166
- shock-associated protein 165
- substance 164
- substances control act 165
- syndrome 164

toxicity
- - determined by phase 1 studies, dose limiting 60
- criteria, common 54

toxicologic 163
toxicology 163
toxin
- black widow spider 37
- botulinum 35, 36
- exfoliating 72
- toxic shock syndrome 166

Toxocara canis
- excretory/secretory antigen 161

toxoids
- diphtheria, acellular pertussis, and tetanus 56

toxoplasmin
- skin test antigen 166

trabecular
- bone index 160
- bone volume fraction 160

trabeculoplasty
- argon laser 19

trace 164
tracheal 164
tracheal gas
- insufflation, continuous 54

tracheal sound 164
tracheitis
- bacterial nosocomial 33

tracheo
- esophageal fistula 161
- tomy set 165

tracheostomy 164
tract
- geniculo-hypothalamic 79
- lateral tegmental 102
- optic 126
- paraventriculospinal 140
- rubrospinal 147
- upper gastrointestinal 171

traction 168
- cervical 54
- intermittent cervical 90
- manual 113
- thioredoxin 164
- trx skeletal 152

traction-absorbing wiring 160
trademark
- registered 148

traditional
- Chinese medicine 160

training
- anxiety control 13
- asthma care 13
- basic aid 29
- exercise 71
- gait 82
- internittent hypoxic 91

train-of-four (EMG) 163
tranquilization
- rapid 147

transaminase
- alanine 18
- glutamic pyruvic 82

transarterial
- embolization 159

transbronchial
- injection 160

transbullar
- injections 160

transcatheter
- arterial chemo-embolization 159

transcortical
- sensory aphasia 165

transcranial
- electrical stimulation 161
- magnetic stimulation 163

transcranial doppler 160
transcriptase
- reverse 147

transcription
- factor 1, thyroid 166
- factor antibody, anti-microphthalmia 55
- factor, microphtalmia 108
- reverse 147

transcutaneous
- electrical nerve stimulation 161
- pacing 160

transdermal 161

transesophageal
- echocardiogram 161
Trans-European
- Network-Integrated Broadband Communications 161
transfer
- admision-discharge 14
- egg 65
- factor, resistance 148
- fluorescence resonance energy 76
- ratio, magnetization 113
- resistance 147
- ribonucleic acid threonine 164
- system, osteochondral autograft 121
- to 179
- zygote intrafallopian 177
transferred to 166
transferrin
- carbohydrate-deficient 43
- saturation 164
transform
- diffraction radon 62
- discrete wave 65
transformation
- zone, atypical 25
transforming
- growth factors 161
- sequence, thyroid 166
transfusion
- blood autologous 10
- intrauterine 95
- system, baylor rapid autologous 34
transgenic
- line of mice 19
transhepatic
- cholangiogram 162
- cholangiography, percutaneous 139
transient
- amplifying cells 159
- electric nerve stimulation 161
- erythroblastopenia of childhood 161
- global amnesia 161
- ischemic attacks 162
- job disability 162
- myeloproliferative disorder 163
- receptor potential 164
- receptor potential channel proteins 164
- synovitis of the hip 165
- tachypnea 166, 167
- tic disorder 166
transistor
- thin-film 161
transit
- time 166
transition
- protein 163
transitional
- care unit 160
- sleep 164
transjugular
- intrahepatic portosystemic shunt 162
- intrahepatic portosystemic stent shunts 162
transketolase 164
translator's work bench 167
translid
- binocular interactor 160
translocation
- 1 gene, plasmacytoma variant 140
- gene, T-cell 166
transluminal
- angioplasty, percutaneous 139
- coronary angioplasty, percutaneous 139
- extraction atherectomy 161
transmembrane 163
- regulator, cystic fibrosis 43
transmetatarsal
- amputation 163
transmisison
- coefficient 181
transmissible
- gastroenteritis 161
- venereal tumour 167
transmission
- disequilibrium test 161
- electron microscopy 161
- scanning electron microscopy 165
transmural
- perioperative myocardial infarction 163
transmyocardial
- revascularization 163
- revascularization, percutaneous 139
transoesophageal
- echo-Doppler system 161
transperineal
- urethral resection 163
transplant 165, 168
- autologous bone marrow 9
- bone marrow 33
- cadaveric renal 51
- generation, late 102
- peripheral stem cell 138
- popliteal vein 140
transplantation
- allogeneic stem-cell 18
- antigen, tumor-specific 166
- post-liver 133
- renal 147
- unrelated donor bone marrow 172
transplantations
- liver, orthotopic 123
transport
- high albumin 83
transporter
- glucose 79
- phosphate-specific 139
transposition
- anterocolic 13
- great vessels 161
- of great vessels 161
transrectal
- ultrasonography 164
transsexual 164
transthoracic 166
- echocardiography 166
transthyretin 167
transtracheal 166
- aspiration 166
- insufflation 167

- selective bronchial brushing 165
transurethral
- incision of the prostate 167
- microwave thermotherapy 167
- needle ablation (prostatic) 167
- prostatectomy 167
- resection 167
- resection of bladder 167
- resection of bladder tumor 167
- resection of the prostate 167
- ultrasound-guided laser induced prostatectomy 167
transvaginal
- cone 167
- ultrasound 167
transverse
- left occiput 101
- magnetization decay curve 163
- right occiput 144
- section 164, 165
- sinus 164
- spinal sclerosis 165
- thoracic diameter 166
trauma
- blunt abdominal 29
- center, regional 147
- closed craniocerebral 40
- life support 24
- life support, basic 35
- life support, prehospital 132
- score 164
- score, revised 148
- scores, revised 148
- surgery 164
- syndrome, acute cervical 13
- syndrome, acute lumbar 19
traumatic
- brain injury 160
- joint disease 162
treadmill
- score 164
- stress test 166
treatment 149, 168
- /therapy, cognitive behavioral 39
- acute intensive 18
- episode data set 161
- goal 81
- hospital 87
- methylphenidate 111
- nerve 121
- orthopedic 126
- outpatient 124
- plan 164
- planning, biological 35
- planning, radiation 148
- versus control 167
- versus treatment 167
Treitz
- ligament 101
tremor 15
- rest 147
treponema
- pallidum 163
- pallidum, immobilization test 163
- pallidum, microhemagglutination 107
treponemal
- antibody absorption test, fluorescent 76
- Western blot 167
trial
- randomized controlled 142
triamcinolone
- acetonide benzoyl-beta-amino-isobutyrate 160
triangular
- fibrocartilage complex 161
tribromoimidazole 160
tricalcium phosphate ceramic 160
triceps
- jerk 162
- reflex 162
- skinfold 165
- surae 164
tricho
- rhinophalangeal syndrome 164
- rhino-phalangeal syndrome type II 164
- thio-dystrophy 166
Trichostrongylus colubriformis 174
tricipital
- skinfold thickness 166
tricuspid
- insufficiency 162
- valve replacement 167
tricuspid stenosis 164
tricyclic antidepressant 160
trifluoro
- acetic acid 161
- thymidine 161
triggered activations 160
triglycerides 161
- liquid form 102
- liver 102
triiodothyronine 159
- resin uptake 164
- rT3 reverse 147
- total 166
trimethoprim 163
- sulfamethoxazole 163
trimethylamine N-oxide 163
trimmer
- gingival margin 80
trinitrotoluene 163
triphenyltetrazolium
- chloride 166
triphosphates
- nucleotide 121
triple
- strength 164
- sugar iron 165
- sugar iron agar 165
- sugar urea (agar) 166
- voiding cystogram 167
triprenyl
- phenol, stachybotrys microspora 155
tris(hydroxymethyl)amino-methane 164
trisodium
- edetate 165
- phosphate 165
tritiated thymidine 167

triturate
- tablet 166
trivalent
- botulinic antitoxin 9
trivalent oral polio vaccine 163
trivittatus 167
trophoblast
- intermediate 95
trophoblastic
- disease, gestational 82
- tumor, placental site 139
tropical
- spastic paraparesis 165
- splenomegaly syndrome 166
- sprue 164
trough whole blood 168
trpc
- osm 127
true vocal cord 167
trunk
- brachiocephalic arterial 30
- rotation, lower 102
trx skeletal traction 152
trypsinogen
- bovine 35
trypticase
- soy (plate) 164
- soy agar 165
- soy broth 165
- soy yeast 166
tryptone
- soy broth 165
tryptophan 164, 175
- oxygenase 164
- rich prealbumin 164
tsp 164
T-tube cholangiogram 166
tubal
- ligation, bilateral 35
- ligation, postpartum 136
tube
- (s), eustachian 71
- cathode-ray 51
- defect, neural 121
- endotracheal 71
- gastrostomy 82
- jejunostomy 96
- nasogastric 117
- nasotracheal 121
- pressure equalization 131
- slide agglutination test 165
- thoracostomy 166
tubercle
- tibial 166
tuberculin
- old 126
- original 126
- test 166
- units (in Mantoux test) 167
tuberculoid
- (in Ridley-Jopling Hansen disease classification) 166
- borderline 35
tuberculosis 160
tuberous
- sclerosis 164, 165
tubo-ovarian
- abscess 163
tubular
- acidification defect, renal 147
- acidosis, renal 147
- necrosis, acute 24
- undulating row photobioreactors 167
tubule
- distal convoluted 57
- distal straight 63
- proximal convoluted 129
- proximal straight 139
tubules
- proximal straight 139
tubuloreticular
- structure 164
tumor
- bladder 35
- blood flow 160
- brain 35
- breast 35
- carotid body 39
- gene, brain 34
- germ cell 78
- granular cell nerve sheath 78
- growth factor alpha 161
- growth factor beta 161
- infiltrating lymphocytes 162
- liposclerosing myxofibrous 102
- malignant mixed mesodermal 109
- multiple 103
- necrosis factor 163
- necrosis factor, recombinant 148
- nodes, metastases 163
- of low malignant potential, mucinous 109
- of the jaws, central mucoepidermoid 48
- of the kidney, rhabdoid 148
- placental site trophoblastic 139
- primitive neuroectodermal 134
- skin test 166
- specific 164
- specific antigen 165
- specific cell surface antigen 166
- specific glycoprotein 165
- specific tissue antigen 166
- specific transplantation antigen 166
- suppressor gene 127
- surface antigen 165
- therapy, interstitial 95
- thrombus 166
- yolk sac 177
tunica vaginalis testis 167
tuning fork 161
turbidity
- reducing unit 164
- thymol 166
turing-wave bifurcation 168
turkey virus hepatitis 167
turn, cough, deep breath 160
Turner syndrome 164
turnip crinkle virus 161
turnover
- rate, red blood cell 148
- time 166
twice 181
- a day 32
- a night 32
- a week 33, 160, 167
twitch
- response, single 158

two
- components 32
- hours 181
- point discrimination 129
tympanic membrane 163
tympanum membrani 163
type
- and crossmatch 160
- and hold 161
- and screen 165
- gastric 82
- gastric and intestinal, mixed 113
- intestinal 95
- specific 164
- specific antibody 165
- specific M protein 165
typhoid
- fever, drug resistant 62
tyrosine 168, 177
- kinase 162
- kinase gene, developmentally regulated EPH-related 62
- kinase involved in signal transduction 177

U

ubg urobilinogen 169
ubiquitin
- activating enzyme 169
- B 169
- C 169
ulcer 168
- Buruli 36
- decubitus 58, 63
- duodenal 63, 64
- gastric 82
- peptic 139
ulcerative
- colitis 169
- dermal necrosis 170
- dermatosis 170
- gingivitis, acute 25
ulna 168
ulnar 171
- collateral ligament 169
- deviation 170
- neuropathy at the elbow 171
ultimobranchial body 169
ultra
- audible 168
- centrifugal 169
- distal radius bone mineral density 170
- filterable platinum 171
- filtrate 170
- filtration 170
- filtration pressure 170
- filtration rate 170
- fine 170
- high frequency 171
- high molecular weight polyethylene 171
- high-density-polyethylene 171
- lente (insulin) 168
- violet radiation 172
ultrarapid
- opioid detoxification 171
ultrasonic
- arteriography 168
- attenuation, broadband 36
- cardiac output 169
- cardiography 169
- encephalography 170
- flow detector 170
- frequency 170
- nebulizer 172
ultrasonography
- intravascular 96
- transrectal 164
- ultrasound 172
ultrasound 171, 172
- Doppler 64
- Doppler sonography 170
- endoscopic 71
- guided laser induced prostatectomy, transurethral 167
- head 87
- high intensity focused 85
- therapy 172
- transvaginal 167
- ultrasonography 172
ultraviolet 172
- blood irradiation 169
- index 172
- irradiation 172
- laser therapy 172
- light 172
- light illumination 172
umbilical
- artery 168
- artery catheter 168
- cord 169
- cord blood culture 169
umbilicus 168, 171
unable to locate 172
unaided visual inspection 172
unauthorized
- absence 168
uncertain 168
- etiology 170
unchanged 72, 169, 179
unclassifiable 169
unconditioned
- response 169
- stimulus 170
unconjugated
- bilirubin 169
- estriol 170
unconscious 169, 170
uncontrolled
- variable 170
uncoupling protein 169
undenaturated
- bacterial antigen 169
under
- developed under nourished 170
- elbow 170
- observation for 171
underdeveloped 170
underlying
- cause of death 169
underweight
- undernourished 172
undetermined 170
- diagnosis 63
- origin 170
undifferentiated
- (unclassifiable) connective tissue disease 170
- B-cell lymphoma 169
- cells 169

- connective tissue disease 170
- leukemia 25
unequal ventilation index 172
unerupted 168
unesterified
- fatty acid 170
unfolded
- protein response 171
unfractionated
- heparin 171
unidentified
- bright object 169
- bright signal 169
- endosteal marrow cell 170
- growth factor 171
unifactorial analysis 170
unified
- atomic mass unit 168
unifocal
- eosinophilic granuloma 170
uniform
- clinical data set 169
- data system 170
- effective health benefits 170
uniglandular disease 171
unilamellar vesicles 158
unilateral 171
- absence of excretion 168
- absence of pulmonary 169
- cleft of lip and palate 169
- facet dislocation 170
- strabismus, divergent 64
uninvolved epidermis 170
unipolar 171
- limb lead on the left arm in electrocardiography 27
- limb lead on the left leg in electrocardiography 26
- limb lead on the right arm in electrocardiography 27
- recurrent depression 171
unit 66, 168
- allergenic 25
- Angstrom 25
- antitoxin 25
- arbitrary 25
- basic structural 35
- cardiac rehabilitation 52
- cells, colony-forming 43
- clerk 169
- clinical research 52
- colony-forming 43
- comprehensive cardiac care 40
- dose 170
- epidermal proliferative 70
- immunizing 95
- intensive care 90
- intensive coronary care 89
- international 95
- of analysis 168
- respiratory care 142
- special care 150
- spleen colony-forming 44
univalent 180
universal
- application (residency) 168
- electron microscope 170
- feeder 170
unknown 168, 171, 181
- factor 170
unlicensed
- assistive personnel 168
unna boot 169
unprotected sexual intercourse 171
unrelated
- donor bone marrow transplantation 172
- donors 171
unsatisfactory condition 169
unsaturated
- vitamin B12 binding capacity 169
unscheduled
- deoxynucleic acid synthesis 170
unsharpness 168
- absorbtion 168
- geometric 170
unstable
- angina 168
- angina pectoris 169
unstable angina 172
unstimulated short-time cultures 172
untreated
- cells 169
unusual
- childhood illness 169
up 179
- to date 172
upper 168, 179
- abdomen surgery 169
- airway obstruction 168
- airway resistance 169
- airways 168
- arm 168
- arm, left 102
- back 169
- body obesity 169
- collateral ligament 169
- confidence limit 169
- control limit 169
- esophageal sphincter 170
- esophagus 170
- explosive limit 170
- extremities, both 36
- extremity 170
- extremity, left 102
- extremity, right 148
- flammable limit 170
- gastrointestinal 171
- gastrointestinal biopsy 171
- gastrointestinal bleeding 171
- gastrointestinal hemorrhage 25, 171
- gastrointestinal series 171
- gastrointestinal tract 171
- half 168
- left quadrant 171
- lid 171
- limits of normal 171
- lobe (lung), left 102
- lobe (lung), right 148
- motor neuron (signs) 171
- outer quadrant, left 102
- quadrants, both 36
- respiratory disease 171
- respiratory tract infection 172
- right quadrant 172
- third 168
upper airways
- reconstruction, multilevel 113

upstream
- activation site 169
- sequence, differential 64
uptake
- radioactive iodine 142
- triiodothyronine resin 164
upward gaze 171
uracil 168
uranium 168
urea 168
- and electrolytes 170
- blood 36
- clearance 169
- cycle enzymopathy 169
- formaldehyde foam insulation 170
- nitrogen, blood 36
- nitrogen, urinary 172
urease
- test, rapid 148
uremic
- medullary cystic disease 171
- syndrome, hemolytic 87
ureteral
- back pressure 169
- occlusion, bilateral 36
uretero
- bladder junction 169
ureteropelvic
- junction 171
ureterovesical
- junction 172
urethogram
- retrograde 148
urethra 168
urethral
- and cervical 169
- and skene glands 36
- catheter in 169
- catheter out 171
- catheterization 169
- dilatation 170
- discharge 170
- pressure, maximum 113
- resection, transperineal 163
- syndrome, acute 25
- valve, anterior 25
urethritis
- nongonococcal 117
urethrotomy
- direct-vision internal 64
uric
- acid 168
- acid creatinine (ratio) 168
- acid nitrogen 168
- acid riboside 169
- acid, blood 36
uridine 168, 171
- cytidine kinases 169
- diphosphate 170
- diphosphate glucose 170
- diphosphate glucuronic acid 170
- diphosphate glucuronosyl transferase 170
- diphosphate kinase 170
- diphosphate-glucuronosyltransferase 171
uridylic acid 168
urinalysis 168
- routine 148
urinary
- abnormalities, asymptomatic 25
- acid phosphatase 169
- aldosterone 168
- alkaline phosphatase 169
- amylase 168
- bladder 169
- catheter 169
- catheter in 169
- catheter out 171
- chorionic gonadotropin 169
- concentration 168
- coproporphyrin 169
- coproporphyrin test 169
- C-peptide 169
- fat bodies 170
- follicle-stimulating hormone 170
- formaldehyd 170
- free cortisol 170
- output 171
- pregnancy test 171
- stress incontinence 172
- tract infection 172
- urea nitrogen 172
urine 168, 171, 180
- activity, urokinase 172
- albumin excretion 168
- analysis 168
- clean catch 42
- collection device 169
- concentrate 169
- culture 169
- diphosphoglucose 170
- diribose phosphate 170
- filtration rate 170
- mid stream specimen 113
- midstream 113
- midstream specimen 113
- osmolality, desmopressin test 58
- osmolality, early morning 70
- output 171
- passed 139
- pregnancy 140
- protein electrophoresis 171
- protein-to-creatinine ratios 171
urobilin 169
urobilinogen
- ubg 169
urogastrone 171
urogenital 171
- diaphragm 171
urogram
- intravenous 96
urography
- intravenous 96
urokinase
- like plasminogen activator 171
- like plasminogen activator receptor 171
urokinase urine activity 172
urological
- care table 170
urology 168, 172
uronic acid 168
uroporphyrinogen
- decarboxylase 170
ursodeoxycholic acid 170
use
- concentration, maximum 113
users
- injection drug 90

usual
- and customary 169
- body weight 169
- childhood diseases 169
- customary, and reasonable (fees) 170
- diseases of childhood 170
- ductal hyperplasia 170
- interstitial pneumonia 171
- state of health 172

uterine
- activity interval 168
- activity unit 169
- aspiration 168
- bleeding, abnormal 25
- bleeding, dysfunctional 64
- blood flow 171
- compression syndrome 170
- contraction, regular 148
- contractions 169
- delivery 170

uterus 168

utilization
- medical care 105
- organophosphate 124

utterance
- mean length 109

uveitis
- acute anterior 7
- anterior 25
- glaucoma-hyphema 171
- glaucoma-hyphema plus vitreous hemorrhage (syndrome) 171

UV-irradiated
- blood, autotransfusion 26

uvula 168

uvulopalatopharyngoplasty 171

uvulopalatoplasty
- Bovie-assisted 28

V

vaccine
- associated feline sarcoma 172
- bacille Calmette-Guérin 31
- hemophillus influenzae type B polysaccharide 83
- human diploid cell 84
- inactivated poliovirus 94
- multivalent influenza 108
- oral polio 124
- oral poliovirus 124
- polio, trivalent oral 163
- tetravalent, rhesus rotavirus 145

vaccinia
- virus Ankara 114

vacuum
- aspiration, electric 71
- aspiration, manual 113
- distillation gas chromatography 173

vagal
- nucleus, dorsal 64

vagina bleed 140

vaginal 172
- administration of conjugated equine estrogens 173
- birth after cesarean 173
- bleeding 173
- delivery, normal spontaneous 121
- delivery, spontaneous 158
- examination 173
- examination, sterile 159
- hysterectomy 173
- hysterectomy, intrafascial 95
- hysterectomy, total 167
- intraepithelial neoplasia 172
- irrigation 173
- outlet, relaxed 149
- tape, tension-free 167

vaginitis
- virus, bovine 37

vaginosis
- bacterial 36

vagus
- nerve, pharyngeal branch 132

valine 172
- codon 82, 83

valproate 174

valproic acid 172

valsalva
- aneurysms, sinus 158

value
- added, economic 71
- added, market 113
- critical serum chemistry 53
- diethylamine shift 63
- predictive negative 135
- protein nutritional 135

valve
- anterior urethral 25
- aortic 26
- area, aortic 26
- atresia, aortic 26
- bicuspid aortic 29
- closure, aortic 26
- defects, aortic 26
- defects, mitral 114
- dual switch 63
- mitral 108, 113
- opening, aortic 27
- orifice, aortic 27
- replacement, aortic 27
- replacement, double 64
- stenosis, aortic 27

valvular
- heart disease 173
- heart disease, acquired 26
- heart syndrome, acquired 26

vancomycin
- resistant enterococcus 174

vanillylmandelic
- acid 174

vannielii
- methanococcus 114

vapor
- extraction, of soil 158

variable 180
- region gene, immunoglobulin 91
- region I 174
- screw placement 174

variance 181
- analysis 20

variant
- major interspecific 108

variations
- DNA sequence 63

variceal
- hemorrhage, esophageal 71

varicella
- zoster immune globulin 175
- zoster virus 175

varicose veins 175
variegated
- aneuploidy, mosaic 114
vas
- ligation, bilateral 36
vascular
- arcade, marginal 113
- cell adhesion molecule 173
- cell adhesion molecule (endothelial cell adhesion molecule) 173
- dementia 172
- dementia, pre-senile 140
- diameter, changes 57
- disease, allograft 26
- disease, arteriosclerotic 24
- disease, arteriosclerotic peripheral 24
- disease, atherosclerotic 26
- disease, hypertensive 88
- disease, peripheral 140
- encephalopathy, subcortical 159
- endothelial cell growth factor 173
- imaging system, digital 64
- imaging, digital 64
- injury, pelvic 140
- insufficiency, chronic 55
- occlusive disease, arteriosclerotic peripheral 22
- peripheral 140
- permeability factor 174
- plexus, deep 64
- radiology, interventional 95
- reactivity, digital 64
- resistance index 174
- resistance, iliac 95
- resistance, intestinal 95
- resistance, intrarenal 96
- resistance, peripheral 140
- resistance, pulmonary 140
- resistance, systemic 159
- resistance, total systemic 166
- response, reduced 149
- test, thermal 167
vasculitis
- activity score, birmingham 36
- allergic 26
vasoactive
- intestinal peptide 173
vasoconstrictor substance 173
vasodilator
- active 26
vasoinhibitory peptide 173
vasomotor
- nephropathy, acute 27
vasopressin 14, 27
- abnormal 27
- aqueous 27
- deamine-4-valine-D-arginine 64
vasotocin
- arginine 27
VASP
- homology, enabled 71
vastus
- lateralis deep 64
- medialis obliquus 174
vector 179
- analysis, activity 26
- augmented 26
- electric field 65
- major injury 108
vehicle
- deep submergence 63
- privately owned 135
vein 172
- graft 173
- graft, saphenous 159
- harvest, endoscopic 71
- occlusion, branch 36
- occlusion, central retinal 52
- patch, distal 64
- pressure, draining 64
- pressure, neck 135
- thrombosis, periprostatic 140
- varicose 175
velocardiofacial
- syndrome 173
velocity 168
- air 26
- angular 181
- capillary blood cell 39
- constant linear 47
- diastolic septal 63
- dynamic 181
- end diastolic 68
- index, Doppler 64
- integral, diastolic 64
- mean 113
- nerve conduction 116
- peak systolic 139
- profile, Doppler 64
- prosthetic flow, diastolic peak 64
- time profile 174
- volume 168
velum
- anterior medullary 19
vena
- cava, inferior 95
- cava, right superior 147
- cava, superior 158
venacavography
- digital subtraction 63
venereal
- disease 173
- tumour, transmissible 167
venereology
- and dermatology, diploma in 64
venipuncture
- direct 64
venography
- digital subtraction 63
- magnetic resonance 111
venom
- black widow spider 37
- phoneutria nigriventer spider 135
venous
- anomaly, developmental 64
- blood gas 173
- bypass, aortocoronary 13
- catheters, central 55
- congestion, pulmonary 140
- hemoglobin saturation, mixed 159
- impedance plethysmography 173
- insufficiency, deep 64
- invasion 172
- oxygen tension, mixed 140
- pressure 174
- pressure, ambulatory 27
- pressure, central 55

- pressure, cerebral subarachnoid 53
- pressure, resting 149
- reflux index 174
- thromboembolism 174
- thrombosis, deep 64
veno-venous
- haemofiltration, continuous 55
- hemodialysis, continuous 55
ventilation
- /perfusion scan 174
- acute conditioned neurosis 11
- ambulatory care network 11
- artificial 26
- assist-controlled mechanical 11
- assisted 26
- high-frequency oscillatory 85
- index, unequal 172
- intermitt. mandatory 92
- intermittent positive pressure 93
- maximal isocapnic 108
- maximum volume 114
- maximum voluntary 114
- non-invasive 117
- perfusion ratio 174
- synchronous intermittent mandatory 152
- time, total 167
ventilator 173
ventral
- areas, medullary 114
- part of the lateral pulvinar 140
- posterolateral 174
- posteromedial 174
ventricle
- anteroventral third 27
- left 102
- right 148
ventricular
- arrhythmias, malignant 113
- assist device 172
- assist system, left 102
- beat, premature 140
- conduction, aberrant 26
- contraction, premature 140
- dysplasia, arrythmogenic right 23
- ejection fraction 173
- ejection fraction, left 102
- end-diastolic pressure, left 102
- failure, acute left 19
- failure, left 103
- failure, right 149
- fibrillation 173
- flutter 173
- heart disease 173
- hypertrophy, left 103
- hypertrophy, right 149
- inotropic parameter 173
- muscle 174
- premature contractions 174
- pressure, diastolic 64
- pressure, right 149
- response interval 174
- response, double 64
- rhythm, accelerated 27
- sense, blanked 37
- septal defect 174
- shortening fraction, left 103
- single-chamber synchronous pacemakers 175
- single-chamber systems, fixed-rate 175
- tachycardia 174
- tachycardia, paroxysmal 140
- tachycardia, polymorphic 140
- volume, total right 164
ventriculo
- atrial 172
- atrial conduction 172
- atrial pacing, sequential 158
- graphy, contrast 55
- peritonial derivations 64
ventriculography
- radionuclide 144, 149
ventrolateral
- hypothalamus 174
- outflow 174
venule(s)
- high endothelial 85
verbal order 174
verified
- not 180
verotoxin
- producing enteropathogenic escherichia coli 174
vertebra
- second lumbar 98
- third lumbar 98
vertebrae
- cervical 40, 55
- dorsal 55
- lumbar, load 101
- thoracic 55, 159
vertebral
- bone density 173
- defects, anal atresia, tracheoesophageal fistula with esophageal atresia, and radial and renal anomalies 173
vertebrobasilar insufficiency 173
vertex 175
vertex presentation 175
vertical 173
- deviation, dissociated 64
- jump 174
- ramus osteotomy 174
- releasing incisions, mandibular lingual 109
- sagittal split osteotomy 174
- shear 174
vertigo
- benign paroxysmal positional 34
very
- late antigen 4 174
- long-chain acyl-CoA synthetase 174
- low density lipoprotein 174
vesicle
- epithelium, seminal 158
vesicles
- apical membrane 19
- dense-cored 63
- seminal 151
vessel
- angioplasty, multiple 114
- average density 26

- density, average 26
- diameter 173
vessels
- transposition great 161
vessel-to-tissue noise ratio 174
vestibular
- disorientation test, brief 36
- membrane 174
- nucleus, medial 113
vial
- multiple dose 105
vibrational
- energy redistribution, intramolecular 95
vibrations
- double 64
Vibrio
- ABE 9
- non-cholera 116
vibroacoustic
- stimulation 172
video
- assisted thoracic surgery 173
- plotter, digital 64
view
- reprojection, intermediate 95
villi
- mature intermediate 108
villonodular
- synovitis, pigmented 140
villous
- edema, significant 159
- sampling, chorionic 55
vincristine
- doxorubicin and dexamethasone 172
- ifosfamide and epirubicin 173
- procarbazine, prednisone, adriamycin 124
vindesine 64
vinyl
- acetate - maleic acid - vinyl chloride copolymer 174
- acetate, ethylene- 71
- polysiloxane putty impression material 174
violence
- programs, domestic 64
- related injuries 174
viral
- avian erythroblastosis oncogene 173
- capsid antigen 173
- feline sarcoma oncogene 173
- hepatitis, acute 26
- oncogene 174
- particles, defective 64
- phenotype, syncytium-inducing 152
- protein specific to HIV virus 81, 127
- respiratory infection 174
- respiratory infection, acute 27
- simian sarcoma oncogene 174
viral replication
- initiation factor in the translational step of 68
viroid
- apple scar skin 24
- dapple apple 56
virtual
- reality, immersive 95
virus
- associated hemophagocytic syndrome 172
- barley yellow dwarf 37
- beet western yellow 37
- blue tongue 36
- bovine alimentary papilloma 29
- bovine vaginitis 37
- bovine virus diarrhea 36
- cassava latent 47
- cauliflower mosaic 47
- coxsackie B 39
- digitaria streak 63
- drosophila S 63
- drosophila X 65
- enteric cytopathogenic, bovine orphan 67
- enteritis, duck 64
- enterocytopathogenic human orphan 67
- Epstein-Barr 67, 70
- friend derived murine immunosuppressive 74
- gibbon ape leukemia 79
- gross leukemia 79
- hepatitis A 83
- hepatitis B 83
- hepatitis C 84
- herpes 88
- herpes like 86
- herpes simplex 87
- herpes zoster 88
- hog cholera 84
- human herpes 85
- human lymphotropic 87
- human papilloma 87
- Kaposi sarcoma herpes 97
- Marek disease 105
- master seed 113
- modified vaccinia, Ankara 114
- murine leukemia 109
- necrosis, hypodermal and hematopoietic 91
- psittacosis-lymphogranuloma-trachoma group 133
- receptor, gibbon ape leukemia 79
- replication, baboon 37
- replication, inhibitor 95
- sin nombre 155
- types I, human T-cell lymphotropic 87
- varicella-zoster 175
- west nile 176
viruses
- Sendai 151
viscosity
- absolute 181
- minimum immobilizing 108
visible
- angle, minimum 114
vision
- binocular single 35
- color 55
- colored 173
- left eye 174
- right eye 174
- test, Allen 27
visit 174
- group, ambulatory 26

- home 88
- hospital 88
- office 127

visiting
- medical officer 174
- nurse 174
- nurse service 174

visual
- acuity 172
- acuity, distance 64
- acuity, mesopic 114
- analogue scale 172
- angle, min of 113
- cortex, associative 26
- efficiency, binocular 36
- evoked response 173
- field 173
- impact performance 173
- motor gestalt test, Bender 36

visualization
- four dimensional 74
- three dimensional 64

visually
- evoked potentials 173
- handicapped, division for 64

vital
- capacity 173
- capacity, forced 77
- capacity, timed 167
- signs 174
- signs absent 174
- signs stable 174

vitamin 174

vitamin B12
- binding capacity, unsaturated 169

vitamins
- prenatal 135

vocal
- cord dysfunction 173
- cord paralysis, bilateral abductor 29
- cord, true 167
- sequencing, auditory 27

vocational
- practice nurse 174
- rehabilitation index 174

Vogele-Bale-Hohner
- head holder 173

Vogt-Koyanagi-Harada's disease 174

voice
- order 174
- response, interactive 95

void 173

voided 180

voiding cystourethrogram 173

volar
- intercalary wrist instability 174

volcanic
- ash, Montserrat 114

volcano
- megabalanus 114

volt
- foot, automated 26
- right, automated 27

voltage
- mean integrated 108

voltmeter
- digital 64

volume 174
- administration, massive 113
- alveolar 172
- and tension 174
- aortic valve stroke 27
- atomic 25
- capacity, total 167
- cerebrospinal fluid 54
- clinical target 54
- controll, automatic 26
- critical closing 42
- decrease, apoptotic 26
- effective arterial blood 67
- expansion, small 159
- expansion, sustained 159
- extracellular fluid 67
- hippocampal formation 85
- index 173
- mean platelet 111
- of distribution, apparent 26
- packed red cells 174
- pair, distributed 64
- plasma 140
- recorder, pulse 140
- regulatory increase 174
- second compartment 172
- third compartment 172
- tidal 174
- velocity 168
- ventilation, maximum 114

voluntary
- apnea, duration 64
- hyperventilation, eucapnic 71
- interruption of pregnancy 173
- ventilation, maximum 114

vomiting
- and diarrhea 64
- and nausea 20, 121
- anticipatory 26
- nausea 121

von Willebrand
- disease 175
- factor 175

vrille 174

W

waist
- above 27
- below 37

Waldenström's
- macroglobulinemia 176

walking
- cast, long leg 100
- cast, short-leg 154

wall
- alveolar 27
- anterior 27
- motion, regional 149
- stents, endoluminal colonic 68
- thickening, systolic 159

ward 175

warfare
- atomic 27
- bacteriological 37
- biological 37
- chemical and biological 39

warfarin
- low-dose 99

warm
- and dry 175
- pink, dry (skin signs) 176

warning
- system, disaster 65
warthin-like
- papillary carcinoma of the thyroid 176
washing
- bronchoalveolar 29
washout
- bladder 37
Wassermann 175
waste
- incinerator, hazardous 88
- index, hazardous 88
water 22, 86
- activity 27
- deionized 64
- distilled 64
- immersion, head-out 88
- intake, high 88
- MPP 176
- multipurpose phantoms 176
- titration alkalinity 160
watery
- diarrhea, hypokalemia, and achlorhydria 175
wave
- latent, systolic 152
- length 181
- number 181
- transform, discrete 65
Weakener of white 176
weapon
- biological 37
Wechsler
- adult intelligence scale 175
- intelligence scale for children 175
wedge
- pressure, pulmonary 140
- pressure, pulmonary capillary 129
- pulmonary capillary 129
week(s) 175
Wegener's granulomatosis 175
weight 176, 180
- atomic 25, 27
- bearing as tolerated 175
- bearing to tolerance 175
- body 33
- breast meat 34
- by volume 176
- daily 64
- dry 64
- fat 77
- fetal 77
- gain, total 168
- infarction 96
weighted
- hemodynamically 88
- imaging, hemodynamically 88
- Play-the-Winner 176
welders and caulker/burners 175
well
- and alive 27
- developed 175
- developed well-nourished 175
- differentiated lymphocytic lymphoma, diffuse 65
- nourished 175, 176
west nile virus 176
western blot 175
wet
- bulb globe temperature 175
- corn bran 175
- corn gluten feed 175
wet bulb temperature 167
wheelchair 175
wheezing
- first time 77
when awake 175
while awake 175
whirlpool 175
white 175
- blood cell 175
- blood cells 175
- blood count 175
- carneau pigeons 175
- carneau pigeons, randomly bred 142
- cell count 175
- cells 175
- collar 175
- female 175
- leghorn, hybrid 88
- male 176
- matter signal hyperintensities 176
- woman 176
- women, diabetic 65
whole
- blood 175
- blood acetaldehyde assay 175
- body bone mineral content 175
- canine blood 175
- cell 175
- cell/recombinant B subunit cholera vaccine 175
- cord blood cells 175
wide
- excision 175
- local excision 175
widened 179
widowed 175
width 179
Wilms tumor gene 176
window
- occipital acoustic 121
- temporal acoustic 160
wire
- Kirschner 97
wistaria
- floribunda within functional limits 175
with 37, 175
- or without 180
- relation to 176
withdrawal
- abrupt 27
- alcohol 27
- latency, hindpaw 88
- opiate 124
within 176
- functional limits 175
- normal limits 176
without 65, 121, 149, 176, 180
- corrective lenses 157
- glasses 157
without correction 151
Wolff-Parkinson-White 176
woman
- black 37
- diabetic black 56
- diabetic white 65

- non-pregnant normotensive 118
- white 176
word
- fluency 175
- recall,delayed 65
- test, dichotic 65
worker
- children's social 54
worker's
- compensation benefits 175
workers'
- compensation board 175
working cell bank 175
workup 176
worse
- than 180
wound 175
- dressing emulsion 175
- gun shot 82
- infection, surgical 159
- multiple fragment 106
wounds
- thoracoabdominal 160
wrist
- instability, volar intercalary 174
Wulong Dan 175

X

x
- number of days 176
- number of gestation weeks 176
- number of hours 176
- number of months 176
- number of weeks 176
xanthogranuloma
- necrobiotic 121
xanthoma
- papular 140
xeroderma
- pigmentosa 176
x-linked
- progressive retinal atrophy 176
- recessive nephrolithiasis 176
x-linked progressive
- retinal atrophy 176
x-ray 141, 176
- abdominal 28
- absorptiometry, dual energy 59, 65
- chest 55
- diffraction 176
- in plaster 176
- prototype network, digital 65
- prototype, digital 65
xylose
- lysine, deoxycholate agar 176

Y

Y chromosome 177
yard 177
year 177
- of birth 177
years 177
- of age 177
- of potential life lost 177
- old 177
yeast artificial chromosome 177
yield
- breast meat 34
- fat 77
yields 179
yolk sac tumor 177
youth
- exchange scheme 177
- risk behaviour survey 177
ytterbium 177
yttrium 177
- aluminum-garnet (laser) 177
- tyrosine, pyrimidine nucleoside 177

Z

zalcitabine 58
zero
- administrative initiative 177
- base budgeting 177
- end-expiratory pressure 177
- insertion force 177
zeta
- sedimentation rate 177
zidovudine 28, 177
zigzag in-line package 177
zinc 177
zirconium 177
Zollinger-Ellison 177
- syndrome 177
zone
- avascular 27
- basement membrane 33
- tolerance, high 88
zonisamide 177
zoological
- spongiform encephalopathy 177
zoster
- associated pain 177
- immune globulin 177
- immune plasma 177
Zucker diabetic fatty 177
zygote
- intrafallopian transfer 177
ZZ genotype 177

Notes

Notes

Notes

Notes

Medical Spanish pocket plus

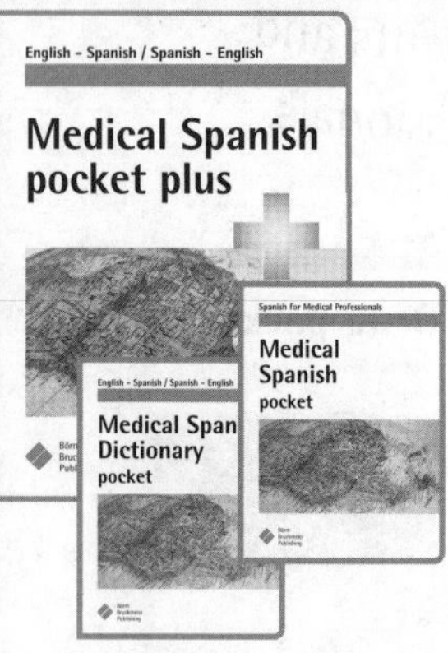

Medical Spanish pocket plus
ISBN 1-59103-213-X, US $ 22.95

- Includes contents of both **Medical Spanish pocket** and **Medical Spanish Dictionary pocket**
- Vital communication tool
- Clearly organized by situation: interview, examination, course of visit
- Accurate translations for almost every health-related term
- Bilingual dictionary contains medical terminology specific to Mexico, Puerto Rico, Cuba and other countries

Also available as PDA software!

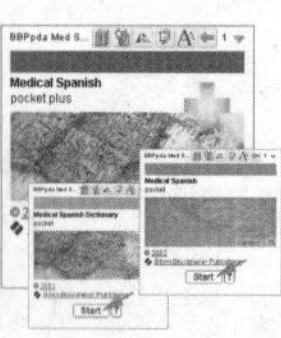

Medical Spanish pocket plus for PDA (2487 kb), $ 24.95

Medical Spanish Dictionary pocket for PDA (2343 kb), $ 16.95

Medical Spanish pocket for PDA (670 kb), $ 16.95

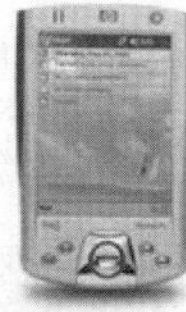

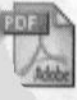

Table of Contents, Text samples, PDA demo files... **www.media4u.com**

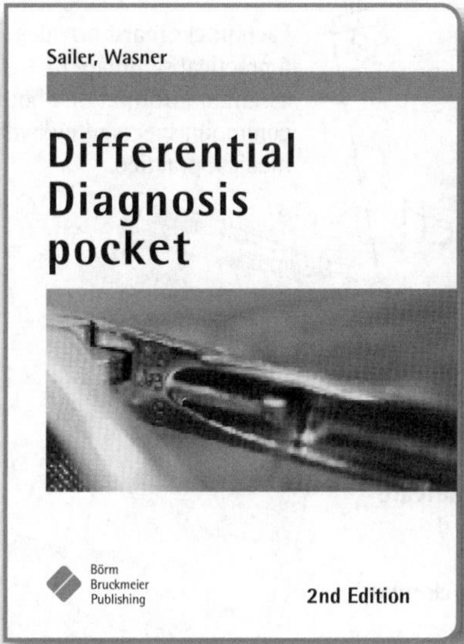

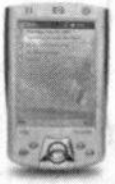

pocketcards

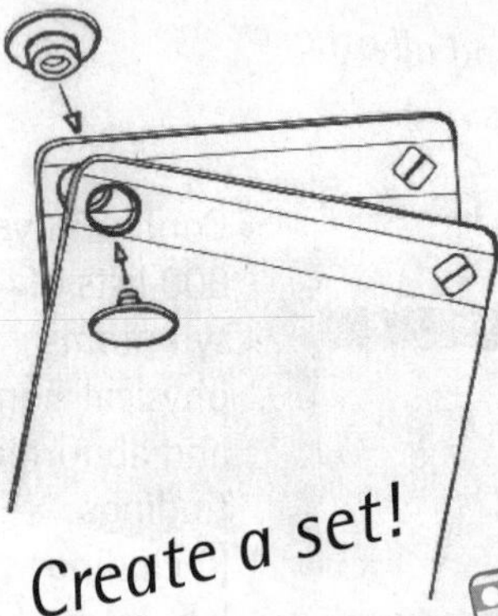

pocketcards cover vital medical information: pocket-sized, printed in color on white plastic.

Each **pocketcard** provides a practical summary of essential information about common aspects of everyda medical practice.

Create a set!

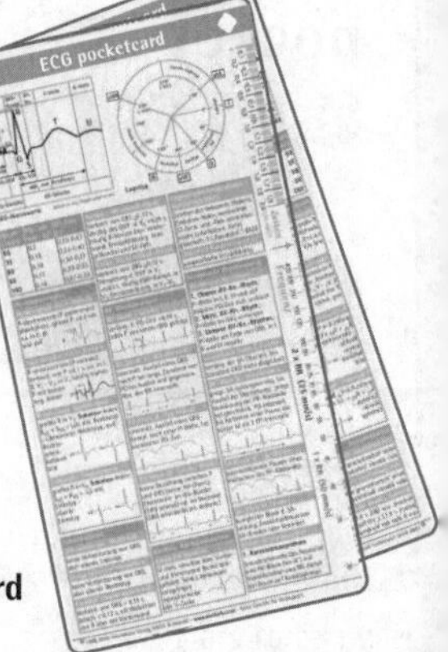

- → **Antibiotics pocketcard 2006**
- → **Antifungals pocketcard**
- → **BLS / ALS pocketcard**
- → **ECG pocketcard**
- → **ECG Evaluation pocketcard**
- → **ECG Ruler pocketcard**
- → **ECG pocketcards**
- → **Emergency Drugs pocketcard**
- → **H & P pocketcard**
- → **Medical Abbreviations pocketcard**
- → **Medical Spanish pocketcard**
- → **Neurology pocketcard**
- → **Normal Values pocketcard**
- → **Periodic Table pocketcard**

www.media4u.com

Orde

Börm Bruckmeier Publishing
PO Box 388
Ashland, OH 44805

Phone: 888-322-6657
Fax: 419-281-6883

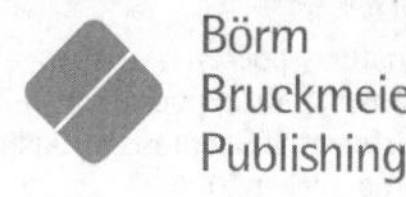

Name	E-mail	
Address		
City	State	Zip

Subtotal

Sales Tax, add only for: CA 8%; OH 6.25% — + Sales Tax

Shipping & Handling for US address: — + S&H

UPS Standard: 10% of subtotal with a minimum of $5.00
UPS 2nd Day Air: 20% of subtotal with a minimum of $8.00

= Total

Credit Card: ❑ Visa ❑ Mastercard ❑ Amex ❑ Discover
Card Number
Exp. Date Signature

For foreign orders, quantity rebate, optional shipping and payment please inquire: service@media4u.com

-orm Bruckmeier Products

pockets

	COPIES	PRICE/COPIES		PRICE
Anatomy pocket		X US $ 16.95	=	
Canadian Drug pocket 2006-2007		X US $ 14.95	=	
Differential Diagnosis pocket		X US $ 14.95	=	
Drug pocket 2006		X US $ 12.95	=	
Drug pocket plus 2006-2007		X US $ 24.95	=	
Drug Therapy pocket 2006-2007		X US $ 14.95	=	
ECG pocket		X US $ 12.95	=	
EMS pocket		X US $ 14.95	=	
Homeopathy pocket		X US $ 14.95	=	
Medical Abbreviations pocket		X US $ 16.95	=	
Medical Classifications pocket		X US $ 16.95	=	
Medical Spanish pocket		X US $ 12.95	=	
Medical Spanish Dictionary pocket		X US $ 14.95	=	
Medical Spanish pocket plus		X US $ 22.95	=	
Normal Values pocket		X US $ 12.95	=	
Respiratory pocket		X US $ 14.95	=	

pocketcards

Antibiotics pocketcard 2006		X US $ 3.95	=	
Antifungals pocketcard		X US $ 3.95	=	
BLS/ALS pocketcard		X US $ 3.95	=	
ECG pocketcard		X US $ 3.95	=	
ECG Evaluation pocketcard		X US $ 3.95	=	
ECG Ruler pocketcard		X US $ 3.95	=	
ECG pocketcard Set (3)		X US $ 9.95	=	
Emergency Drugs pocketcard		X US $ 3.95	=	
H&P pocketcard		X US $ 3.95	=	
Medical Abbreviations pocketcard Set (2)		X US $ 6.95	=	
Medical Spanish pocketcard		X US $ 3.95	=	
Neurology pocketcard (2)		X US $ 6.95	=	
Normal Values pocketcard		X US $ 3.95	=	
Periodic Table pocketcard		X US $ 3.95	=	

= Subtotal